HEALING GOTHAM

HEALING GOTHAM

New York City's Public Health Policies for the Twenty-First Century

Bruce F. Berg, PhD

Associate Professor, Political Science
Fordham University
Bronx, New York

Johns Hopkins University Press
Baltimore

© 2015 Johns Hopkins University Press
All rights reserved. Published 2015
Printed in the United States of America on acid-free paper

2 4 6 8 9 7 5 3 1

Johns Hopkins University Press
2715 North Charles Street
Baltimore, Maryland 21218-4363
www.press.jhu.edu

Library of Congress Cataloging-in-Publication Data

Berg, Bruce F., author.
Healing Gotham : New York City's public health policies for the
twenty-first century / Bruce F. Berg.
p. ; cm.
Includes bibliographical references and index.
ISBN 978-1-4214-1599-4 (pbk. : alk. paper) — ISBN 1-4214-1599-2 (pbk. : alk. paper) —
ISBN 978-1-4214-1600-7 (electronic) — ISBN 1-4214-1600-X (electronic)
I. Title.
[DNLM: 1. Health Policy—New York City.   2. Urban Health—
New York City. WA 546 AN7]
RA566.4.I3
362.1'042097471—dc23   2014016736

A catalog record for this book is available from the British Library.

*Special discounts are available for bulk purchases of this book. For more information,
please contact Special Sales at 410-516-6936 or specialsales@press.jhu.edu.*

Johns Hopkins University Press uses environmentally friendly book materials,
including recycled text paper that is composed of at least 30 percent post-consumer
waste, whenever possible.

For Noah, Samara, Adam, and Ellis
and their health

CONTENTS

I am greatly indebted to Fordham University and its Office of Research for providing me with the necessary release time to conduct the research for the manuscript and its initial writing.

Staffers at the New York City Department of Health and Mental Hygiene were particularly helpful in the early research for this project. New York City Council public hearings and press conferences by Mayors Rudolph Giuliani and Michael R. Bloomberg provided a wealth of information on public health policy and the politics of public health in New York City.

My wife, Abbey, proofread major sections of the manuscript, asked appropriate questions, and provided encouragement throughout the project.

At Johns Hopkins University Press, I am grateful to Kelley Squazzo for her decision to support the project.

Finally, I would like to thank the town of Lucca, Italy. This manuscript was born in Lucca. The beautiful Tuscan town provided both the creative environment that allowed me to develop the topic as well as a wonderful distraction whenever I needed a diversion.

HEALING GOTHAM

INTRODUCTION

Public health is one of the oldest functions of statecraft, dating back to the ancient Romans, if not before. Centuries of political system involvement in public health as well as the advancement of knowledge about various disease and health conditions have produced a range of public policy tools that governments use to address community health issues. Although the specific community health conditions in need of political system action have changed since ancient times, many of the same tools continue to be employed by political systems, in addition to newly developed ones, in pursuit of public health solutions. What factors determine which public policy tools are chosen by political systems to address community health issues?

Public health and urban public health are practically synonymous. There were no community health issues until there were communities of a sufficient size to produce health problems on a scale necessary to be addressed by the state. The growth of cities produced congestion, population density, and the detachment of people from their supply of food and water. These conditions in turn produced health problems that could not be resolved by individuals acting alone. As a result, some of the first demands placed on newly emerging urban political systems were related to the public health needs of those living in the newly formed urban societies. And although the needs have changed, urban societies have continued to produce public health problems that require attention by the political system.

Municipal governments in Europe were well ahead of their American counterparts in addressing public health issues, but this was mostly because many of these cities developed centuries before those in America. Cities in the United States, copying their European counterparts, quickly caught up in using the relevant policy tools. When the industrial revolution simultaneously created a common set of community health problems in both Europe and America, cities in the United States imported public health tools from Europe, which allowed them not only to catch up but in some cases to surpass European municipalities. By the end of the nineteenth century, New York City had a public health infrastructure as developed as any in Europe. In time, it became one of the most extensive in the world.

This study examines New York City's public health enterprise and the tools it employs in responding to contemporary public health problems. More specifically, it examines those tools the city has adopted to deal with the public health problems caused by lead-based paint, asthma, HIV/AIDS, West Nile virus, and obesity. It also attempts to explain their adoption and use in light of the major forces that influence contemporary urban politics and policy making in the United States.

Public Health Defined

The goal of public health is to prevent disease and injury and to promote health through organized community effort (Patel and Rushefsky 2005, xii). Public health has several dimensions that distinguish it from other elements of the delivery of health care. First, because the focus of public health is aggregate health benefits, public health focuses on the health of populations, not single individuals. Second, because public health, by definition, views the health of all individuals in the community as critical to the health of each individual, the political system, with its ability to mobilize collective action at the community level, is seen as an appropriate macrostructure to address public health issues. If necessary, the political system has the authority not only to allocate costs and benefits through public policy among individuals and groups but also to use coercion to modify the behavior of individuals and groups in a manner conducive with public health goals (107).

Unlike medical care, public health focuses on community action and treatment more than the direct care of the individual by a physician. The interaction between patient and physician is initiated primarily when the patient contracts a condition in need of attention. The nature of this interaction does not give the physician a major role in prevention. In contrast, public health focuses much more on prevention than cure in that it promotes "community action to avoid disease and other threats to the health and welfare of individuals and the community at large" (Duffy 1990, 1). For those who view public health as a discipline separate from the practice of medicine, possibly the greatest difference between the two has been the success of public health in its contributions to overall societal health. Public health advocates argue that over the past century, approximately thirty years have been added to mean individual life expectancy. Over twenty of these additional years are attributable to public health interventions as opposed to medical interventions. The public health interventions would include "the construction of water and sewer systems, draining mosquito infested swamps and addressing spoilage, quality and nutrition in our food supply" (Clinton 2004).

Because of its focus on prevention, public health policy frequently envelops policy areas that include environmental and housing policy, food, and nutrition. In addition, public health, because of its focus on the community roots of health and disease, is far more willing to address the class or socioeconomic basis of health and disease since public health practitioners never view the human body as independent of its larger environment.

Despite public health's emphasis on prevention and medical care's focus on cure, public health and individual medical care have experienced an evolution of convergence for the past century (Patel and Rushefsky 2005, 3). The advancement of knowledge about health and disease has resulted in the medical establishment recognizing that, in many cases, the prevention of disease through community action or preemptive care is both possible and more efficient than curing disease once it appears. At the same time, public health officials have come to realize that not all diseases are community based and that community health would be enhanced if all individuals had access to quality medical care. Since the advent of bacteriology in the mid-nineteenth century, the public health community has realized that medical research may provide the roots of both prevention and cure for some public health conditions. In the mid- to late nineteenth century, the merger of the medical profession with public health was responsible for major strides in reducing the incidence of tuberculosis and other infectious diseases (Duffy 1968b, 238).

The Tools of Public Health Policy

Public policy comprises actions taken by political systems in response to problems articulated by members of the system or outside forces acting on them. The specific actions that political systems take constitute the tools used by public policy makers to address public problems. Over time the political system has used a slowly expanding number of tools in crafting public policy solutions, including grants, taxes, inspection, screening, monitoring, regulation, the direct provision of services, and education (Birkland 2005, 174–177). They can be distinguished by such criteria as the imposition and locus of cost, the degree of individual coercion required, and the necessity of enforcement in order for the policy to be successful.

Public health policy was probably one of the first policy areas in history where the state used "public regulation of private property and personal behavior" as a mechanism to "protect people from unnecessary hazards to their health" (Fee, in Rosen 1993, xxvi–xxvii). As a substantive subfield of domestic public policy, public health policy has employed many of the same tools used by other subfields of public policy.

Official statements of public health policy, including the tools employed to address public health conditions, can be found either in legislation or in bureaucratic regulations and statements of practice emanating from legislative or local charter mandates. In some cases, all or most of the tools being used can be found in a single piece of comprehensive legislation. New York City's childhood lead paint poisoning law is a good example. In other cases, however, where the disease or condition is due to multiple or unknown factors, the methods being used to address the disease may be the product of multiple pieces of legislation, multiple government agencies, and various bureaucratic practices. In 2010 the World Health Organization (WHO) issued a statement on "health in all policies," which recommended that governments best address public health when all areas of public policy "include health and well being as a key component of policy development" (WHO 2010). New York City's campaign against obesity and, to a lesser extent, the programs attacking childhood asthma and HIV/AIDS adopted this type of framework. As a result, policy tools to address these conditions were found across a wide range of public policy arenas, including the public schools, parks and recreation, housing, and transportation.

Table 1.1 displays policy tools employed by the public health community. With most public health issues, governmental authorities must first measure the extent of a public health problem or condition. Once these measurements reach a certain threshold, indicating a sufficient prevalence or intensity, the political system can assess the extent of the problem. To do so, public health policy makers must engage in surveillance—that is, "the ongoing systematic collection, analysis and interpretation of data on specific health events affecting a population" (Thacker and Stroup 1994). Because not every public health threat produces an immediate physician visit or hospitalization that can be easily counted, and not all who suffer from a condition may be aware of it or willing to divulge it, public health officials at times have to be pro-active in their attempts to measure the existence and prevalence of a problem.

Surveillance tools include inspection, screening, monitoring, and reporting. In ancient Rome, public markets were inspected by public officials for cleanliness and health, and inspection is still a major public health tool. New York City officials inspect various facilities open to the public, from restaurants to day care centers. More recently, the advance of medical technology has allowed public health authorities to screen individuals for specific illnesses or conditions. Screening in a rudimentary sense also dates back many centuries, such as when authorities went house to house to identify the plague or other contagious diseases. In some cases, governmental authorities mandate that specific groups be screened for specific conditions. New York State mandates newborn screening for various conditions, including hearing disorders and HIV. Monitoring, another assessment tool, takes place through periodic inspections or screening over time. Recently, the New York City school system has implemented Fitnessgram, which includes periodic body mass index (BMI) measurements used to track obesity.

Epidemiology studies diseases in populations. By measuring and comparing "trends and changes in disease occurrence and characteristics," policy makers can develop a response (Joseph 1992, 147). For new diseases, surveillance of the population through testing or monitoring is the only way public authorities can

TABLE I.I
Public Health Policy Tools

Surveillance
    Screening, performed by public or private actors
    Monitoring of individuals, businesses communities
    Mandated reporting by physicians and hospitals
    Inspecting businesses
Education
    Target
        Public
        At-risk groups
        Those who have access to at-risk groups (e.g., teachers)
        Communities
        Physicians/hospitals / health care providers
    Source
        Public agencies
        Private actors (e.g., businesses)
Regulation
    Target
        Individuals
        Businesses, nonprofit corporations
    Thresholds
        Blood lead levels, particulate matter, sulfur content in fuel
    Incentives
Direct provision of public services
    Target
        Individuals
        Communities
    Means of supply/distribution
        Public agencies
        Healthcare providers
        Community based
        Organizations
Rights
    Positive rights: guaranteeing individuals specific elements of public health
    Negative rights: protection from government intervention
Liability
    Assignment of accountability for harm
Grants/subsidies
    Financing provided by one level of government to another

understand the pattern of the disease and possibly protect vulnerable at-risk populations.

Finally, when physicians, hospitals, or other public and private health workers are the primary source of contact with individuals' public health, authorities have required those health workers to report the incidence of specific diseases or conditions to public health agencies. As early as the mid-nineteenth century, authorities in New York City and elsewhere sought regulations requiring physicians to report selected diseases of their patients (Patel and Rushefsky 2005, 109). The beginnings of this primitive system of surveillance had only limited success because some physicians were reluctant to stigmatize their wealthier patients by reporting their conditions and usually faced no sanctions for not doing so. Today, the Centers for Disease Control and Prevention (CDC) has developed, in conjunction with state and local departments of health, a much more comprehensive and reliable system of reporting. At the local level, however, the city's Board of Health can also designate diseases as reportable and communicates with physicians and hospitals to facilitate reporting.

Once the existence and extent of the public health problem has been assessed, officials must determine whether and how to intervene. One approach is based on the assumption that a perfectly working market with mobile, all-knowing, and utility-maximizing consumers and suppliers would produce far fewer public health problems. That is, all-knowing individuals would behave in ways that decrease their own exposure to public health problems. Many conditions, however, can inhibit the market. From a public health perspective, individuals often lack the information to behave in a public-regarding way. And even if they possess the knowledge, they might behave in ways that maximize their own self-interest but not service the interest of public health. For instance, factories create a great deal of self-interested activity as well as benefits for their workers and the public. But these same factories may engage in a level of pollution that exposes the public to unhealthy air and water through a negative externality. Prior to the promulgation of environmental protection laws, factories were not required to assess their impacts on the air as a cost of doing business and therefore never had to address this issue. The role of public policy is either to repair the market or to attempt to replicate the ends that would be achieved if the market were working and individuals were all-knowing, public-regarding actors. If one of the market imperfections or failures is the lack of knowledge, public education through the supplying of information addresses that failure.

A second related set of assumptions is rooted in Richard Thaler and Cass Sunstein's concept of libertarian paternalism (Thaler and Sunstein 2008). The goal of public health policy to a great extent is to "influence people's behavior in order to make their lives longer, healthier and better" (8). Thaler and Sunstein believe that "the emerging science of choice" whereby individuals can be "nudged" to make better choices for themselves is what makes libertarian paternalism viable (7). That is, they believe that since all choices are biased by a structured environment, sound-choice architecture can induce individuals to make better choices for themselves.

Thaler and Sunstein are aware that market models do not always structure choices in a way that are beneficial to the individuals, especially when individuals lack information. They note that, in dealing with the sale of goods and services, "companies have a strong incentive to cater to people's frailties and to exploit them" (79). They are also aware that in making self-interested choices, individuals will frequently opt for present benefits in exchange for less certain future costs even if the costs may be greater, unless they are made aware of the magnitude of the risk (79).

Decades, if not centuries, before Thaler and Sunstein developed their approach to public policy, policy makers were relying on information as a way to influence individual choices. The use of education in public health policy has also evolved over centuries. Of key importance today is that, through technology and mass communication, governments can disseminate information far more effectively than the early public health policy makers were able to do. In the early twentieth century, New York City's Department of Health placed information about tuberculosis on the back of streetcar transfers (Duffy 1968b, 541). At that time, short of sending public health workers door to door, this was the most effective means of mass communication.

There are, however, differences between Thaler and Sunstein's approach and public health policy making. Most important is that public health officials have no reservation about proposing and using more coercive measures if the "nudge" is not effective in achieving public health goals. Officials have on occasion fallen back on less coercive tools, such as education, when they get political pushback on the use of more intrusive methods. To many officials, an outright ban on cigarettes would be preferable to supplying the public with information and regulating advertising. But the tobacco industry has been able to keep this proposal off the political system's agenda. Thaler and Sunstein draw a distinction between libertarian paternalism and pure paternalism, embodied by product bans, and public health officials make this distinction as well.

In changing behavior through education, Thaler and Sunstein (2008, 34) are well aware of "status quo bias" and the challenge of getting individuals to change old but unhealthy habits. In promoting the supply of information as a way to change behavior, they argue that, because people learn from others, peer pressure is critical in breaking old habits. As a result, communities, not just individuals, must be educated.

Possibly the most visible example of this approach is the Federal Trade Commission's decision in the mid-1960s to require the surgeon general's health warning on packs of cigarettes. More recently, New York City public health authorities have attempted to combat obesity by having restaurants posts caloric content on menus. The assumption is that, given this knowledge, citizens will act in their own best interest by not smoking and eating less. One of the challenges authorities face in educating the public about health threats or conditions is reaching the target population. Frequently, they solicit the cooperation of schools or community groups.

Public education as a tool of public health policy has multiple dimensions, such as who is being educated. In the case of smoking, when the entire public is the target, public service announcements on radio, television, and the internet and posters on bus shelters and mass transit are used. In some cases, public health authorities target smaller segments of the population for education, including teachers, physicians, and other professionals who have been deemed more effective in communicating with the public. Authorities may also seek to educate professionals to assist them in identifying cases or helping them prevent or treat those who have an illness or condition of public health concern. If a focus on specific communities or neighborhoods where the incidence of a condition or disease is prevalent is more appropriate, targeted mass media techniques can be used, but perhaps more effective are community-based organizations or government agencies, such as social service agencies or libraries located in affected communities. This is especially the case in seeking to educate individuals in low-income neighborhoods or ethnic enclaves where language or cultural barriers may inhibit the community's receiving a mass education message.

A second dimension is the cost of providing the information. When the public health agency provides the education, the cost is borne by the public through taxation. When the New York City Department of Health and Mental Hygiene (DOHMH) produces posters or public service announcements, this cost becomes part of its budget, subject to the city's budgetary process, where the mayor and city council are the primary actors and where public health officials might have to compete with other agencies for necessary funds. At times, however, as in the case of smoking, a tactical decision is made that education may be more effective if supplied at the point of the public health threat. In the late 1960s, the mandate to place a warning on their cigarette packs imposed a direct production cost on cigarette manufacturers and not the public.

When public health education mandates that private actors supply information to the public, the costs become political as well as economic. At this point what appears to public health officials as mass public education appears to private actors as regulation. Private actors, not wanting to bear the cost of providing such information, will push back. Just as important, the private provision of public information is also costly to private actors because, in most cases, as in the case of cigarette manufacturers, the substance of the education being provided is not in their interest either. Cigarette manufactures were being mandated to pay for the provision of information that would induce the public to smoke less.

When public education has not worked, or when public officials conclude that it will not work, more coercive methods, including regulations and mandates, have been used. They assume that, even given all available information, individuals or firms might not act in their own best interest or in the best interest of the community. The use of regulations or mandates developed as far back as ancient Rome, where authorities regulated public markets in order to ensure the safety of food being sold. Over time, these regulations evolved into licensure laws for those establishments selling foodstuffs to the public.

Today, regulations or mandates have two significant components: targets and thresholds. Regulations can apply to the public, as with smoking regulations. Over the past several decades, policy makers have been successful in limiting where individuals can smoke as a way to reduce the harm caused by smoking and to influence individuals not to smoke at all. Regulations can also apply to selected publics, such as physicians, hospitals, or businesses. If mandated at the federal level, they can also apply to state and local governments. Many regulations come with thresholds that establish goals that must be met. Thresholds, although frequently the result of political compromise, have their roots in some determination, based on medical or health knowledge, on what level of regulation is needed to have an impact on reducing harm or enhancing public health. Over the past several decades, air and water quality regulations have included thresholds that have attempted to reflect current definitions of healthy water and air, as well as the best practicable technology for achieving those thresholds.

Regulations and mandates are coercive tools of public policy because they mandate that individuals or firms behave in specific ways. Possibly the most coercive measure is the quarantine. In prior centuries, cities isolated persons believed to have communicable diseases in order to protect the rest of the public, and the practice is still employed on occasion today (Rosen 1993, 39). Quarantine limits individual mobility to the point of sequestering people in their homes or a hospital until they are deemed no longer a threat to public health.

Regulations are accompanied by penalties or fines for noncompliance. Penalties are effective only if they can be consistently and effectively enforced. In the absence of enforcement, regulations appear to targets as incentives or disincentives with the risk of being apprehended as part of the calculation of compliance. Occasionally, governments offer incentives, instead of regulations, to induce responsible behavior. Given the difficulties of using incentives to target the public, they are primarily aimed at businesses.

While much of public health involves inspection, monitoring, and regulation, public health authorities frequently have to address public health concerns by dealing directly with the public through the direct provision of services. One of the most significant examples is vaccination. As far back as the early 1900s, New York City's Department of Health produced and supplied smallpox vaccine to hundreds of thousands of New Yorkers (Leavitt 1995, 106–108). In the mid-1990s, the Department of Health again played a major role in polio vaccinations. During the AIDS crisis, public health officials distributed condoms to at-risk populations.

As in the case of education, public health policy makers at the local level frequently rely on community-based organizations to deliver services. These organizations have the ability to tailor services to specific communities as well as to act as intermediaries between the macrostructure of the political system and families in their communities. As a result, there is a greater chance that the service will be accepted and utilized if delivered by groups with whom the community is familiar.

Grants or subsidies are also common. Although their use goes back at least a century when health dispensaries in New York City received subsidies from the state to deliver health care to immigrants and the poor, the federal government in the mid-twentieth century popularized the practice (Patel and Rushefsky 2005, 23). The expansion of the U.S. Public Health Service in the post–World War II era, the passage of Medicaid, and the proliferation of federal health grants during the Johnson, Nixon, and Ford administrations resulted in state and local public health activities being supported by federal funds. Today, intergovernmental assistance is employed in areas including AIDS, obesity, lead-based paint poisoning, and even West Nile virus.

Although the local role in public health policy is primary, local inaction can have national implications. Thus, federal fiscal assistance is an attempt to make sure that state and local governments have the resources to respond to emerging public health problems. At the same time, federal assistance serves to motivate states and their local governments to adopt a specific method by lowering its cost through an intergovernmental subsidy.

In the twentieth century, medical and social science research began to establish links between environmental or product hazards, along with their sources, and harm to human health. Responses to these threats have involved both rights and liability.

The concept of rights, as an aspect of policy, occupies a unique position in American politics. The Constitution gives most Americans procedural rights to participate in American politics. In addition, the Constitution, and more specifically the Bill of Rights, created what many scholars have called negative substantive rights. These negative rights give citizens the right to be free of government restraint and coercion (Stone 2002). From a public health perspective, the existence of broad negative rights sets up a potential constraint on public health policy that occasionally needs to rely on the coercive power of the state in order to protect the community from actions by a few individuals or firms that harm community health. In addition, the constitutionally implied right to privacy also potentially interferes with the activities of officials who need to gauge the health of individuals before they act. What the Constitution has not done is create positive substantive rights, or entitlements. While most Americans are guaranteed the right to participate in a process, they do not have the right to be free of disease, to be well educated, or to be nutritiously fed. On occasion, however, state and local public policies do create these rights. In the early 1980s, the New York State courts established a right to shelter for those who were homeless. And New York City's most recent lead-based paint poisoning law establishes a right for children to live in homes that are lead safe.

The creation of substantive rights implies that someone is responsible for assuring that the right, or entitlement, is delivered. In public health, failure to deliver on a substantive right may result in real harm to individuals. The establishment of liability allows individuals and groups to realize their rights by suing businesses and others for harm done as a result of the production of the hazard (Patel and Rushefsky 2005, 129).

Although inertia, tradition, and the legacy of the public health enterprise may explain public health policy choices today, the urban public health enterprise and the problems it faces are more complex than was the case centuries ago. Factors that explain public health policy choices have become more complex as well, although they are not totally divorced from similar choices made centuries ago.

The Determinants of Urban Public Health Policy: Two Analytical Frameworks

What forces or factors influence the choice of public health policy tools by New York City's political system? This study focuses on four factors as possible determinants of public health policy choices: the state of knowledge about the public health conditions being confronted; the role of economic development and those forces promoting it; the intergovernmental context within which the city's political system exists; and the increasing racial and ethnic diversity of the city. These four factors have their roots in two distinct analytical frameworks. The importance of knowledge as a change agent in public policy making has its origins in the rational model and, as applied to public-sector policy making, concepts of imperfect information as a form of market failure. The other three determinants examined in this study all come from the study of urban politics and the evolution of theory and approaches to the study of urban politics and public policy in the later quarter of the twentieth century.

While the two analytical frameworks can be viewed as rivals, they are also complementary pieces of a larger puzzle. The application of knowledge through the formulation and implementation of public health policy tools is constrained by factors indigenous to the urban political process. This dynamic is most visible in examining contemporary public health policy in New York City.

Framework One: The Rational Model and Market Failure

Medical or health policy making, as practiced by physicians and public health professionals, primarily involves the application of or the search for knowledge in an attempt to resolve individual or community health problems. In this regard, health policy making takes on many of the characteristics of the classic and often maligned rational model. Policy makers are isolated and freed from outside forces to seek all possible solutions. Within obvious resource constraints, they conduct research to arrive at a solution.

Although the rational model can be traced back to Jeremy Bentham's discussion of utilitarianism, more recent iterations have their basis in the works of decision theorists David Braybrooke and Charles Lindblom (1963), Herbert Simon (1965), and Graham Allison (1971). The rational model assumes that individuals or organizations are aware of their preferences and the values that can be attached to them in such a way that these preferences can be ordered. Given their preference orderings and with perfect information, individuals and organizations have the ability to assess alternatives to achieve their goals, thereby maximizing their utility. In its pure form, the model assumes that, given clear goals, perfect information, and no time constraints, decision makers can achieve the most optimal solution to the problem they are facing.

Public microeconomists realized that the conditions for a perfectly working rational model were rarely, if ever, present. They developed the concept of market failure to explain market malfunction when those perfect conditions were not present. One of the principal factors in market breakdown is imperfect information, a lack of knowledge about the effects of one's choices on oneself as well as the larger group. Some public microeconomists used market breakdown as a rationale for government intervention. The public sector can attempt either to supply individuals through education with the information to make them more rational decision makers or to create through regulation a societal outcome similar to that which would have been achieved had individuals and organizations been able to make decisions with perfect information.

Information, or knowledge, is central to the rational model and to correcting market failures. Because the value of knowledge in public policy making is hardly in dispute, the central concerns of this framework are to what ends the knowledge is applied, the constraints that stand in the way of the application of knowledge, and what happens when policy is made with less than perfect knowledge.

Public policy interventions are most efficacious when they are based on knowledge about how the intervention will solve the problem it is meant to address. Most policy makers are constantly looking for knowledge to guide them in their choice. In the public health field, this knowledge comes from medical or health research on the cause of conditions and diseases or research that attempts to address cure or symptoms when causes are not discoverable. Urban political systems do not always accept such knowledge and the policy tools that the research knowledge might imply. In a policy-making process with multiple interests each pursuing a different policy result, knowledge may simply serve as one additional actor in the process. Moreover, incomplete knowledge or professional disagreements regarding knowledge add to the politicization of expertise in the policy-making process.

Medical or health knowledge dictates whether a specific health condition or disease can be prevented, whether it can be cured once it has been contracted, or in the absence of a cure whether the individual can be treated to lessen if not eliminate the debilitating symptoms of the disease. Without such knowledge, the tools chosen by policy makers will be based to some degree on ignorance, resulting in a much lower probability that the policy intervention will be efficacious. Existence of knowledge on how to prevent a disease or condition from occurring, and its translation into a successful policy intervention, will obviate the need to seek a cure or treatment. In the absence of knowledge on prevention, health research seeks to find a cure, or at least a treatment to deal with the symptoms.

To prevent a disease or condition from occurring, one must know its cause or etiology. If one succeeds, then one can decrease or eliminate its incidence or prevalence in the population. Incidence is "the rate of new cases of a disease in a defined population over a defined period of time," usually a year (Schneider 2011, 66). It is usually calculated by dividing the number of cases reported to local authorities by the population at risk. "Prevalence is the total number of cases existing in a defined population at a specific time" (66). This type of data is typically obtained through a population survey.

It is possible that one might know the cause of the disease but be unable to prevent it. Knowing the cause or etiology, however, will assist in finding and implementing a cure for those who have contracted the disease or condition. Finally, the symptoms of the disease can be treated without ascertaining the cause. In treating a disease or condition, short of curing it, one needs only to address the negative manifestations of the disease. This can be accomplished in the absence of knowledge about cause or etiology. Thus, when knowledge about the cause or cure for a disease or condition does not exist, or is under debate, policy makers or private practitioners can still take measures to address symptoms. In many urban communities, the causes of asthma are multifactorial and still being debated. This state of causal uncertainty may exist for quite some time. Yet medical knowledge does exist to ease asthma's most negative manifestations and prevent hospitalization.

The existence of knowledge about prevention, cure, and treatment, however, in no way guarantees that it will be employed. Societal forces at times will thwart attempts by policy makers to use tools based on medical or health knowledge because either they have not yet been convinced as to the validity of such knowledge or they believe that the employment of tools based on this knowledge will be disadvantageous to their own interests. In their attempts to get communities to adopt fluoridation of the water supply, public and dental health authorities learned that good science does not always result in public acceptance. "Invariably a few reputable scientists or other professionals can be found to dispute the accepted medical/health views in question, thus encouraging the doubtful and the many uninformed who object on completely specious grounds" (Duffy 1990, 290). On occasion, conflicts over the nature of medical or health evidence or knowledge "mask disagreements over policy issues, values and interests" of principal actors attempting to influence policy decisions (Patel and Rushefsky 2005, 146).

Even when there is consensus among researchers and experts, public acceptance of policy tools based on medical or health knowledge may lag. In these cases, disagreement is usually not based on disputes over the state of medical or health knowledge but more on a group's disagreement with the policy prescription implied by the knowledge. Medical research in the late 1980s developed the knowledge to stop the spread of HIV/AIDS, but public health officials were unable to entirely stop the spread of the disease because of the behavior of some gay males and intravenous drug users. In part this was due to the intransigence of the gay community, reluctant to surrender its rights to the public health establishment. This continued to be the case even after knowledge about the cause of HIV/AIDS was affirmed. And the tobacco industry has fought each and every attempt to further regulate smoking, regardless of the availability of knowledge affirming the dangers of tobacco.

The force of medical or health knowledge is a very influential factor, even once it gets thrown into the policy-making process. For years, policy analysts have expressed skepticism about "speaking truth to power," but in the field of health and medical research the political process and its actors have probably yielded to the influence of this type of knowledge more than they have in most other policy-relevant fields of knowledge (Wildavsky 1979). Deference to professional knowledge declined in most professions throughout the later decades of the twentieth century. Compared to most professions, however, the decline in deference to the medical profession and medical knowledge probably lagged; and despite the decline in professional prestige and public deference assigned to physicians, the medical profession maintained a residual amount of public deference and respect especially in the application of medical knowledge to health problems. This was due, in part, to the fact the health practitioners operate within both the private sector, where they have considerable autonomy, and the public sector, where they are simply one of many actors.

There are at least two ways in which the presence or absence of knowledge will influence the choice of policy tool. First, the state of existing knowledge will determine whether the tool being chosen will address prevention, cure, or treatment. If there is insufficient knowledge about the cause of a disease, the choice will focus on cure or treatment of symptoms. Second, the greater the professional, medical, or health consensus is on the cause or etiology of the disease, the greater the influence of knowledge will be on the choice.

Framework Two: New York City and the Evolution of Urban Political Theory

Urban political systems are fraught with constraints that block the direct application of policy knowledge. Urban public health policy, despite its roots in medical research and private policy making, is no exception. Forces that underlie urban political systems and public policy making can at various times either constrain or encourage the application of public health knowledge. The three forces that are discussed in this study are the role of economic development and those forces promoting it, the intergovernmental context within which the city's political system exists, and the increasing racial and ethnic diversity of the city. Prior research has already established that these forces significantly affect New York City's policy-making processes (Berg 2007). The roots of these three determinants lay within both the evolution of theories and approaches to the study of urban politics and public policy and the recent history of New York City.

Throughout much of the middle decades of the twentieth century, academic analyses of urban politics were dominated by two grand theories: pluralist or process approaches, and elitist or structuralist approaches. By the end of the 1970s, both had been rejected by mainstream scholars of urban politics. Pluralism was rejected primarily because it failed to recognize structural elements in the urban political economy that favored business and development interests. Elitism, including its Marxist and neo-Marxist relatives, was rejected for being too structural. It simply failed to explain most cases where business development interests either failed or were forced to compromise within political arenas in which inclusive processes gave other groups a stake in policy decisions.

Out of these rejections, smaller midlevel theories arose. These included regime theory (Stone 1989; Elkin 1985), the growth engine approach (Logan and Molotch 1996), and the application of corporatism to the urban political environment (Savitch 1988). What these three approaches shared was an acknowledgment of the primacy of economic development interests to the urban political economy without the orthodoxy of prior structuralist approaches. Unlike the rejected grand theories, these approaches were not claiming to explain the entire urban political milieu, nor were they claiming that business and development interests dominated urban public policy making in all aspects of urban life. But in their emphasis on urban economic development they did deemphasize other critical aspects of urban politics, including the role of race and ethnicity as well as the extent to which urban political systems were being influenced by politics at higher levels of government. The search for comprehensive approaches to understand the urban political environment continues.

As urban political theory evolved in the late twentieth century, so did the political lives of cities. And New York City's political system was at the forefront of this evolution. This evolution was directed by several trends. First and foremost among these trends was globalization. For New York City, and other cities in the Northeast and upper Midwest, globalization began with the loss of significant manufacturing employment beginning in the 1970s. Manufacturing employment had been a major source of well-being for unskilled and uneducated New Yorkers. Over the past three decades of the twentieth century, manufacturing employment decentralized to other parts of the country and other parts of the globe as consumer markets expanded.

In addition, the advent of multinational corporations and the rise of global markets and competition reduced the autonomy of nation-states. As a result, cites were left to fend for themselves as corporate capital became more mobile and national governments lost control of their economies to global forces. New York City fared better than many other American cities as it became a center of global finance and producer services responding to the needs of corporate headquarters centered in a small number of "global cities" (Sassen 2001). But New York City's status as a global city did little to help its working- and lower-class populations and newly arriving minority groups, whose members were forced to take low-paying service jobs because of the absence of manufacturing employment.

The national government's declining global economic autonomy in the late twentieth century was matched by a decline in the national government's willingness to assist state and local governments at home. From the New Deal to the early 1980s, a liberal regime in Washington had produced grant programs to assist urban areas with growing populations and problems, as well as direct aid programs to the city's low-income residents. In an almost symbiotic federal-local relationship, New York City's own liberal regime devoured much of the federal grant opportunities. Federal funds supported a significant number of city programs, including many in the public health arena.

The high water mark for the federal government's fiscal support of New York City occurred in the mid- to late 1970s. Not only did the federal government play a significant role in bailing the city out of its 1975–76 fiscal crisis, but also in 1977 federal aid constituted 20 percent of city spending. In that year, federal aid to the city matched state aid to the city (Berg 2007). From that point on, however, federal aid declined as the liberal regime that dominated national politics gave way to conservative-neoliberal regimes. Some federal grants were eliminated, others had their budgets cut significantly, and still others were collapsed into block grants. Although the city remains dependent on federal aid, this aid to the city is now approximately half of what it was as a percentage of city spending. Lost federal aid has made the city more dependent on its own revenue raising ability and made it more difficult for the city to respond to emerging problems.

At the same time, however, the city remains dependent upon and influenced by the state and federal levels of government. Federal aid is still a significant component of the city's budget, and state aid to the city has been maintained at its previous levels. Despite the aggregate intergovernmental funding loss, the city is still subject to unfunded or semifunded mandates coming from both state and federal levels. That is, the federal and state governments dictate city policy choices across various policy areas even though the money to fund these policies and programs is not being supplied. Some of these mandates fall within the public health policy area. Thus, the federal and state levels continue to influence city public health policy through mandates and some financial assistance.

Beginning in the 1970s, the city's ability to raise its own revenue was damaged by the exodus of manufacturing employment and the income that manufacturing jobs produced for the city's residents. This was exacerbated by the out-migration of many middle-class, tax-paying city residents seeking to escape city problems and the in-migration of low-income minority groups, dependent on city services and assistance. While the city has always been a haven for immigration, the rate and diversity of immigration that occurred in the later part of the twentieth century and early twenty-first century was unprecedented. Over time, civil rights laws, Supreme Court rulings, and the city's own liberal regime empowered these new groups to make demands on the city for service delivery at levels equivalent to what other groups in the city were receiving. And while Mayors Giuliani and Bloomberg cite immigration as a major source of economic innovation and adrenaline for the city's economy, the level of diversity still poses an incredible challenge for any service delivery bureaucracy, including public health, attempting to meet the needs of the city's entire population.

By the end of the twentieth century, the city found itself buffeted by three factors. First, because of the need to raise its own revenue, the city was forced to compete in the global economic environment. The promotion of economic development was viewed as the most politically palatable avenue to achieve revenue stability and growth. The city could no longer rely on increasing intergovernmental transfers, and in the political environment of the time, raising taxes was not viable. Second, despite declining intergovernmental revenues, the city still found itself as a unit of local government in the federal system. It continues to be dependent on funds from the state and federal levels, and its public policy choices continue to be affected by state and federal mandates, some of which directly affect public health policy. Because of its size and influence, the city has some ability to influence what goes on at higher levels of government, but for the most part the arrow of influence is one way, coming from the state and federal levels. Third, while New York City's position as the most ethnically and racially diverse city in the country and maybe the world is certainly a source of economic and cultural vibrancy, this diversity also poses challenges for the city. Diversity creates problems and constrains the way in which the political system can respond to them.

Economic Development and Urban Public Health Policy

Urban economic development and those who promote it have a complex relationship with public health policy. Although much of the city's early and continuing concerns with public health had a strong humanitarian focus, the city's early and continuing focus on public health was also linked to economic development. As an emerging center of business, cities had to provide a venue that was safe, and being free of disease was part of that concept. As a manufacturing center, the city also had to ensure that entrepreneurs and industrialists had access to a healthy work force as well (Lieber and Opdycke 1995, 910–911).

In many instances, successful economic development enhances public health. But economic development is unique in its relationship with urban public health in that some of the activities that encompass economic development exacerbate urban public health problems. Complicating this relationship further, in those instances where economic development creates public health problems, individuals and businesses benefiting from those activities may actively oppose any public health policies that attempt to curtail or prohibit their activities.

Economic development promotes public health in a variety of ways. On a political system level, economic development is one of the most (if not the most) palatable ways for a political system to raise revenue necessary for funding public health programs. At a stable level of taxation, increased economic activity increases the productivity of land and labor, allowing the political system to raise more revenue without raising taxes. For elected officials, taxes are the least preferred method of raising revenue, given their unpopularity with the public. And as a source of revenue, intergovernmental financial assistance is at best unreliable and at worst declining over time. As a result, economic development that increases political system revenue, without increasing tax rates, enables those political systems to engage in more public health activities.

Economic development also promotes public health at the individual or community level by raising the collective or individual standard of living. Economic development takes unemployed individuals and employs them. It takes low-income individuals and increases their purchasing power. An increased standard of living gives individuals access to amenities, such as increased leisure time or household goods, which enhance public health in most cases. Economic development can also enhance individual and community education, making individuals more aware of public health issues and giving them the time, ability, and political wherewithal to address problems in their neighborhoods.

But urban economic development can also create public health problems for the community, necessitating action by the political system. Urban populations are sufficiently removed from food production that they have lost the ability to assess food quality prior to ingestion. In the nineteenth century, simple economic activities such as the slaughtering and sale of beef created public health issues that local communities could not address without government intervention. Without refrigeration, the sale of beef became an economic activity that needed monitoring to assure the community that the beef sold was edible. In addition, regulations were needed to limit areas where slaughterhouses or butchers could dump waste products. At first public government established and regulated markets, and later it licensed butchers (Duffy 1968a, 420–439).

Toward the end of nineteenth century and into the twentieth century, the industrial revolution increased the scale and intensity of economic activity. Problems of industrial waste and air and water pollution arose, which produced health problems affecting the community. Not all economic activity produces public health problems. But in urban areas, the mere concentration of economic activities may have adverse impacts on public health through the creation of traffic congestion and the need for waste disposal. Most of the retail and office operations that populate midtown Manhattan are not directly involved in production that pollutes the environment; but the densely populated economic activities of midtown produce air pollution and a place a significant demand on the city's waste disposal infrastructure.

Globalization as an artifact of economic development has produced public health challenges. More rapid and less expensive global transportation is responsible for many individual, communal, and global benefits. But giving people and things greater ability to travel globally means that local or regional public health threats in some parts of the world have the potential to become public health threats all over the world. Disease, harmful food, and other dangerous products now move across the globe with minimal restraints.

Not only does economic development activity harm public health, but also those who benefit from harmful activities may use their resources to oppose or thwart attempts by others, through public policy, to address the harm that has been done. Negative externalities of economic development are a significant cause of public health problems. Dilemmas for political systems arise in assessing the benefits versus the harm of economic development.

Over the past two centuries many industries directly or indirectly harmed public health through the despoiling of public resources, such as air and water. Initially, industries and those engaging in economic development activities used these resources for free and produced negative externalities in the creation of air and water pollution. The public paid for this production through the degradation of its environment and poor health, for which it was not compensated. Public demands for government action resulted in laws and regulations that limited the ability to exploit public resources without paying for them. Naturally, actors who at some point receive a good for free and are subsequently asked by the political system to pay for it, or have its use restricted, will use their resources to oppose those laws and regulations from being enacted and implemented. Industries and businesses that benefit from the creation of public health harms will seek to suppress any regulation of their behavior. If this fails, those affected businesses will seek regulations with compliance thresholds that will not damage their firms' profitability.

In some cases, economic development interests oppose the employment of public health tools not because they created the problem that the tool is seeking to address but simply because the tool is bad for business. Throughout the nineteenth century, business interests in many urban areas fought the use of quarantines to stop the spread of contagious disease because quarantines were often an impediment to economic activity (Patel and Rushefsky 2005, 78). As a result, public health problems attributable to, or having a negative impact on, economic development are more difficult for political systems to address, particularly when the economic development activities responsible for the problem are concentrated and organized.

Intergovernmental Relations and Urban Public Health

Most fields of domestic policy in the United States are affected by federal, state, and local relations; public health policy is no exception. The United States is a federal system where, according to constitutional principles, the federal and state governments both are sovereign and share power. Local governments are legally creatures of the states. Over the past century, however, local governments and particularly large cities have gained a great deal of political influence at the state level, primarily due to reapportionment that took place in the middle of the twentieth century. In addition, local governments and large cities in particular have gained considerable political influence at the federal level, although the precise amount of this influence has waxed and waned over the past several decades. The federal system, based on the legal relationship between the federal and state governments, has evolved overtime into a three-way intergovernmental partnership with local governments at times playing an equal role to the federal and state levels. This is certainly the case in urban public health policy where cities have dominated policy making over the centuries.

Public health is by definition a function most appropriately addressed by local governments. Unlike medical care, the focus of public health is the community, a concept most synonymous with local governments. The state and federal governments may have a role in public health policy, but the point of diagnosis and implementation, where the policy tools are administered, is at a level of government that has knowledge of and is proximate to the community.

In fact, the origins of public health policy exist at the local government level. Even in the United States, local governments, and more specifically large urban political systems, were addressing public health concerns before the United States was formed. The entry of states and the federal government into public health in any significant way did not occur until the middle to late nineteenth century. Although local governments still play the primary role in the formulation and administration of public health policy, they do receive major assistance and regulatory guidance from the federal and state governments. How did the present intergovernmental public health policy relationship evolve?

In the case of New York City, the origins of state and federal involvement in the city's public health policy making are different. New York State became involved in the city's public health policy making as early as the first half of the nineteenth century. Public health advocates at the city level felt they were stymied in their efforts to implement public health reforms by the corrupt and patronage-based political machine that controlled the city's political system. In their frustration, the advocates frequently appealed to the state legislature in Albany to intervene in city affairs regarding public health policy. Although the state legislature was at times reluctant to act, on a number of occasions it intervened by establishing offices at the local level with public health responsibilities. This intervention culminated in the state legislature's passage of the Metropolitan Health Bill in 1866, recognized by many as the first major piece of public health legislation in the United States and certainly the first comprehensive piece of urban public health policy (Duffy 1968b). In most of these early interventions into city public health policy making, New York State officials were not acting on their own initiative. State entry into city public health policy was due to the forces of political reform and public health advocates in the city seeking state intervention.

One public health historian has stated that, "before the twentieth century, the federal government demonstrated more interest in farm animals than in public health" (Duffy 1990, 239). Aside from establishing a program that would address the medical needs of seaman, the federal government deferred to states and their local governments on issues of public health until well after the Civil War. In response to a yellow fever epidemic in 1798, Congress passed a law requiring all federal officials to observe state quarantine laws (Duffy 1968a, 139). Throughout the nineteenth century, all federal activity in the area of public health was either deferential to state and local policies or weak and ineffectual (Duffy 1990, 162–172).

Beginning in the twentieth century both state and federal governments began to take a more active role. A primary rationale for increased activity by these levels of government was the goal of achieving uniformity. The transportation revolution of the twentieth century and the subsequent increased mobility of the population produced the recognition that public health problems did not respect local or even regional political boundaries. One local political system's failure to address a public health concern may well have negative spillover effects for neighboring jurisdictions and even those thousands of miles away. Large port cities such as New York realized this as early as the late eighteenth and early nineteenth centuries. Many of these cities adopted policies, especially during epidemics or epidemic threats, of inspecting ships before they were allowed to dock and quarantining anyone suspected of having a disease. New York in particular was also forced to adopt public health policies to deal with the health issues that could result from the continuous waves of immigrants that the city experienced throughout the mid- to late nineteenth century.

Throughout the early decades of the twentieth century, states established health boards and then comprehensive departments of health. These state boards made recommendations to the local governments, such as appointing a health officer. Many of these recommendations ultimately became mandates. States also began to provide their local governments with a range of services related to public health policy, including state laboratories (Duffy 1990, 232). These state-based services were particularly valuable to small cities, towns, and rural areas, which lacked the economies of scale to establish their own public health infrastructure. The state-local public health policy relationship was very much dependent on the indigenous state political culture and the tradition of state-local relations, with some states taking greater control of public health policy making and others ceding much of the authority to their local governments.

The federal government's goals of uniformity in public health policy were somewhat similar to the states. In the twentieth century, the transportation revolution transformed local health problems into national health problems. With individuals moving more freely about the country, it became impossible for a single state or local jurisdiction to address a disease that took on epidemic characteristics, and participation by the federal government was necessary. Moreover, once the federal government became a primary purchaser of health care services, through Medicare and Medicaid, problems such as obesity or cigarette smoking that might have remained local, or even individual, became national in scope. The federal government became an interested party when its budget was being affected by these problems.

By the twentieth century, attitudes about activist government and the role that the federal government should play in domestic policy making were changing. A more positive attitude was best reflected in the New Deal policies of President

Franklin D. Roosevelt and the Great Society programs of President Lyndon Johnson.

Unlike the state-local relations in the area of public health policy, it was not until the second half of the twentieth century that the federal involvement in public health policy included mandating states to take certain actions. Before that time the federal government lacked the constitutional authority as well as the political will to impose the utilization of specific public health policy tools on the states. The United States Public Health Service (USPHS), established in 1902, had far less draconian methods to engage the states and their local governments. They sought to assist states with their quarantine activities especially in those cases where the epidemic threats were of a foreign nature. The USPHS also sought to assist states in collecting data on public health problems so that governments at all levels could better understand the nature and extent of the problems with which they were dealing. Similar to the state-local relations, the USPHS established a laboratory in Washington, D.C., that began to conduct public health research. During the 1918 swine flu pandemic, the USPHS "organized the states to address the issue" and assisted states in mobilizing physicians (Duffy 1990, 241–243).

Unable to coerce states to act on behalf of public health and on a host of other issues as well, the federal government developed the use of the grant-in-aid during the first half of twentieth century. Grants are public policy tools that subsidize a directed activity at the state or local level. That is, they lower the cost of an activity (i.e., the selection of a specific public policy tool) in the hopes that the recipient will take the grant and engage in the desired tool selection. Over time, this became one of the primary ways by which the federal government was able to both assist state and local governments to achieve their public health goals and induce some state and local governments, through financial assistance, to take action that they would not otherwise have taken.

One of the first federal grant programs to further public health goals was the 1922 Shepherd-Towner Act, which made federal moneys available to states for maternal and infant hygiene (Patel and Rushefsky 2005, 87–88). Elements of Shepherd-Towner became part of the 1935 Social Security Act, the backbone of FDR's New Deal. Also included in that piece of legislation were funds given to the USPHS to assist state and local governments in further developing a public health infrastructure (Duffy 1990, 258).

During World War II, the federal government stepped up its own public health mission, and in the postwar era it increased aid to the states as well. In 1943 the USPHS was reorganized to include the office of surgeon general, the National Institutes of Health, and an office focused on state services. In 1944 the functions of the USPHS were clarified to include the training of public health professionals who would serve at all levels of government. In the years immediately following the end of the war, Congress passed legislation funding the construction of hospitals across the country through grants to the states. The Centers for Disease Control (CDC) was also created (Patel and Rushefsky 2005, 17). In the past fifty years, the federal government's role in public health policy has been strengthened through establishment of grants-in-aid for a wider variety of public health issues, increased funding for these programs, and the issuance of regulations to promote public health. Chief among these programs are Medicaid and Medicare, whose passage during the Johnson administration gave millions of Americans access to health care. While these two programs were not public health programs per se, by giving health insurance to many low-income Americans, pressure was removed from local public health agencies, which viewed health care to low-income individuals as an emerging public health function.

Over time, many states and their local governments have come to rely on federal grants for funding public health activities. During those periods when federal public health funding declines, state and local activities are severely affected.

Similar to states, the federal government also issues mandates. Mandates impose behavior on individuals, firms, or state and local governments. In a few cases mandates might be accompanied by grants or tax incentives that subsidize the desired behavior. Mandates imposed on state and local governments direct the choice of a public policy tool. In the 1970s, federal air and water quality standards established thresholds and directed governments on how to achieve them. In fact, the federal government has been criticized for mandating the specific choice of a public policy tool rather than simply setting a regulatory threshold and allowing state and local governments the freedom to decide how to achieve it (Koch 1980).

Quite possibly the most significant public health mandate issued by the federal government was achieved as a result of attacks on cigarette smoking in the 1960s by the surgeon general and the Federal Trade Commission. This mandate, imposed on tobacco companies, directed those firms to place a warning on their products advising the public of the health hazards of cigarette smoking. The smoking case represents both the potential influence and impact of the federal government in the area of public health and the limits of federal intervention. Through its regulatory powers and its ability to control interstate commerce, the federal government now has the power to address threats to public health, such as tobacco, in a most effective way. The limits placed on the surgeon general and the Federal Trade Commission by Congress in the 1960s resulted in only a modest cancer warning being placed on the cigarette pack. This and the subsequent failed attempts by the Food and Drug Administration (FDA) to regulate tobacco as a drug demonstrate that constituency politics at the federal level can prevent truth from speaking to power as it can at any other level of government (Fritschler 1975).

The federal government's role in public health has increased significantly over the past century. This role, however, is still secondary to the state and local levels, which have both an affinity and a proximity to their communities, making them far more effective and appropriate formulators and implementers of public health policy. Commenting early in the 1990s, one historian described that the role of the federal government "is to set minimum standards of public health and encourage states and communities to meet or exceed those standards, to assist training public health personnel, to gather statistics, to aid with emergency health problems, to provide advice and counseling, to help educate the public and to promote research in areas ranging from biomedicine to social welfare" (Duffy 1990, 306). The terrorist attacks in 2001 and later Hurricanes Katrina and Sandy shifted the funding for federal public health significantly toward emergency preparedness. As a result, there is probably less federal funding available today for other public health issues.

The impact of intergovernmental relations on urban political systems should affect urban public health policy making in several ways. First, urban public health policy makers are more likely to adopt a policy tool if it is subsidized through a grant from a higher level of government or if it is mandated by a higher level of government. Second, because of New York City's history at the forefront of public health policy making, the city's adoption of specific policy tools may be followed by their adoption and support at the federal and state level.

Racial and Ethnic Diversity and Urban Public Health

Racial and ethnic diversity affect urban public health policy in various ways. And to the extent that the diversity is due to a large immigrant base, the impact of racial and ethnic diversity on public health policy is even greater. The public health policy choices of New York City, the most diverse city in the country and one of the most diverse cities in the world, are significantly affected by the extent and nature of its racial and ethnic composition.

New York City owes much of its current racial and ethnic diversity to its legacy and inertia as a city attractive to immigrants and to its position as a regional, national, and global economic center. As centers of economic activity, cities have always been magnets attracting individuals and groups, citizens and noncitizens alike, searching for employment and economic betterment. Throughout its evolution from a manufacturing center to a service and commercial center and most recently to a global financial center, New York City has retained its attractiveness as an immigrant city. As the city became a center for immigration and for global commerce, public health concerns increased. Immigrant health became so important that by the end of the nineteenth century, the federal government had become involved in setting up an immigrant health screening facility on Ellis Island. The federal activities were in conjunction with the city's already established function of using quarantines for those "suspected of carrying disease" (Lieber and Opdycke 1995, 911). Concerns about immigrants bringing disease into the city, or country, also had significant racial and ethnic overtones, depending on the group involved (Rosner 1995, 2).

New York City's racial and ethnic diversity and its history as a city of immigrants affect its public health policy choices in several ways. First, urban political systems that experience waves of immigration have had to maintain a vigilant public policy to address public health threats potentially brought into the cities by newly arriving immigrants. As a result, racial and ethnic diversity does not necessarily influence the choice of policy tools, but it does expand their number by broadening the range of public health issues with which an urban political system will have to deal. While immigrant groups are not responsible for most of New York City's public health problems, throughout the city's history they have been linked with specific public health issues. In the nineteenth century, New York City officials had to contend with the threat and sometimes reality of immigrant groups arriving with yellow fever, smallpox, and cholera. These threats resulted in the city developing quarantine facilities and specialized hospitals to isolate those infected individuals, including newly arriving immigrants who threatened the public's health. More recently, in 2003, the outbreak of severe acute respiratory syndrome (SARS) in China heightened concerns among New York City's public health establishment due to the extent of Chinese immigration to New York City.

Second, diverse political systems have to manage their diversity not only to assure successful public policy formulation and implementation but also to promote a social and political civility. On a most basic level, ethnically and racially diverse political systems must contend with language literacy issues and settlement patterns to formulate citywide public policy. This is the case in all areas of public policy, not just public health. Residents must understand public policy directives to respond appropriately; thus political systems must speak in their language. Discussing immigrant reaction to public health measures in the nineteenth century, John Duffy (1968b, 191) notes that, being "unable to comprehend the reason for many health measures and generally suspicious of officialdom," the immigrants "often hid their sick and paid only lip service to the principles of public and personal hygiene."

When racial and ethnic groups live in enclaves, as many immigrant groups do, public policy must cater to enclave settlement patterns, as well as enclave social organization and leadership. Moreover, diverse cultures have varying attitudes not only toward government involvement in the community but also toward lifestyle issues that may be related to public health problems. At the outset of the AIDS crisis, local leaders in some communities of color were reluctant to participate in the public health campaign against AIDS because of their antipa-

thy toward homosexuals and intravenous drug users. As a result, racial and ethnic diversity does not so much influence which policy tool is adopted but the
way such tools are deployed across diverse communities. Without this acknowledgment of and response to diversity, urban political systems will fail to achieve
desired public policy results in these communities.

Third, to be effective in reaching diverse communities, public health tools
must be employed in culturally competent ways. Not only do the habits and customs of diverse racial ethnic communities pose a challenge for public health authorities seeking to employ a policy tool across the entire city, but these habits
and customs may themselves be a source of public health concern. Over the centuries, New York City has experienced waves of immigration from multiple con-
tinents. Each wave brings new groups with their own customs and attitudes. Not
only are new groups at times suspicious of governmental health authorities,
but they may engage in behaviors or customs that, while acceptable in their
countries of origin, may be a source of public health concern. As the childhood
lead-based paint poisoning problem was being addressed in the 1990s and early
2000s, there was concern that some immigrant groups from Central America
were using lead-based pottery in their homes, exacerbating the problem. Even
today, residential housing patterns that might produce overcrowding, unhealthy food and nutrition habits, and a group's adversarial relationship to the
medical establishment may contribute to public health problems.

Finally, the incidence of public health problems and their differential impact
on specific racial and ethnic groups may also pose a challenge for public policy
makers. Many public health problems have a disproportionate impact on communities of color. This may be due to discrimination, past or present, or to the
fact that in New York City, as in many other cities, there is a strong relationship between low-income communities and communities of color. These communities lack access to quality health care that might otherwise enable them to
protect themselves from many public health threats. Also, because of poor housing, infrastructure, and community resources, these communities are typically
more exposed to public health threats (NYC Department of Health and Mental Hygiene 2004). Another contributing factor is lack of political resources that
would, on some occasions, give these communities the wherewithal to fend off
noxious facilities that are sometimes the source of public health concerns.

In the extreme, there is the possibility that the group's high incidence of a disease or condition is due to the policies of the political system itself. Public policies, either purposefully or inadvertently, frequently place facilities that produce
harmful environmental effects in one part of the city. This is done to keep them
away from residential areas, especially those where upper-income groups have
settled. Many groups who cannot afford upper-income housing must settle in
those parts of the city where these harmful facilities exist. They are exposed to

the foul air and toxins that negatively affect health. Because low-income groups that end up living in these unhealthy parts of the city are predominantly minority, this condition is termed environmental racism. To the extent that environmental racism and its public health impacts become politicized, the political system will be the target of demands by those affected groups for the adoption of specific tools to alleviate the inequitable distribution of public health harms.

"For decades, some low-income communities of color in New York have borne a disproportionate burden of polluting infrastructure" (Bautista 2010). In 1989 the New York City Charter adopted a "fair share" clause whereby agencies placing noxious facilities in communities were mandated to analyze each designated community's share of city facilities. Community boards and borough presidents were also supposed to have a say in final location decisions, although their input was merely advisory and not determinative. Although the intent of the charter fair-share program was laudable, in the end there was little change in city practices on the siting of facilities. Moreover, the city charter could address only city facilities. Those facilities sited by other levels of government, such as the state-controlled Metropolitan Transit Authority, were never included in the city's analysis (Bautista 2010).

Much of New York City's political history can be explained through the arrival, mobilization, and political participation of racial and ethnic groups. Concomitantly, these groups have been the source of many of the most significant articulated demands placed on the political system. As a result, although the identity of the racial and ethnic groups has changed over time, the fact that public health policy and its impacts on New York City's population can, in part, be explained through race and ethnicity is nothing new. It does, however, serve to increase the role that race and ethnicity play in city politics and at times serves to exacerbate intergroup tensions and decrease civil harmony.

Why New York City?

New York City is the ideal setting in which to study urban public health policy. First, as the country's largest urban area, New York City has had to address a wide range of public health issues. Because of its dense settlement patterns, the size and diversity of its population, housing stock, transportation patterns, and point of entry for millions of immigrants, the city's environment is conducive to practically every public health issue experienced by major cities in the United States. The history of urban public health issues and policies is very much reflected in the city's public health history.

Second, from its early days, the city has developed the political culture supportive of political system involvement in addressing public health issues. The city's continuous but ever changing immigrant base, initially from Europe through the middle of the twentieth century but becoming more global after that, has resulted in a political system dominated by a liberal set of political attitudes less fearful of government intervention than most other urban political systems in the country. This liberal political culture has produced approximately 150 years of public health interventions by the city and state political systems. As evidence of New York City's political culture supportive of public health intervention, the city's comprehensive effort to address public health issues is the oldest of all urban areas in the United States, dating back to the middle of the nineteenth century with the establishment of the Metropolitan Board of Health. New York City had a working Department of Health before any other large city, and it was the first in the country and one of the first in world to have its own laboratory facilities engaging in bacteriological research and the production of vaccine (Leavitt 1995).

Throughout the twentieth century, the city's public health enterprise was complemented by an expanding city medical health enterprise. Beginning with the New Deal's creation of neighborhood health clinics through the administration and partial financing of Medicaid and the administration of a network of city-funded and city-administered hospitals and allied health centers, the city of New York became involved in the delivery of health and medical services to individuals on a massive scale. Because of New York State mandates requiring local government cost sharing in the financing of Medicaid, the city was paying more than $2 billion in Medicaid costs by 2000. In addition, New York City's Health and Hospitals Corporation administered eleven acute care hospitals, several outpatient clinics, and two long-term care facilities (NYC Health and Hospitals Corporation 2003). Most but not all of the recipients of the city's delivery of individual health and medical services were those in poverty. In addition, with the merger of the city's Department of Health and Department of Mental Health, Mental Retardation and Alcoholism Services in 2001, the city Department of Health was also delivering services to those suffering from alcoholism and substance abuse. The city did receive considerable state support in these efforts.

The city's health enterprise has become so expansive that at least four agencies participate in the implementation of public health policy on a full-time basis, and other agencies are intermittently involved. The Department of Health and Mental Hygiene oversees primary disease monitoring, prevention, and control functions of the typical local health department. The Health and Hospitals Corporation oversees the municipal hospitals and allied health facilities. In addition to overseeing the city's water system, the Department of Environmental Protection is responsible for carrying out the Federal Clean Water Act and Clean Air Act. This includes the maintenance of the city's wastewater treatment facility. In addition, the agency deals with hazardous materials and toxic site issues, as well as enforcing the city's noise code (Kirk 2002, 150). The Department of Sanitation collects and manages the city's solid waste. The agency's responsibilities include the disposal of asbestos and medical waste as well as the operation of waste transfer stations (312).

The status of the city's public health enterprise as the oldest and one of the most progressive of urban political systems in the United States is well recognized (Duffy 1968a; 1968b; 1990). This does not mean that on every public health issue New York City is ahead of every other city, but it does mean that the city has been at the forefront on most public health issues facing urban political systems in the United States.

Third, because of the public health problems the city has faced, together with a political culture conducive to a political system response to most problems, the city public health policy tool box is more extensive than most urban political systems. This is of critical importance since public health policy tools constitute the dependent variable in this research. The city's public health infrastructure and its policy tools serve as a referent for the study of urban public health in this country. Cities with little variation in their choice of tools would offer insufficient variation in the dependent variable.

Finally, although an examination of New York City's public health policy behavior does not allow for claims of external validity to other cities, it does provide a referent for the study of how an urban political system can respond. As such, this study assesses how the state of medical or health knowledge, the pressures that economic development place on an urban political system, intergovernmental relations, and increasing ethnic and racial diversity influence a city's public health policy choices across five public health problems.

The Cases Discussed in this Study and Methods

Over the past several decades, New York City's political system has addressed numerous public health challenges. In order to compare and contrast the tools adopted by public health policy makers within the analytical frameworks discussed in this introduction, it is not possible to deal comprehensively with every major challenge. The five public health issues considered here—lead-based paint poisoning, asthma, HIV/AIDS, West Nile virus, and obesity—reflect the public health issues currently being addressed. They include communicable diseases, problems caused by environmental degradation, and issues of lifestyle and behavior. Some of the problems focus specifically on public health problems faced by children. Missing from this study are long-standing public health challenges including tuberculosis and smoking, and more recent ones such as emergency preparedness.

Each chapter focuses on the public policy tools employed by the city to combat the public health issue in question. Analysis examines what role medical or health knowledge, economic development issues, intergovernmental relations, and racial and ethnic diversity have played in the city's use of each tool.

Interviews with selected officials in the New York City Department of Health and Mental Hygiene were conducted early in the research process, but the interviews were focused primarily on the location of sources rather than on substance. Where an interview produced relevant information on policy substance, it is cited in the text.

For the chapters on HIV/AIDS and childhood lead-based paint poisoning, I relied heavily on the New York City Municipal Archives for the early histories of the city's responses. By the mid- to late 1990s, I was able to obtain documents from New York City agencies, especially the Department of Health and Mental Hygiene, either directly or from their websites. I also relied on documents from New York State and the federal government, particularly the New York State Department of Health and U.S. Centers for Disease Control and Prevention.

I was able to collect videos of mayoral press conferences and city council hearings starting in the mid-1990s. These became a primary source of information on policy tools. For each of the five diseases discussed, I was able to view and review from 50 to 150 hours of press conferences and hearings. The press conferences and hearings provided formal statements of policy and testimony by experts in the field, city agency officials, representative of the mayor, and citizens. They offered information on the choice of tools and their implementation and a critical assessment of both. Secondary sources, primarily local newspapers, provided additional interpretation and depth.

CHAPTER TWO

LEAD POISONING IN CHILDREN

Policy toward childhood lead-based paint poisoning is an area where there is no uncertainty or debate on the cause of the problem. The solution was derived with no debate within the public health community. The singular challenge was for political officials to legislate and promulgate a law that would address the problem in an effective manner. In addition, true to the legacy of public health policy, lead-based paint policy has been dominated by local policy makers, with limited participation by the state and federal officials.

New York City's policy on childhood lead-based poisoning evolved over several decades and involved multiple pieces of legislation. In addition, from the time that its health impacts could be accurately measured, the childhood victims of this condition in the city have been disproportionately minority. Despite this, the development of lead-based paint policy in the city has not been influenced by racial politics. Instead, economic development concerns have been the primary forces involved in the debate. The decline in childhood exposure to lead and the consequent decline in lead poisoning, much of it due to public health policy, should be viewed as one of public health's more significant success stories. Legislation has firmly established a child's right to lead-safe housing in most housing categories in the city.

The new law has an impact not only on health but also on housing. Landlords, the real estate industry, and even the city government itself, as a major owner of aging residential housing, all have an interest in keeping lead-based paint abatement costs as low as possible. As well-organized and influential interests in the city's political system, these actors have attempted to affect policy development in this area.

Since the science behind lead-based paint poisoning is clear and no longer a subject of debate, the primary focus of policy is prevention through abatement of the source. Rather than primary prevention, however, the political system initially opted for a strategy of secondary prevention: treatment and cure for those children diagnosed with lead-based paint poisoning. That is, rather than eliminate the source of poisoning before it occurred, public policy addressed the source of lead poisoning only after a child had been tested and shown to have elevated blood lead levels (Bellinger and Bellinger 2006). In 1982 New York City adopted legislation that promoted primary prevention, but the legislation was never implemented or enforced. All subsequent legislation at all levels of government has focused on secondary prevention.

The principal policy tool being used in these efforts is regulation of those who own residential dwellings. The points of controversy within the regulatory regime are measures that define when action must be taken. Rights, regulations, and their accompanying thresholds also play a role in assigning liability. If, in the absence of regulatory compliance, negative health impacts occur, courts are asked to assess liability. Education is also employed: landlords must know their responsibilities, and tenants must be aware of landlord obligations in order for the policy to work.

Scientific research on the incidence of lead poisoning as well as its harmful effects on children played a significant role in getting the issue on the public agenda. At the same time, research and the resulting knowledge about lead poisoning predated public policy at the city, state, and federal levels by many years.

The Science and Etiology of Lead-Based Paint Poisoning

Knowledge about lead-based paint and its harmful effects evolved throughout much of the twentieth century. Childhood lead poisoning was first identified in 1892 in Australia where it was associated with some childhood deaths. During the 1940s, research "demonstrated the persistence of severe residue in children who had recovered from acute lead poisoning" (Needleman 1998, 1871). Throughout the first half of the twentieth century, lead poisoning could be diagnosed only by its most severe symptoms or death, due to prolonged or severe exposure. By the 1970s and 1980s, research had not only confirmed its effects at high blood lead levels (BLLs) but also demonstrated its harmful effect on child IQ and behavior at lower levels. "Population-based epidemiological studies revealed the existence of what was labeled subclinical lead poisoning" (Bellinger and Bellinger 2006, 854). Although the damage being produced by the poisoning was not severe enough to produce symptoms sufficient to meet current diagnostic criteria, the damage was still severe enough to have measurable impact on the child's IQ (Bellinger and Bellinger 2006).

Lead in the bloodstream could not be detected through a blood test until the 1940s. Nevertheless, well into the 1960s childhood lead poisoning "was diagnosed in its early clinical stages only by the suspicious and informed physician" (Berney 1993, 5). The symptoms were often mistaken for other conditions and diseases (Rabin 1989, 1669). Innovations in screening technologies in the 1970s made lead blood level screening much less expensive with results being "obtained on site in a few minutes" (Berney 1993, 14).

Children "absorb and retain more ingested lead" than adults (Medley 1982, 67). Because of their higher rate of metabolism and greater level of physical activity, children also inhale more lead, relative to their weight, than adults. Most importantly, once lead has entered their bodies, children do not process it as well as adults. In adults, skeletal tissue holds ingested lead. In children, "lead present in bone can readily reenter the circulatory system where it becomes available to vulnerable soft tissue" (67). Lead also attacks the developing brains and central nervous systems in children more virulently than it does adults. Some research has suggested that "children who do not get enough calcium and iron may be more susceptible to the lead in their environment, whatever the source" (Johnson 2003b, B2).

Initially, it was thought that lead in the bloodstream at levels of 60 micrograms per deciliter or higher were needed to cause harm. In fact, children with BLLs in excess of 100 micrograms not only had brain disorders, but in many cases x-rays of the stomach showed visible lead-based paint chips (American Academy of Pediatrics [AAP] 2005, 1037). "Children with blood lead concentrations greater than 60 micrograms may complain of headaches, abdominal pain, loss of appetite, display clumsiness, agitation, and/or decreased activity" (AAP 2005, 1039). More recent research suggests that harm (e.g., impairment of neurocognitive functioning) can begin at BLLs as low as 6–15 micrograms per deciliter (Florini and Silbergeld 1993, 33). Physicians recommend that if lead-based paint is in the environment, children should be tested even if they are not exhibiting any of the overt symptoms of poisoning. And the AAP (2005) currently recommends medical intervention for children who have BLLs of 10 micrograms per deciliter. In 1991 one in eleven children in the United States had blood lead concentrations greater than 10 micrograms (AAP 2005). In 2012, the Centers for Disease Control recommended lead level limits of 5 micrograms per deciliter, and this is the level at which New York City currently initiates services (Hartocollis 2012; NYC Department of Health and Mental Hygiene [DOHMH] 2011).

Prolonged exposure to high levels of lead can result in brain dysfunction, coma, convulsions, and death. Moderate levels of exposure can affect the central nervous system, harming cognition (AAP 2005, 1037). Research reported in the 1980s suggested that even low levels of exposure to lead were far more harmful than initially thought, producing problems with speech, fine motor coordination, and short attention span. One study showed deficits of four to six points on intelligence tests at blood lead levels as low as 10–25 micrograms per deciliter (Berney 1993, 9, 26). "Teachers reported that students with elevated tooth lead concentrations were more inattentive, hyperactive, disorganized and less able to follow directions" (AAP 2005, 1038).

The standard treatment for lead poisoning at elevated BLLs is chelation, the intravenous administration of an amino acid that decreases lead in the bloodstream (NYS Comptroller 2007, 26). Although there is conclusive evidence that chelation can reduce BLLs, the evidence that reduced BLLs through chelation will decrease earlier diagnosed cognitive impairments is inconclusive. More recently, succimer, a drug administered orally has also been used, but the research on the drug's impact on measures of cognition is inconclusive (AAP 2005, 1039–1043). Some have argued that if the child is removed from the source of the poisoning, he or she "can recover from the effect of lead poisoning" (Hsu 1997, B4). Other research suggests that "even minute exposures to lead accumulate in the body, producing effects that may endure long after the exposure ends" (Florini and Silbergeld 1993, 35).

Although not all childhood lead poisoning comes from lead-based paint, its primary sources throughout the twentieth century were paint and gasoline. The removal of lead from gasoline in the 1990s resulted in a significant decrease in mean childhood BLLs and left lead-based paint as the primary source of lead poisoning in children (Needleman 1998, 1871). Although it was initially thought that most children obtained high BLLs by eating paint chips peeling off household walls, more recent studies suggest that children are exposed to "fine lead dust that forms as painted surfaces chip and peel . . . Children get this lead dust on their hands by crawling or playing on contaminated carpets or floors" (Morrison 1998, 16). The dust is then inhaled or ingested.

Incidence of Lead-Based Paint and Lead-Based Paint Poisoning

According to the National Safety Council, lead-based paint can be found in approximately two-thirds of homes built before 1940 and approximately half of all homes built between 1940 and 1960 (Brody 2006). Lead-based paint poses a health problem in those residences where it is peeling or cracking and falling from ceilings or walls. This occurs primarily in low-income neighborhoods where housing is deteriorating or not well maintained (Middlekauff 2001). In the city, cases of lead-based paint poisoning were most prevalent in neighborhoods with pre–World War II housing that was once occupied by wealthy families but had trickled down to low-income families. Before the health effects of the paint were known, wealthy families had painted their homes with lead-based paint because it was light and durable. When the housing was later occupied by lower-income families, the lead-based paint was painted over. Because of poor maintenance, the old lead-based paint became exposed and began to crack and peel, creating a health hazard (Gaiter 1981). In 1994 a government study reported that low-income children were "four times more likely to have elevated levels of lead in their blood than" high-income children (Purdy 1994).

In 2006, with approximately one-quarter of all children nationally exposed to lead in their homes, more than 400,000 were found to have BLLs that were "deemed hazardous to normal mental and physical development (Brody 2006). When the federal government lowered the level of lead exposure considered safe, it significantly increased the incidence of the problem (Purdy 1994).

TABLE 2.1
New York City Lead Poisoning Cases and Screening, 1949–2008

Year	Bloods Screened	EIBLL Defined as Intervention Worthy	EIBLL Cases	EIBLL ≥ 45 μg/dl	EIBLL ≥ 10 μg/dl
1949			3		
1950			1		
1951			21		
1952			19		
1953			25		
1954			86		
1955			125		
1956			100		
1957			97		
1958			116		
1959			171		
1960			146		
1961			173		
1962			198		
1963			338		
1964	4,049		509		
1965	4,766		601		
1966	4,279		466		
1967	4,175		467		
1968	4,707		725		
1969	10,023		727		
1970	87,007	≥ 60 μg/dl	2,649		
1971	115,816		1,925		
1972	100,182		944		
1973	124,092		761		
1974	124,900		494		
1975	111,954	≥ 40 μg/dl	1,595		
1976	103,016		984		
1977	96,385		652		
1978	111,430		802		
1979	123,873		931		
1980	136,683		976		
1981	136,163		1,538		
1982	134,433		1,259		
1983	146,171	≥ 30 μg/dl	1,193		
1984	170,588		960		
1985	20,467		1,195		
1986		≥ 25 μg/dl	1,284		
1987			1,043		
1988			793		
1989			890		
1990			662		
1991			701		
1992			809		
1993		≥ 20 μg/dl	1,909		
1994			1,969		
1995			1,709	125	21,575

Year	Bloods Screened	EIBLL Defined as Intervention Worthy	EIBLL Cases	EIBLL ≥ 45 µg/dl	EIBLL ≥ 10 µg/dl
1996			1,377	88	16,103
1997	297,531		1,149	86	12,936
1998	303,710		1,061	73	10,817
1999	295,584	≥ 15 µg/dl	893	61	8,146
2000	319,312		817	47	7,194
2001	306,389		653	39	5,638
2002	297,177		628	41	4,876
2003	304,130		587	40	4,234
2004	298,039		764	32	3,834
2005	312,845		875	20	3,190
2006	317,173		800	16	2,722
2007	398,121		620	31	2,270
2008	409,254		536	15	1,634
2009	413,518		512	21	1,634
2010			448		1,429
2011			342		1,183

Sources: Andrew Kerr. 1970. Project Plan for Lead Poisoning Control. Policy Planning Council Project Management Staff. March 13; New York City Department of Health. 2012. Health department announces number of childhood lead poisoning cases dropped 17%, achieving new historic low in New York City (press release). October 1; New York City Department of Health and Mental Hygiene. 2001. Preventing Lead Poisoning in New York City: Annual Report, 2001; New York City Department of Health and Mental Hygiene. 2009. Preventing Lead Poisoning in New York City: Annual Data Report, 2009; New York City Department of Health and Mental Hygiene 2011. Report to the New York City Council on Progress in Preventing Childhood Lead Poisoning in New York City.

Note: Indication of environmental intervention blood lead levels (EIBLL) is defined as at least one blood lead level test in a child (younger than 18 years of age) producing a result of 15 micrograms (or greater) of lead per deciliter.

Table 2.1 reports the number of blood samples screened for lead poisoning as well as the number of reported environmental intervention blood lead levels (EIBLL) for each year from 1949 to 2011. EIBLL refers to the blood lead level "at which environmental and case coordination services for children with lead poisoning are initiated" (NYC DOHMH 2011, 1). The current EIBLL threshold is 15 micrograms per deciliter but the DOHMH provides services to all children who test above 5 micrograms per deciliter (NYC DOHMH 2011). All data come from the Department of Health, now the Department of Health and Hygiene. For blood samples screened, some years have no available data. Before the 1960s, such data were not compiled. Even with the missing years in the 1980s and 1990s, it is apparent that by the late 1990s more than 300,000 children in the city were being screened for lead poisoning each year.

The reporting of cases of EIBLL is complicated because over time the Centers for Disease Control and Prevention (CDC) kept lowering the EIBLL threshold as research produced more knowledge about the effects of lead poisoning and as testing was able to detect lead in the blood at lower levels. The increased number of EIBLL cases and the fluctuation in the number of cases yearly may be due as much to increases in the number of children being screened as well as changes in the EIBLL threshold as to any real increase (or decrease) in cases. Over time, however, the number of cases of lead poisoning did decline. Beginning in the mid-1990s, blood samples tested in New York State began to record cases at extremely high levels ($\geq$ 45 micrograms per deciliter) and at lower levels than the CDC threshold ($\geq$ 10).

New York City began screening for lead poisoning in the late 1960s, but physicians were reporting cases of lead poisoning to the Department of Health (DOH) as early as 1950, when one case was reported to the DOH. By the 1990s the AAP and the CDC recommended universal BLL screening for all children one and two years of age. Later as BLLs for children in the United States began to decline, recommendations were reduced to targeted screening of specific populations. According to the AAP, any child with a BLL in excess of 10 micrograms should be rechecked periodically (AAP 2005, 1041).

According to former commissioner of health, Mary McLaughlin, in New York City 143 cases were reported between 1950 and 1954, with 80 cases (her numbers) in 1954. There were 39 deaths among the 143 cases, a 27.3 fatality rate (McLaughlin 1956, 3711). Over time the fatality rate fell not only because of increased reporting, especially of low-exposure cases, but also because improved and more rapid blood testing allowed the medical community to catch high-exposure cases earlier. By the late 1960s, more than 700 cases per year were being reported (Berney 1993, 13). The number of new cases per year went well over a thousand for many years during the 1970s, 1980s, and 1990s. The number of new reported lead poisoning cases in the city did drop below a thousand in the late 1990s (Lambert 2000a; Strasburg 2002).

Child health advocates however, have disputed the city's statistics, arguing that more than 136,000 children had contracted lead poisoning in the five-year period between 1995 and 2000, and that in 2000 more than 6,000 newly identified cases of lead poisoning were reported to the city, most of them among minority children. Some of the statistical discrepancy was due to the use of different thresholds of lead-based paint exposure (Cardwell 2002; Goldstein 2003). From the early 1990s to the present, the DOH used a BLL of 20 micrograms per deciliter as the threshold for taking action in a home but 10 micrograms per deciliter as the reportable lead poisoning threshold when communicating with the CDC. Because many children at risk for lead poisoning were never screened, estimates of the incidence of lead poisoning were often little more than educated guesses (Public Advocate for the City of New York 1998, 4).

TABLE 2.2
Racial Profile of New York City Children with EIBLL, 2001–2008 (%)

Group	Population Composition	2001 EIBLL ($n=653$)	2005 EIBLL ($n=875$)	2008 EIBLL ($n=536$)
White	23	5	9	13
Non-Hispanic Black	29	42	31	28
Asian	9	18	18	23
Hispanic	34	34	40	34
Other	4	1	2	2

Sources: New York City Department of Health. 2001. Preventing Lead Poisoning in New York City: Annual Report, 2001; New York City Department of Health 2005. Preventing Lead Poisoning in New York City: Annual Report, 2005; New York City Department of Health. 2008. Lead Poisoning in New York City: Annual Data Report, 2008.

Note: Indication of environmental intervention blood lead levels (EIBLL) is defined as at least one blood lead level test in a child (younger than 18 years of age) producing a result of 15 micrograms (or greater) of lead per deciliter.

The close association between race and class in New York City in the second half of the twentieth century meant that any condition that fell heavily upon lower-income New Yorkers was going to be felt disproportionately among racial and ethnic minorities. In 1999 the eight New York City health districts with the highest rates of lead poisoning were all in Brooklyn and Queens, constituting what many had been calling the "lead belt," populated mostly by minorities (New York Public Interest Research Group 1999). The data in table 2.2 suggest that the racial breakdown of childhood lead poisoning is approximate to each group's composition in the population with the exception of Asians, who appear to suffering disproportionately as of 2008.

In 1991 the U.S. surgeon general "declared lead poisoning the principal environmental health hazard afflicting American children," with lead dust from lead-based paint being the primary cause (Molloy 1992). But the CDC was reluctant to recommend mandatory BLL testing of all children "since a vast majority of children from middle and upper income families would not test above the 10-microgram level" (Brody 2006). Throughout the late 1980s and early 1990s, there were more than one thousand lead poisoning claims against private landlords and the city, costing landlords and the city millions of dollars (Beller 1994).

Throughout much of the 1990s, more than 80 percent of homes of children who tested at the BLL threshold where the city Department of Health took action had a discoverable lead hazard in the home (Public Advocate of the City of New York 1998, 6). As a result, policies to attack poisoning from lead-based paint were targeted as the cause of the harmful health effects, and the only immediate treatment for lead poisoning was to remove the child from the hazard.

New York City's Lead-Based Paint Programs

Table 2.3 displays the tools used by the city to combat childhood lead poisoning. New York City's public policy on lead-based paint evolved over five decades. What became apparent during the period was that public policy on lead-based paint was affected as much by housing policy as public health policy. Today, the city's programs dealing with lead-based paint are implemented jointly by the city's Department of Health and Mental Hygiene (DOHMH) as well as the city's Department of Housing Preservation and Development (HPD).

In 1959 the city amended its health code granting "discretionary authority" to the DOH "to order the removal of lead-based paint from inside residential dwellings" (Pedro 2000, 565). The same code amendments banned the use of lead-based paint in residential dwellings. Through the late 1960s, the city had no systematic method for identifying cases of childhood lead-based paint poisoning. Although increased lead poisoning screening produced more cases throughout the 1960s, in those parts of the city where children were deemed to be most at risk for lead poisoning, fewer than 10 percent of them were screened in any year. Screening and case identification took place through referrals from city child health stations, home visits by public health nurses, and hospitals. Children suspected of lead poisoning were referred to the city's Social Hygiene Clinic for a blood test (NYC DOH 1969, 17). The DOH attempted to educate health professionals about the need for early detection of lead poisoning. Lead poisoning was suspected as a result of either specific behavior patterns observed by health professionals or reports by parents that the child placed plaster or paint chips in his or her mouth. In these cases, physicians were encouraged to perform blood tests and send specimens to the DOH laboratory (Eidsvold et al. 1974).

These case-finding activities on the part of the city, however limited, did result in a significant increase in the number of reported cases. Between 1950 and 1954, 1955 and 1959, and 1960 and 1964, 152, 609, and 1,364 new cases, respectively, were identified (NYC DOH 1970a, I-9a).

If a blood test reported a BLL of 60 micrograms or greater, the parent was contacted to bring the child back to the health station. In addition, a public health nurse was sent to the home to see whether there were other children who might also be suffering from lead poisoning. The DOH's Bureau of Sanitary Inspection also went to the home to inspect "the premises for loose paint chips and plaster" (NYC DOH 1969, 18). In some cases, posters were placed in those buildings where a case of lead poisoning had occurred after children chewed plaster or paint (NYC DOH 1954). Paint samples, if found, were sent to DOH laboratories and analyzed for lead content. If they contained lead, the landlord was notified of a health violation (NYC DOH 1969, 18). Before 1970, however,

TABLE 2.3
Public Policy Tools Addressing Childhood Lead Poisoning

MONITORING AND SCREENING

New York City and New York State

Collect incidence and prevalence data

New York State

Mandates universal screening for children ages 1–2

Certifies blood lead level testing facilities

EDUCATION (RELEVANT PUBLICS)

New York City

Department of Health and Mental Hygiene

Informs relevant communities of the existence of the law through education and out-reach activities

Department of Housing Preservation and Development

Provides outreach and education to communities, owners, and contractors regarding lead-safe work practices

Department of Health (educating tenants)

Requires landlords to provide written notice to tenants of landlord's obligation to inspect for and repair lead-based paint hazards and the tenants' obligation to provide access to apartments

Requires landlord to inform apartment occupants of the results of the inspection and provide them with a written report

New York State

Coordinates lead safety-training programs for contractors and subcontractors

Educates health care providers on medical management of lead poisoning

Federal government

Researches and disseminates expertise on BLL thresholds (CDC)

Educates health care providers regarding management of children exposed to lead poisoning

REGULATIONS (LEAD PAINT DETECTION AND REMEDIATION)

New York City

Department of Health and Mental Hygiene

Sends letter to families educating them about lead poisoning and advising further follow-up testing when child is tested at 5 micrograms per deciliter

Inspects an apartment whenever a child is identified with a BLL of 15 micrograms per deciliters or higher

Certifies to HPD for abatement if landlord fails to act

Inspects the corrected area of an apartment when a violation is reported post remediation

Department of Housing Preservation and Development

Landlords

Inspects every apartment with a child under 7 in multiple-unit buildings with three or more apartments

Inspects annually and when apartments turn over

Defines lead paint area as 1.0 milligrams per square centimeter

TABLE 2.3 (continued)

Details household lead paint hazards requiring action by landlord:
> Friction surfaces that could produce a hazard by rubbing (includes lead dust)
> Impact surfaces that could produce a hazard by being hit
> Chewable surfaces (windowsills)
> 40 micrograms per square foot on floors
> 250 micrograms per square foot on windowsills

Requires prompt action when hazards are found:
> 50 days to correct hazard
> 21 days to correct hazard after violation is reported or found by DOHMH or HPD
> Fines of up to $250 a day for each violation, up to a maximum of $10,000

Abatement activities
> Prohibits dry scraping and sanding of paint
> Requires federally certified workers for abatement or containment
> Temporarily relocates family when work cannot be completed safely
> Provides written notice to DOHMH within 10 days of beginning abatement work

Postabatement activities
> Has dust clearance test conducted by an independent third party where remediation area is more than 100 square feet

New York State
> Sets standards for contractors performing lead abatement

Federal government
> Enforces compliance of state lead-based poisoning abatement standards with rules promulgated by Title VI of the Federal Toxic Substances Control Act
> Residential Lead Based Paint Hazard Reduction Act (1992): Requires abatement of lead paint hazards in federally owned residential properties and housing receiving federal assistance

REGULATIONS (HEALTHCARE PROVIDERS)

New York State
> Requires physicians / health care providers to perform blood tests on children and send the sample to state-certified laboratory for testing

SERVICE PROVISION

New York City
> Department of Housing Preservation and Development (HPD)
>> Addresses problems when landlord fails to act
>> Inspects buildings whenever DOHMH reports a child with an elevated BLL (including intact surfaces)
>> Performs inspections in response to tenant complaints
>> Performs inspections for all city-owned housing (with children under age 7)

New York State
> NYS Department of Health: Oversees case management of children with elevated BLLs

Nonprofit groups
> Provide lead-safe housing

LIABILITY
Landlord
> Repairs harm done, especially when regulations have not been followed, in multiple-unit buildings with three or more apartments (includes the city for city-owned housing)

FINANCIAL ASSISTANCE
New York City
> Department of Finance: Provides city tax credits to landlords for abatement activities in low-income housing

New York State
> Provides funding for local health departments for education and outreach activities, coordinating referrals for home visits with affected families by health department personnel
> Provides Medicaid for lead screening for eligible children

Federal government
> Department of Health and Human Services: Preventive and Health Services Block Grant (to state)
> (Federal) Healthy Communities Program: Provides preventive environmental health services to targeted geographic areas with a high rate of undocumented health needs
> Maternal and Child Health Block Grant (to state): Provides federal funds for lead paint poisoning prevention
> Housing and Urban Development Lead Based Paint Hazard Control Program and Lead Hazard Reduction: Provides funds for contractor certification training in lead-based paint hazard abatement
> Housing and Urban Development-Community Development Block Grant: Provides funds for lead abatement activities
> Housing and Urban Development: Provides funds to address lead-based paint hazards in selected high lead poisoning neighborhoods and for one- and two-family homes, to lead awareness packages distributed through local hardware stores, and to inspect visually and lead safe work practices education programs for owners and contractors
> (Federal) CDC Childhood Lead Poisoning Prevention: Provides federal grant funds monitoring of blood lead levels, follow-up care for those with elevated blood lead levels, and community and professional awareness and education

there was no mandate that the landlord had to address the violation (NYC DOH 1970a, I-17-18).

In the city, increased publicity contributed to more children being screened and added pressure on the political system to respond in a more comprehensive manner. In the late 1960s, the *Village Voice* ran a series of articles on lead poisoning that described the deaths of young children and the housing conditions that could produce lead poisoning. In East Harlem, a Puerto Rican group, the Young Lords, began to conduct its own door-to-door testing program using a urine test that could detect the presence of lead but not the precise level (Eidsvold et al. 1974, 957).

In 1969 the city announced its first comprehensive lead poisoning prevention program. To coordinate the new programs, the city established the Lead Poisoning Control Unit within the city's DOH (NYC Office of Chronic Disease Services 1969), which was given responsibility for "data collection, sanitary inspection, citywide health education, and interagency coordination" (Eidsvold et al. 1974, 957).

The program included expanded public education and screening to find cases at "the incipient stage before poisoning occurs" (NYC Office of Chronic Disease Services 1969). Primary responsibility for education and case finding was given to the city's district health centers. Initial case finding activities were focused on children ages one to six years living in areas of the city with high concentrations of deteriorated housing. Case finding involved the operation of screening facilities at health centers and the incorporation of testing into health care facilities at the community level. It also involved education about lead poisoning and screening at Head Start, day care centers, and health fairs and through neighborhood organizations and door-to-door outreach (Eidsvold et al. 1974, 957).

As a result of these efforts, the number of screenings increased. Compared to 1969 where slightly more than 10,000 children were screened, more than 55,000 children were screened in the first eight months of 1970 and approximately 100,000 children were screened in 1971. The screenings in 1970 and 1971 yielded 1,772 and 1,925 cases of lead poisoning respectively, more than double the number of cases found in 1969 for each year (NYC DOH 1970b; Eidsvold et al. 1974, 957).

In addition, as part of the 1969 initiative, the city implemented a program to remove loose paint and plaster in those homes where child lead poisoning occurred and changed the city health code to require "the covering of lead contaminated walls in cases in which there is a child with poisoning and lead in the paint or plaster on the walls of more than 1%" (NYC Office of Chronic Disease Services 1969). Before 1970, the city health code empowered the DOH to act but did not mandate that it act, nor did the code give the department sufficient power or resources to respond when there was no compliance with its directives. The new health code, Section 173.13, mandated that the DOH "shall order the removal of paint . . . and the refinishing . . . or covering of such surfaces" when any person living in that dwelling has a BLL of 60 micrograms or higher and if there is paint containing "more than 1 percent of metallic lead" on any interior surface (NYC DOH 1970a, I-18). "If the landlord fails to comply with the repair order within five days after it is served, the amended code states that the Health Department 'shall request that the (NYC) Housing Development Administration to execute the order' " (I-19).

The lead poisoning initiatives implemented in 1970 represented a significant improvement over prior policy in education, case finding, and abatement. But the 1970 initiatives did not come close to solving the problem of childhood poisoning due to lead-based paint. In many parts of the city where children were deemed to be most at risk, less than one-fifth of the children were screened in the first four years of the program (Eidsvold et al. 1974, 960).

The program's most significant flaw was that the city could not order housing corrections until a child was poisoned. The law was additionally weakened by poor enforcement. In 1980 the Department of Housing Preservation and Development's (HPD) lead-based paint repair program "failed to correct the lead hazard in one third" of the residences in which a reported lead-poisoned child lived (Alfaro et al. 1982). As a result, some lead-poisoned children, after being released from the hospital, returned to the home that was making them ill. Even when the Housing Development Administration did act, mandated repairs were "limited to the area from which the positive sample or samples" were collected (Eidsvold et al. 1974, 958). This meant that, even though an entire dwelling might have lead-based paint covering its interior, only one wall, a ceiling, or a window-sill might be treated by the Emergency Repair Program of the Housing Development Administration (Eidsvold et al. 1974, 958).

With the failures of the 1970 program apparent, in 1982 the city council enacted a law that placed greater emphasis on preventing lead-based paint poisoning. Local Law 1 of 1982 amended the city's administrative code establishing "the presumption that peeling paint in any pre-1960 building contained impermissibly high levels of lead and imposed on landlords the affirmative duty of ameliorating these conditions" (Pedro 2000, 567). Under the law, a lead-based paint hazard was defined as the existence of paint with 1 percent or more lead (NYS Comptroller 2007, 31). The law made peeling lead-based paint a housing code violation (Alfaro et al. 1982). In effect, the law established a right to lead-free housing for children in any pre-1960 building.

The 1982 lead legislation represented a more comprehensive solution to the problem of lead-based paint poisoning, but neither city officials in the executive branch nor the real estate industry wanted this legislation. The city viewed it as too expensive to implement, especially given the city's fiscal position at the time. And real estate interests and developers argued that the legislation would depress housing rehabilitation in the city. For the most part Local Law 1 was ignored (Chachere and Rodriquez 2004).

According to the law, all housing built before 1960 was presumed to have lead-based paint interiors, and the law required that "landlords remove or cover all lead-based paint in all dwelling units where children 6 years old or younger reside" (Freudenberg and Steinsapir 1986). If a landlord had knowledge that a child lived in a dwelling built before 1960, the 1982 law required that he "abate all lead-based paint in the unit, regardless of whether or not such paint constituted a hazard" (Bluemel et al. 2005, 218). Because the law established an affirmative duty for landlords to address lead-based paint in pre-1960 buildings whenever a child six years or younger lived in a dwelling, it created an expansive, yet vague, area of liability for the landlord. According to some, "building owners were not only responsible for remediation of the lead hazard, but could also face civil penalties if a child was found to be lead poisoned" (NYS Comptroller 2007, 31). Yet when the courts applied a reasonableness standard to the actions of landlords, the issue became vague. Did a landlord take reasonable actions to "prevent and repair hazardous lead conditions" and what does reasonable mean when the landlord has a continuous responsibility (Pedro 2000, 570).

The law applied to all city dwellings "in which three or more families reside" (Bluemel et al. 2005). City housing officials estimated that more than 200,000 apartments would have to be inspected and repaired (Kennedy 1996). According to the 1982 law, applicable lead surfaces in need of treatment were defined as any surface with a lead reading of 0.7 milligrams per square centimeter or greater. This represented a more stringent standard than was currently being recommended by the federal government (Bluemel et al. 2005). Although the 1982 law did not specifically address the issue of lead dust, the city health code incorporated current federal standards at 40 micrograms per square foot of floor space and 250 micrograms per square foot of windowsill space (New York City Coalition to End Lead Poisoning [NYCCELP] 2003a).

Landlords did not like the law because of its comprehensive approach of removing all lead-based paint and the consequent costs involved. As a result, most landlords ignored the law even in light of court rulings mandating action (Pedro 2000). Reflecting a conflict of interest, some city officials also did not like the law because the city was a major landlord and would have to incur significant costs to comply with the law as well (Public Advocate for the City of New York 1998, 3). Nor was the city enforcing the law on private landlords (Bluemel et al. 2005). Therefore they rejected a policy of total remediation and continued to enforce a policy similar to what had existed before the 1982 law was passed. More children were screened, and more cases were being found, but abatement, compliance, and enforcement were minimal.

Throughout the 1980s and 1990s the city was sued on several occasions by the victims of lead-based paint poisoning and their advocates for failing to enforce its own law (*New York Times* 1985). Advocates argued that the city was ordering the removal of lead-based paint only when it was peeling in dwellings built prior to 1960, and in some cases only in the specific area of the apartment where it was exposed (Hevesi 1991). In 1986 Hunter College's Community Environmental Center reported that between 1983 and 1985 only 2,375 lead-based paint violations had been issued by the city under the 1982 law and that few of them had resulted in remedial action by landlords or enforcement by the city (Freudenberg and Steinsapir 1986).

In 1987 the New York Coalition to End Lead Poisoning (NYCCELP) sued the city alleging noncompliance with Local Law 1. The ruling in the case established that the 1982 law applied to all interior lead-based paint, even if it was not peeling or chipping (Pedro 2000). Finally, in 1989, in response to a suit filed in 1985 by Bronx Legal Services on behalf of families harmed by lead-based paint, the state courts mandated that the city expand its program to eliminate lead-based paint in "thousands of apartments" (Hevesi 1989). The courts also directed the city's Department of Housing Preservation and Development "to issue regulations addressing how it will respond to complaints of the possible presence of lead-based paint" (*Citylaw* 1996). In effect, the courts were ordering the city to enforce the law the city had enacted in 1982. In apartments built before 1960 where peeling paint was found, all lead-based paint would have to be covered or removed. Despite these rulings, "housing owners continued to ignore the law in the absence of enforcement by the city" (Pedro 2000, 568). The city, as landlord, also continued to abate only where the threat of lead poisoning was obvious.

In 1991, the Dinkins administration recommended that the 1982 law be revised, arguing that the court's strict interpretation of the law made it "too costly to carry out" (McKinley 1992a). Some critics noted that the Dinkins administration opposition to the law was based, in part, on the fact that much of the housing that would have to be inspected and repaired was city-owned housing (McKinley 1992a).

In late 1992 the city council took up a Dinkins administration proposed revision of the 1982 law but failed to produce a new piece of legislation (McKinley 1992b). In 1994 the Giuliani administration, similar to the Dinkins administration, proposed amendments to the 1982 lead-based paint law that would have required the city to address only the most hazardous lead-based paint problems; but again the council took no action (Sengupta 1995).

In 1995 a state appeals court ordered several city agencies to explain why they had not repaired "lead-based paint violations in city-owned apartments or face contempt charges" (Arena 1995). The suit was filed by the NYCCELP. As a result of the ruling, HPD proposed to implement the 1982 law "by establishing a priority-based complaint investigation system" (*Citylaw* 1996). Peeling paint in pre-1960 buildings would receive the highest priority with peeling paint in post-1960 buildings and nonpeeling paint receiving attention only when departmental resources allowed (*Citylaw* 1996). The state courts rejected this plan. In December 1995 a state court found the city in contempt for "failing to issue regulations that adequately govern how the (1982) law should be carried out" (*New York Times* 1995).

In 1997, in response to a suit by lead-based paint poisoning victims and their advocates, a state court judge threatened to jail the city commissioner for Housing

Preservation and Development for failing to enforce the 1982 law. The courts rejected the attempt by the DOH to limit the city's responsibility to abatement if the lead-based paint had 1 milligram of lead per square centimeter rather that statutorily established standard of .07 (*Citylaw* 1997).

In late June 1999 the council passed a new lead-based paint law, Local Law 38. The new law significantly weakened the 1982 law. Because the 1982 law had never been fully enforced, though, the new law simply codified current practice. The new legislation adopted the position that the removal of all lead-based paint was not only unnecessary but also potentially harmful, owing to the lead-based paint dust that would be unleashed during abatement of intact lead-based paint. As a result, the principle behind the new law was that homes should be lead safe, whereas the principle behind the 1982 law was that homes should be lead free (Herszenhorn 1999). The definition of lead-based paint was raised back to 1 milligram of lead per square centimeter, a less stringent standard than under the 1982 law (Pedro 2000). Under the new law, landlords had no obligation to deal with the presence of lead dust (NYCCELP 1999).

Opponents of the new legislation labeled it "the landlord protection act" (Lombardi 1999). In October 1999 a coalition of child health advocacy organizations and community groups, led by the Northern Manhattan Improvement Corporation, sued the city in state court seeking to overturn the new lead-based paint legislation. They argued that the city could not implement the law, scheduled to take effect at the end of 1999, without an environmental review (Lombardi 1999; Northern Manhattan Improvement Corporation 2011). In July 2003 the New York State Court of Appeals, the state's highest court, struck down Local Law 38. The court ruled that the city council had failed to provide an analysis of the environmental impacts of the legislative changes in moving from the 1982 law to the 1999 law, as mandated by the State Environmental Quality Review Act. Specifically, the court criticized the council and Local Law 38 for failing to recognize that lead dust was a "primary exposure pathway" to lead poisoning (Wasserman 2003). By throwing out the Local Law 38, the court revived the 1982 law (Baker and Archibald 2003). Both the Bloomberg administration and representatives of the real estate industry criticized the court ruling.

A New Law

The decision by the Court of Appeals set in motion an effort by both the city council and the Bloomberg administration to find a suitable replacement for the 1982 law; one that might satisfy the advocates and the courts as well as the real estate and housing industries (Wasserman 2003).

In mid-December, the council passed Local Law 101A by a vote of 44–5 (Chen 2003). Mayor Bloomberg vetoed the legislation several days later. The council overrode the mayor's veto in February 2004. Local Law 101A of 2003 became Local Law 1 of 2004, The New York City Childhood Lead Poisoning Prevent Act.

Similar to Local Law 38, the goal of 101A is lead-safe and not lead-free homes. Local Law 101A did not attempt to address the removal or remediation of lead-based paint that was intact. But there were several key differences between the two pieces of legislation. The central theme of the new law is that "if landlords are going to be permitted to leave lead-based paint in place, they must be pro-active in assuring that the lead remains in a condition that is not hazardous" (Chachere and Rodriguez 2004). Compared to Local Law 38 of 1999, 101A requires landlords and the city to be much more aggressive in inspecting apartments and repairing lead-based paint hazards. Failure to comply can result in fines and expanded liability.

The new law requires landlords to "inspect every apartment with a child under seven years for conditions that may lead to exposure" (NYCCELP 2003b). Under the prior law, the applicable age was under six, so the number of homes that landlords would have to inspect increased significantly. It was estimated that of the "1.8 million city apartments built before 1960, 350,000 units" were estimated to have a child under the age of seven (Hu 2004). After the first year of the program, however, the DOH had the discretion to reduce the inspection age requirement to those homes with children under six years of age (Romano 2004).

Another key difference is that the new law requires landlords to inspect for and correct an expanded definition of lead-based paint hazards. The primary lead hazard is no longer just peeling paint. Friction surfaces that could produce a hazard by rubbing and impact surfaces that could produce a hazard by being hit are also included, as well as chewable surfaces such as windowsills (Romano 2004). The new law also includes lead dust as a hazard that needed to be corrected. Law 101A establishes a lead-based paint dust hazard according to the current federal guidelines of 40 micrograms per square foot on floors and 250 micrograms per square foot on windowsills. But the law also gives the DOHMH the ability to raise the standards (NYCCELP 2003c). Unlike Local Law 1 (1982), Law 101A defines lead-based paint as an area that has 1.0 milligrams of lead per square centimeter. Advocates had wanted a return to the 1982 law definition of 0.7 milligrams (Romano 2003).

The new law requires the landlords to conduct annual inspections of apartments and "promptly correct any hazards" (NYCCELP 2003b). Its language also requires landlords to take action to prevent lead-based paint hazards in addition to correcting them once they occurred (NYCCELP 2003c). The law prescribes how abatement is to be conducted in some instances. Law 101A prohibits the dry scraping and sanding of paint (McIntire 2003). The law requires landlords to hire "federally certified workers to perform lead abatement or containment" (NYS Comptroller 2007, 32). If the landlord is doing the work himself, specific practices are to be followed. When abatement is completed, the new law requires a dust clearance test; in hazard remediation areas of more than a hundred square feet, the dust clearance test has to be conducted by an independent third party (NYCCELP 2003c). Temporary relocation is required when work cannot be completed safely. Other requirements are to "use only firms and workers that are EPA certified" and to "provide written notice to DOHMH within ten days of beginning abatement work" (Bluemel et al. 2005). In comparison to Local Law 38, 101A shortens the time that landlords have to correct lead-based paint hazards before a violation would be cited.

Under the new law landlords are required to "provide written notice to tenants of the landlord's obligation to inspect for and repair lead-based paint hazards and the tenant's obligation to provide access" to the apartment (NYCCELP 2003b). Law 101A gives tax credits to landlords "who undertake lead poisoning prevention activities in low income housing" (NYCCELP 2003b). Landlords are also required to inspect and address lead-based paint hazards when their apartments are rented to new tenants.

The landlord under Local Law 101A is given fifty days to correct the hazard, ten fewer days than under the previous law (NYCCELP 2003c). If the landlord fails to correct the hazard and the violation is found by DOH or HPD, the landlord is given twenty-one days to make repairs. If the landlord fails to correct the hazard in the allotted time, a fine of "up to $250 a day for each violation to a maximum of $10,000" can be imposed (Romano 2004). Law 101A also requires landlords to inform the occupants of the results of the inspection and provide them with a written report and also to keep those reports for ten years. Failure to comply with these reporting requirements is a misdemeanor (NYC Department of Housing Preservation and Development 2004).

In the early 2000s a few nonprofit organizations began to provide a limited amount of lead-free housing to those families with children who had been diagnosed with lead poisoning. This housing provided a temporary refuge while the family's home was been made lead safe (Northern Manhattan Improvement Coalition-Lead Poisoning 2011).

The definition of lead poisoning also changed under the new law. Under the old law, the DOH was required to inspect a home if a child was reported to have a blood level of 20 micrograms per deciliter. In response to updated research, 101A lowered the threshold for DOH action to 15 micrograms per deciliter (NYCCELP 2003c). This increased the number of cases with which DOH would have to deal.

If a child has a BLL above 5 micrograms per deciliter, DOHMH sends the child's family a letter recommending follow-up testing. The mailing also provides the family with information on lead poisoning prevention and reminds families to report peeling paint (NYC DOHMH 2011). In 2007 DOHMH's Lead Poisoning Prevention Program (LPPP) sent out 3,338 of these letters (NYC

DOHMH 2009a). If a child has a BLL above 15 micrograms, the LPPP "initiates case coordination and environmental intervention services" (NYC DOHMH 2009a, 26). Case coordination involves educating the family about reducing the child's exposure to lead as well as educating the child's health care provider about "appropriate medical management" including follow-up testing, which DOHMH tracks (26). If necessary, DOHMH can make referrals to the family on the availability of lead-safe housing. If the child's BLL is above 45 micrograms, DOHMH consults with the child's health care provider so that the child can receive appropriate care, including chelation and hospitalization (NYC DOHMH 2009a). In 2005, twenty-one families were accommodated in lead-safe housing, twenty-two families in 2006, and twenty-three families in 2007 (NYC DOHMH 2005b; 2008; 2009a).

DOHMH environmental intervention, initiated with a BLL of more than 15 micrograms, involves several stages. First, DOHMH sends inspectors to the child's residence. The child's family may also be interviewed to identify the source of the lead poisoning. Second, if a lead-based paint hazard is found, DOHMH contacts the building owner to remediate the hazard. DOHMH monitors this work to make sure the remediation takes place using "lead-safe work practices" (NYC DOHMH 2009a, 26). Finally, if the owner fails to remediate the hazard, DOHMH refers the residence to the HPD to make the repairs (NYC DOHMH 2009a). Since the implementation of 101A, DOHMH inspections of primary residences have declined from 1,294 in 2005 to 829 in 2006 and 636 in 2007. The agency monitored remediation in 4,981 residences in 2005, 4,173 in 2006, and 2,755 in 2007. For those residences in which the owner failed to perform remediation, LPPP referred 324 residences to HPD for remediation in 2005, 200 in 2006, and 159 in 2007 (NYC DOHMH 2005b; 2008; 2009a). Finally, "LPPP also issues orders to correct lead-based paint hazards in homes of non-lead poisoned children and newborns in high risk neighborhoods" (NYC DOHMH 2009a, 22). In 2005, LPPP issued 894 violations for lead-based paint hazards and monitored remediation in 734 dwellings (NYC DOHMH 2005b, 27). In 2007, LPPP issued 739 violations for lead-based paint hazards and monitored the remediation of lead-based paint hazards in 909 residences (NYC DOHMH 2009a). In a few high-risk communities, LPPP has funded the remediation of lead-based paint hazards, including the replacement of residential doors and windows (NYC DOHMH 2005b, 26).

Under Local Law 101A, DOHMH must monitor lead-based paint hazard remediation to assure that it is complying with the city health code's safe work practices guidelines. In conjunction with this responsibility, LPPP "investigates complaints of paint dust and debris from unsafe work practices during repair and renovation work" (NYC DOHMH 2009a, 22). More than three thousand inspections were carried out in 2007 (NYC DOHMH 2009a).

Much of the success of the city's lead poisoning prevention program is dependent on the LPPP's communicating with health care providers. LPPP regularly consults with physicians and health care providers on protocols for the care of lead-poisoned children. They hold professional forums, educate medical students, and distribute literature to health professions. In addition, LPPP has "promoted" the use of an online registry where health care providers can access BLL records of their patients (NYC DOHMH 2009a).

Public education, especially for those communities and families who are most at risk for lead poisoning, is as important as educating health care professionals. LPPP operates a multifaceted education and outreach program. It maintains an information phone line, distributes educational literature, conducts workshops, and participates at community health fairs. In this effort, it coordinates its activities with a variety of community-based organizations, including "clinics, schools, day care centers, faith based organizations, Head Start programs, and Women, Infants and Children (WIC) centers (NYC DOHMH 2009a, 24). LPPP also trains workers in community-based organizations to be cognizant of lead poisoning symptoms and has recruited hundreds of stores that sell paint to participate in the Healthy Homes Hardware Store campaign, a program that publicizes safe work practices (NYC DOHMH 2009a).

Local Law 101A created several areas of lead poisoning policy where DOHMH is required to coordinate its efforts with HPD. First, when LPPP finds a lead-based paint hazard in the home of a lead-poisoned child, it refers the building to HPD for a building-wide assessment of compliance with the law. In 2007, 509 buildings were referred to HPD (NYC DOHMH 2008). HPD inspects buildings whenever DOHMH "identifies a child with an elevated blood level" (NYS Comptroller 2007, 32). HPD also performs inspections in response to tenant complaints. In its role as a housing inspector for all city-owned housing, HPD is now required to inquire about children under seven years anytime an inspection is conducted and to complete a full lead-based paint hazard inspection if a child is present (Romano 2004). Second, LPPP and HPD have collaborated on a U.S. Department of Housing and Urban Development (HUD) grant that provides funding for building owners to remediate lead-based paint hazards in high-risk communities. The project offers building owners forgivable loans for lead hazard remediation (NYC DOHMH 2005b). Third, Local Law 101A gives LPPP the authority to order landlords to remediate lead-based paint hazards in one- and two-family homes even when there is no lead-poisoned child, especially in high-risk communities. "HPD performs similar functions for tenants in dwellings with three or more units" (NYC DOHMH 2008, 24).

As in Local Law 38, DOHMH is required to inspect the corrected area of a home in the case of a violation. They are also required "to certify to HPD for correction" if the landlord failed to act within the allotted time. If the landlord failed to correct the hazards, HPD is ultimately responsible for addressing the problems. The new legislation mandated much more detailed inspections by both HPD and DOHMH, requiring that even intact surfaces be examined (Romano 2003).

One of the most controversial aspects of Local Law 101A was its expanded concept of liability for both landlords and the city. Opponents of 101A were concerned about the impact that this might have on the rehabilitation of housing in the city and the overall supply of housing. City officials and real estate interests were concerned less about a rash of lawsuits on lead-based paint than about rising insurance rates for landlords and how this would affect housing rehabilitation activities. At the time of 101A's passage there was disagreement over its impact on landlord liability. Some analysts have suggested that much of the initial discussion was based on misperception, if not misinformation. Nevertheless, these same analysts suggested that, in the short term, insurance companies might "raise rates based on misperceptions of liability risk" (Bluemel et al. 2005). In addition, under the 1982 law, Local Law 1, the courts ruled that landlords had a continuous duty to inspect apartments for lead hazards and are presumed to know that a hazard exits. Under Local Law 38, the law had been clear that landlords had to inspect apartments only once a year (NYCCELP 2003c).

Mayor Bloomberg's detailed veto message in January 2004 addressed a number of issues with 101A in addition to liability. While the mayor lauded the new law's requirements for dust clearance worker training and testing requirements once hazards had been corrected, his administration had several problems with the legislation that resulted in the veto. First, the Bloomberg administration believed that the regulations on chewable surfaces were unreasonable. Its reading of the law suggested that landlords and the city would have to address every windowsill with lead-based paint since it was a potentially chewable surface accessible to children. The administration believed that the deadline for this type of abatement was too short, and as a result the abatement work might be done by untrained workers resulting in a worsening of the lead poisoning risk through the release of lead dust. Second, the veto message argued that the short time frames the city was given to inspect and remediate did not take into consideration that both DOHMH and HPD might have difficulties gaining access to apartments (NYC Office of the Mayor 2003). Since the legislation did not address access issues, the administration was concerned that the city would be sued.

For instance, the bill requires that HPD inspect a private apartment within 14 days after a violation correction date to determine whether the violation was, in fact, corrected. If HPD cannot perform this inspection because it cannot gain access to the apartment, HPD could conceivably be sued (for its failure to timely conduct this inspection), since the bill fails to address the specific lack of access situation. This type of problem applies to numerous other provisions of the bill as well. (NYC Office of the Mayor 2003)

The mayor's veto message also focused on several areas of expanded liability. First, given increased demands on landlords, such as "difficult and probably unachievable timeframes," concern was raised that increased liability would result in more expensive or disappearing insurance (Bluemel et al. 2005). Under those circumstances the Bloomberg administration feared that landlords might abandon their properties or seek to evict families (NYC Office of the Mayor 2003). Second, according to some, 101A included a presumption that even when landlords and the city had complied with all regulations and made best efforts to investigate and remediate all lead-based paint hazards in a home, they could still be held liable for a new lead-based paint hazard in the home even if never notified of that hazard (Bluemel et al. 2005). Third, the city was not only subject to expanded liability as a major landlord but also exposed because HPD was being given an increased responsibility for abatement with shorter time frames for compliance (NYC Office of the Mayor 2003).

When 101A was passed in December 2003, a spokesperson for the mayor criticized the policy stating that "this misguided piece of legislation would divert precious resources away from the programs which have reduced lead poisoning cases by 80 percent in recent years, stifle our efforts to build more affordable housing and force people into homelessness by driving up housing costs" (Chen 2003). At a press conference shortly after the bill's passage, Mayor Bloomberg claimed that 101A might harm city children more than help them if landlords became reluctant to rent to families with children (Cooper 2003). After the city council overrode the mayor's veto, the city commissioner of health, Thomas Frieden, claimed that "this is about the worst piece of public policy I have seen in 20 years of public health . . . It is the law and we are planning to implement it, but it's not going to be preventing lead poisoning" (Steinhauer 2004).

The Bloomberg administration was not alone in its criticism of Local Law 101A. In a 2004 editorial, the *New York Daily News* noted: "The theory of the law . . . is that landlords will snap to and clean up their buildings under the burden of onerous regulation and well founded fears of lawsuits. Hoping to be proven wrong, we predict two very different results: a slowdown in the considerable pace at which lead poisoning has been declining in the city and a significant drop in the rehabilitation projects." Another critic of 101A noted that since the buildings in question were all built pre-1960, most, if not all, of the landlords had done nothing "illegal, immoral, or even stupid to create the existing problem" (Vitullo-Martin 2003). Yet the new law was holding those landlords responsible even when they followed all of the law's regulations. Moreover, the money that would have to be spent on lead clean up, some of it needless, would no longer be spent on housing rehabilitation. The costs of housing rehabilitation would increase, "reducing the amount of rehabilitation actually done" (Vitullo-Martin 2003).

Implementation of the City's Lead Poisoning Prevention Program

Local Law 101A establishes a right to lead-safe housing for many but not all of the city's children. In doing so, it places the burden of meeting this goal on landlords, such that they bear much of the cost for achieving lead-safe housing for their residents and can be sued if the goal is not met. And environmental justice groups continue to monitor the enforcement of the law, litigating when necessary (Northern Manhattan Improvement Corporation 2011).

In 2005 DOHMH published a plan to meet the national goal of eliminating childhood lead poisoning by 2010 (NYC DOHMH 2005a). This was mandated for those jurisdictions receiving lead poisoning prevention funding from the CDC (NYS Comptroller 2007, 28). The plan focused on three goals: preventing exposure of children to lead-based paint; preventing exposure of children to nonpaint lead sources; and promoting blood lead testing of children, especially those at high risk for lead poisoning (NYC DOHMH 2005b, ii). Educating parents, and in particular immigrant groups, became a major component of the plan. Educating health personnel, especially those in high-risk neighborhoods, about screening children was also a component of the plan. In addition, because of the decline in lead-based paint poisoning and the increased use of lead products by immigrant groups, nonpaint sources of lead poisoning took on increased significance (NYC DOHMH 2005b).

In January 2006 the New York City Independent Budget Office (IBO) published a report examining the first-year implementation of Local Law 101A (Local Law 1 of 2004). First, the IBO report noted that, although HPD had spent more than double the funding on lead-based paint related activities in 2005 than in 2004, it had still spent considerably less than what had been budgeted for the program in that year. Most of the additional funding went for the hiring of more personnel to work on the program. The number of HPD employees working on the program had tripled to more than four hundred with one hundred new inspectors (NYC IBO 2006, 2–3).

Second, the new law had significantly increased HPD's workload. "The number of lead based paint violations issued in 2005 increased 277 percent relative to 2004, to 35,729. At the same time, the percent of violations certified as corrected by landlords fell from 28 percent to 14 percent. The number of lead related emergency repairs increased 83 percent to 1,854" (3). The IBO report noted that the increase in emergency repairs was due to a decline in landlord compliance. Under Local Law 38, the landlord had been able to certify that his own violations had been addressed. Now that violations had to be cleared by a third party, the rate of compliance dropped (5).

Third, some of the increase in HPD workload was due to non-lead-based paint violations found in the course of inspections mandated by 101A. HPD inspectors were required by 101A to perform a room-by-room inspection, not just an inspection of the lead-based paint hazard area. As a result, they were bound to find additional hazards, such as plaster in need of repair and non-lead-based paint that was peeling (4). Fourth, HPD inspections now took longer, and HPD was unable to conduct the same number of inspections per inspector as it was previously. The report noted that, although aggregate HPD inspections per inspection team per day had not declined, the lead inspection teams' average number of inspections per day had declined to three per day compared to HPD's previous average of nine (5).

In the years after the implementation of 101A (Local Law 1), DOHMH reported that a little more than 15 percent of those children who tested at 15 micrograms of lead per deciliter lived in housing built after 1950. More importantly, in those residences of children with high EIBLL, inspectors could not find peeling or deteriorated paint in more than 20 percent of those homes (NYC DOHMH 2005b; 2009a; 2009b). Some of this may be due to new sources of lead poisoning being brought in by newly arriving immigrants. Of course, real estate interests would take this as evidence that a significant number of lead-poisoned children are not poisoned because of lead-based paint, and therefore this needs to be considered in any legal determination of responsibility. Regardless, unknown sources of lead poisoning make the disease less preventable.

Advocates for lead poisoning prevention had a different take on the implementation of 101A (Local Law 1). In 2007 a survey of Bushwick by Make the Road New York, a nonprofit advocacy group, and the New York City Coalition to End Lead Poisoning found many landlords in noncompliance with both city abatement regulations and federal disclosure requirements (Make the Road New York Staff 2009).

Scientific Research and the Evolution of Lead-Based Paint Poisoning Policy

Research on the health impacts of lead poisoning and the links to lead-based paint have not dictated public health policy, but advocacy for laws that restrict the use of lead-based paint and laws that mandate remediation of lead-based paint hazards in the home have followed research documenting the harms of inaction in this area. The paint industry accepted the harmful effects of lead-based paint as early as the 1940s when it began to decrease and then eliminate its manufacture for housing interiors.

The issue of lead poisoning and lead-based paint has clearly not been an area of public policy where lack of knowledge has served as an impediment to government action. Not only is the research conclusive, but given the causes and etiology of lead poisoning and specifically the link to lead-based paint exposure, the conditions and their harmful impacts are completely preventable (Bellinger and Bellinger 2006).

Over the past several decades, two additional areas of research involving lead-based paint and lead exposure have influenced public health policy in this area. First, current research now confirms the harmful effects of lead dust exposure. This research began to appear in the mid- to late 1990s (AAP Committee on Environmental Health 2005). Given this research, it is understandable why 1999 Local Law 38, which did not address lead dust, was such a divisive piece of legislation, why advocates and members of the city council sought to replace it as soon as it was passed, and why the New York State Court of Appeals rejected it because the city council had not performed due diligence in examining the environmental impact of the legislation. Although new research documenting the harms of lead dust ingestion did not affect the choice of the public policy tool chosen to address lead-based paint, it did affect the scope and breadth of the tool, as Local Law 101A specifically made reference to lead dust.

The second area of recent lead exposure research that has had an impact on public policy has focused on the changing definition of BLLs. Over time, research was able to document the harmful effects of elevated BLLs at lower levels of micrograms per deciliter. In the 1960s, 60 micrograms per deciliter of blood was deemed as the threshold. Because of the steady accumulation of "epidemiological evidence demonstrating adverse effects of lead on children's neurodevelopment," the level used to define an elevated blood level, or lead poisoning, was revised downward (Bellinger and Bellinger 2006). It was lowered to 40 micrograms in the 1970s, 25 in the mid-1980s, and 10 in the early 1990s. In 2003 one study found that BLLs of less than 10 micrograms inversely affected children's intelligence test scores. Despite this study, the CDC decided not to lower the intervention threshold, arguing that "no known clinical intervention exists which can lower blood levels to less than" 10 micrograms (NYS Comptroller 2007, 22). But in 2012 the CDC announced a new lower threshold of 5 micrograms per deciliter applicable to children younger than six years of age (Hartocollis 2012). Similar to lead dust, research documenting the harms of lower levels of exposure did not affect the choice of tool being used but did influence the threshold at which intervention through regulation or the treatment of lead poisoning victims was pursued.

The Intergovernmental Role in Lead Poisoning Policy

Both the state and federal levels have had a role in lead poisoning policy. At the same time, however, it is the local level of government that has had the most significant role in public policy making. At best, federal and state policies on lead poisoning and lead-based paint have complemented what New York City accomplished. New York State's primary involvement in lead poisoning policy in New York City is directly related to the state's responsibility for licensing and regulating the practice of medicine and the delivery of health care. As such, the state plays an important role in the lead poisoning blood-screening program as well as case management for those children and pregnant women who have lead poisoning. On most significant policy issues surrounding the lead poisoning and lead-based paint issue, the state has ceded its authority to New York City since the city has its own laws. Of all three levels of government, the city was the first to act in the lead-based paint poisoning issue. The public policy tools of screening, regulation, and education were employed by New York City before the state and federal levels got involved in the issue.

In 1970 New York State passed the Control of Lead Poisoning Act (CLPA). In this legislation, the commissioner of health was given the mandate to develop a statewide plan "to reduce and prevent lead poisoning" (Pedro 2000, 562). The legislation laid out the basic dimensions of the statewide plan, including inspection, detection, and education. An important component of the legislation was the ceding of authority to local health departments (Pedro 2000). This coincided with New York City's initial comprehensive program.

In 1992, more than two decades after the state's initial lead poisoning legislation, and ten years after New York City passed Local Law 1, New York State passed the Lead Poisoning Prevention Act (LPPA). Key components in LPPA, missing from the 1970 legislation, were screening and reporting. But similar to the 1970 legislation, the 1992 legislation ceded much of its authority to local governments, which were deemed more capable of implementing the law. LPPA was designed to oversee and assist county "health programs and activities relating to childhood lead poisoning" (NYS Comptroller 2007, 25).

Under the law, the state department of health is supposed to coordinate lead poisoning reduction and treatment programs across the state, establish a statewide registry of lead-poisoned youth and develop a public education program to address "lead exposure, detection and risk reduction" (NYS Comptroller 2007, 26). In this effort, New York State participates in Leadtrac, an internet database for state and local health department officials "to help improve tracking of affected children moving between health jurisdictions" with regard to periodic BLL tests and case management (NYS DOH 2004, part III).

The legislation also gave the NYS DOH the authority to set standards for contractors performing lead abatement (Pedro 2000). In this effort, the state coordinates a lead safety training program for immigrants and non-English speaking day laborers, who are frequently involved in lead-based paint abatement. The state does receive federal funding from the Environmental Protection Agency for this program.

The most significant function of the state in lead poisoning policy is its screening mandate. In response to LPPA, the state department of health promulgated regulations requiring "screening of all children at both ages 1 and 2" years as well as an annual lead risk assessment of children aged six months through six years, beginning in 1995 (NYS Comptroller 2007, 26). This was the most significant element of lead poisoning policy undertaken by the state. Of course, by 1992 New York City was already screening a large percentage of its at risk population, but there was no universal screening mandate until the state got involved. For those eligible children, BLL testing is paid for by the state's Medicaid program and also by the state's Family Health Plus program, covering low-income children who fall above the Medicaid eligibility level (NYS DOH 2009).

Despite the city's early involvement in screening and the state screening mandate in 1995, the city has never achieved 100 percent screening. Of course, the city at best has indirect control over private physician practice. For 2003 the DOHMH reported testing 84 percent of children before their third birthday (NYC DOHMH 2004b). In 2005, 88 percent of children were tested before their third birthday (NYC DOHMH 2005b). The percentages for 2007, 2008, and 2010 were 90, 92, and 93 percent respectively (NYC DOHMH 2008; 2009a; 2011).

For screening to be as successful as it is, DOHMH embarked upon an educational campaign with multiple targets. DOHMH "intensified educational community outreach efforts, with a focus on high-risk, foreign born communities" (NYC DOHMH 2009a, 21). To further relationships with immigrant communities, DOHMH has "conducted a multilingual radio campaign that encouraged parents to get their children tested for lead and to report peeling paint" (21). Given the high percentage of Medicaid enrollees among lead-poisoned children, DOHMH coordinates much of its educational efforts with the Medicaid Managed Care Organizations in the city, since all Medicaid funded health care in the city is delivered through managed care organizations.

Because of the state's traditional role in licensing the medical profession, much of the 1992 LPPA screening regulations were directed at physician practice and all health care providers. Initially, this involved a significant state effort in educating health care providers, a function that the state continues to fulfill (NYS DOH 2004, part III). According to the state regulations, providers must perform blood tests and send the sample to a state-certified laboratory for testing. The labs must report all results back to the NYS DOH in a timely manner. If the test returns elevated BLLs of 10 micrograms of lead per deciliter or greater, the county health department notifies the health care provider who then follows state regulations in treating the child (NYS Comptroller 2007, 27).

The state has a role in providing health care providers with information on the "medical management of children with elevated BLLs" as well as providing case management or oversight of case management for those children (NYS DOH 2004, part III). In 1992, for children whose BLLs were between 10 and 20 micrograms, health care providers were required by the state to provide "risk reduction education" and nutritional counseling" (NYS Comptroller 2007, 26). Children with BLLs greater than 20 micrograms must receive a complete diagnostic evaluation in addition to medical treatment if deemed necessary by the provider. Elevated BLLs of 20 micrograms or more also required the local health department to inspect the home "or any environment in which the affected child spend eight hours or more per week" (e.g., a day care center) (26). On occasion the state has subsidized the provision of lead-safe housing to those "families of children being treated for elevated BLLs" while the lead hazards in their homes are being abated (NYS DOH 2004, part III).

In 1999 the state expanded its activities with the passage of the Childhood Environmental Lead Poisoning Reduction Act. The law was targeted specifically at New York City (Pedro 2000, 565). The law required that state lead-based paint poisoning abatement standards "comply with the rules promulgated by Title IV of the Federal Toxic Substances Control Act. In accordance with these rules, the commissioner of health had the authority "to approve training activities and certification for lead abatement contractors" (Pedro 2000). In addition, the 1999 law mandated that "owners of multiple dwellings built before 1978 'eliminate all deteriorated paint and perform any repairs necessary to make painted surfaces structurally sound' in units that were either rented or leased for over 100 days" (565). The law required owners to correct lead-based paint hazards within thirty days of notification by the tenant. The law also required landlords to advise tenants of their rights under the law. But the law included no enforcement mechanism (Pedro 2000).

While BLL testing for eligible children is funded by Medicaid, the state does give the city financial assistance to combat lead poisoning at the community level. The NYS Department of Health provides funding for all local health departments across the state involved in lead poisoning prevention and treatment. The funding assists local health departments with education and outreach activities, coordinating referrals for home visits with affected families including home visits by health personnel, "building relationships with local housing agencies and community-based organizations to support remediation" of housing that contains hazards, and promoting training for those engaged in abatement (NYS DOH 2008, 3). The state receives federal Preventive Health and Health Services Block Grant funding. And through competitive grants to local health departments, New York City receives some of this funding through the Healthy Neighborhoods Program. This program "is designed to provide preventive environmental health services to targeted geographic areas with a high rate of documented unmet health needs" (NYS DOH 2004, part III).

Federal involvement in the lead-based paint poisoning issue has served three purposes. First, through the activities of the CDC, uniform thresholds for treatment have been disseminated. Second, by appearing on the agenda of the federal government, lead-based paint poisoning has received national attention from the media and has served as a means of further informing and educating relevant publics as to the problem and possible solutions. In addition, congressional legislation mandated that several federal agencies "sponsor education and outreach activities to increase public awareness of the scope and severity of lead-based paint poisoning" (Tinker and Keiser 1997, 129). Third, through a variety of grant programs, the federal government funds prevention and abatement activities around the country.

In 1971 Congress passed the Lead-Based Paint Poisoning Prevention Act (LPPPA). More than a decade after New York City had banned the use of lead-based paint in residences, Congress, through the LPPPA, banned "the use of lead-based paint in housing owned or subsidized by the federal government" (Pedro 2000, 556). The law defined lead-based paint as having 0.5 percent lead. The law said nothing about lead-based paint in privately owned housing; nor did the act do anything to alleviate lead-based paint hazards in federally subsidized housing that already existed. In 1977 the federal Consumer Product Safety Commission (CPSC) finally ruled that paint for residential use could not contain more than 0.06 percent lead by dry weight (Bellinger and Bellinger 2006).

Two years later, in 1973, Congress amended LPPPA and directed the U.S. Department of Housing and Urban Development to eliminate lead-based paint hazards in all federally subsidized housing. However, not only did HUD not issue regulations to implement this element of the law until 1976 but its program suffered from insufficient funding for years (Pedro 2000). In 1980 the General Accounting Office published a report entitled "HUD Not Fulfilling Responsibilities to Eliminate Lead-Based Paint Hazard in Federal Housing" (Needleman 1998, 1874). The report criticized HUD for not having assessed the state of lead-based paint in federally subsidized housing or developing any methods for dealing with it. During the Reagan administration the funding for this grant was folded into a larger Maternal and Child Health Block Grant. This action decreased the extent to which the funds would be targeted to the elimination of lead paint poisoning (Gaiter 1981).

It was not until 1988 with the Lead Contamination Control Act that Congress authorized the CDC to develop programs to eliminate childhood lead poisoning nationwide. The CDC had assumed responsibility for monitoring the issue as early as 1973. As a result of the 1988 law, CDC created its own Lead Poisoning Prevention Branch, which is responsible for coordinating federal efforts with state and local entities to end childhood lead poisoning. The CDC activities include public and health care provider education; financial assistance to states and localities to help support screening, treatment, and follow-up care; and developing neighborhood-based efforts to address lead poisoning (NYS Comptroller 2007, 22).

One of the CDC's most important roles in eliminating lead poisoning has been educating the professional health provider community. Even before the 1988 legislation the CDC had been assessing research on lead poisoning and publishing what it concluded was appropriate thresholds for medical intervention. Even though research on lead poisoning suggested as early as 1960 that there were thresholds above which lead poisoning and its negative health impacts took place and medical intervention was appropriate, the CDC did not publish its first statement on lead poisoning until 1975. By that time the BLL threshold of concern had declined from 60 micrograms per deciliter of blood to 30 (NYS Comptroller 2007, 22). The CDC's role as the disseminator of medical expertise was critical to advance lead poisoning protocols. Its statements in the 1970s "provided the only concise guide to the identification and management of children exposed to lead" (Needleman 1998, 1874).

As previously discussed, the CDC has the primary role in establishing the threshold limits for childhood lead exposure and has lowered the threshold as recently as 2012. The CDC has also had a role in the issue of screening. In its 1985 report, the CDC lead poisoning advisory committee stated that, "ideally, all children in this age group (9 months to 6 years) should be screened" (quoted in Needlman 1998, 1873). In 1990 the CDC issued its strongest statement on lead poisoning prevention, the Strategic Plan for the Elimination of Lead Poisoning. The report was based on research that documented that the "effects of exposure to even moderate amounts of lead" were "more pervasive and long lasting than previously thought" and that lower threshold levels meant many more children would now be classified as lead poisoned (1872). The report recommended more prevention programs, effective abatement (including lead dust) in high-risk housing, and national surveillance of those with elevated BLLs (1872). Finally, amending prior statements, the CDC recommended universal BLL screening of all children between one and five years of age. A hotline was set up to answer "parents' questions and direct them to help" (1872).

By the mid-1990s, however, the CDC began to back away from its call for universal screening of all children, primarily because of cost considerations. The CDC's strong position of the early-1990s received pushback from the American Academy of Pediatrics and some of its local chapters, the health insurance industry, health maintenance organizations, and some real estate interests. They argued that lead poisoning was a condition whose incidence was high in some areas of the country but not all and therefore universal screening was too expensive (Needleman 1998). A new CDC cost-benefit study in the mid-1990s con-cluded that the "screening of all children in an area would be cost effective only when the expected prevalence of BLLs higher than 10 micrograms per deciliter of blood was greater than 14%" (Needleman 1998, 1873). Subsequent CDC lead poisoning publications focused much more on the conditions under which screening should take place than on managing the condition. Advocates for a comprehensive federal response to lead poisoning have been unsatisfied with the CDC's change in position (1874).

As part of the federal government's Healthy People 2010 initiative, the CDC's lead poisoning division has set a goal to eliminate blood levels higher than 10 micrograms in all children six years of age and younger by 2010. As a result, the CDC called on all state and local governments receiving lead poisoning preven-tion funding to issue plans on how this goal would be achieved. CDC guidelines called on states and localities to address various issues in their plans, including the identification of high-risk populations and neighborhoods and the development of strategies to create lead-safe housing (NYS Comptroller 2007, 25).

In 1992 HUD's role in the lead-based paint issue was expanded with the pas-sage of the Residential Lead-Based Paint Hazard Reduction Act, Title X of the Housing and Community Development Act of 1992. The law required "the abatement of lead-based paint hazards in federally owned residential properties and housing receiving federal assistance" (Pedro 2000, 559). Although one of the stated purposes of the legislation was to end lead-based paint hazards in all resi-dential dwellings, the law did not require abatement. Instead it directed HUD and the U.S. Environmental Protection Agency (EPA) to issue regulations "re-quiring disclosure of known lead-based paint conditions and hazards by persons selling or leasing housing constructed before 1978" (559). The "leasing" aspect of the disclosure requirement meant that landlords would have to "educate tenants by disclosing to them all known facts and documents pertaining to lead-based paint in the dwelling" (Make the Road New York Staff 2009). Failure to comply with the regulations on the part of those selling homes could result in civil or criminal penalties. The law also gave homebuyers the right to test for lead-based paint before they purchased a home (Pedro 2000). Around the same time, both Federal National Mortgage Association (Fannie Mae) and the Federal Home Loan Mortgage Corporation (Freddie Mac) amended its own regulations on lead-based paint in homes. Fannie Mae required a lead test in the home unless docu-mentation could be provided that the homebuyer had complied with applicable state or local laws on lead-based paint hazards. Freddie Mac also included lead-based paint regulations in its loan commitment process (Rechtschaffen 1997).

The 1992 law called for coordinated action among federal agencies, includ-ing the CDC, EPA, and HUD, to eliminate lead poisoning. As a result of this mandate, the EPA created the National Lead Information Center (NLIC). This agency "operates a national hotline and clearinghouse," which promotes "coordination among federal agencies to improve the effectiveness of the NLIC on lead education and outreach efforts to high risk populations" (Tinker and Keiser 1997, 136). The legislation called for "standards and regulations for lead-based paint inspections, risk assessment and abatement" (NYS Comptroller 2007, 23). In this regard, the legislation furthered the use of education as a tool since it encouraged federal agencies to issue best practices for inspection, abatement, and training of those who would be involved in these activities at the state and local levels.

In attempting to influence state and local public policy, a traditional federal tool has been financial assistance. The federal government administers at least ten different grant programs that fund lead prevention, abatement, and education activities; New York City receives funding under many of them. Title X came with authorizations for federal grants to states and local governments for capacity building and federal regulatory compliance (NYS Comptroller 2007, 23–24). Over the years the city has received millions of dollars under the Lead-Based Paint Hazard Control program and the Lead Hazard Reduction program, both administered by HUD under Title X. The HUD grants have funded contractor certification and training in lead-based paint hazard abatement as well as the development of local government expertise and collaboration with other relevant agencies at the state and local levels (Morrison 1998, 17–18).

In 2005 the city received $7.5 million from HUD to address lead-based paint hazards in the Brooklyn neighborhoods of Bushwick, Bedford-Stuyvesant, and East New York, neighborhoods with the highest elevated blood levels in the city. Some of the funding went to HPD to focus on lead-based paint hazards in one and two family homes in these neighborhoods. Some funds went to DOHMH for education and outreach "targeting housing units that have been identified as 'physically poor' by HPD's Office of Code Enforcement" (NYC HPD 2005). Federal funds paid for "lead awareness packages," which were distributed through local hardware stores, and visual inspection and lead-safe work practices education programs for owners and contractors (NYC HPD 2005). Local community groups and development corporations were also included to assist HPD and DOHMH in the outreach effort (NYC HPD 2005).

The city has received funding from the CDC's Healthy Homes / Lead Poisoning Prevention Program (NYC Office of Management and Budget 2009, 65–88). These federal funds, along with the HUD grants, are competitive. The city also receives funding through the Healthy Communities Grant Program, another competitive grant administered through the EPA (United States Catalog of Federal Domestic Assistance 2009). Since the city was involved in lead poisoning prevention and abatement before these grants were initiated by the federal government, no documentation exists that these grants influenced the selection of public policy tools by the city in dealing with lead poisoning due to lead-based paint. For fiscal year 2013, however, total federal spending on the Healthy Homes / Lead Poisoning Program was reduced from $29 million to $2 million, essentially eliminating this funding stream (Dell'Antonia 2012).

In addition to HUD funding that is earmarked for lead-based paint poisoning prevention some of HPD's lead abatement activities are funded by the federal Community Development Block Grant (CDBG), also administered by HUD (NYC IBO] 2006, 2). This formula-based grant received by the city gives it considerable discretion across a wide range of housing rehabilitation and community development activities. CDBG moneys have played a major role in the city's lead-based paint hazard abatement program (2). The federal government also funds approximately 50 percent of the state (and city) Medicaid program that funds much of BLL screening in low-income communities.

Economic Development's Role in Lead Poisoning Policy

Economic development interests often opposed various aspects of lead-based paint poisoning prevention and hazard abatement. In New York City, real estate and developer interests were most prominent, but the lead-based paint industry and the health insurance industry have also been involved.

In the first half of the twentieth century as the lead poisoning issue was evolving as a public issue, the Lead Industries Association (LIA), the peak association for lead-based paint manufacturers, played a major role in opposing those who sought to educate the public about the dangers of lead-based paint and sought to ban its manufacture. At various points, the LIA sought to discredit research that linked lead-based paint with negative health impacts and downplay the number of children who were suffering from lead poisoning (Rabin 1989, 1671–1673). By the time New York City banned the use of lead-based paint in 1959, however, the LIA and the paint industry had found substitutes for lead. Most manufacturers were no longer manufacturing lead-based paint or were marketing non-lead-based alternatives. And the industry was no longer devoting resources to disputing the research or downplaying the incidence of lead poisoning (1673).

Economic development interests also were involved in the CDC decision to back away from a recommendation for universal lead poisoning screening for children. In the late 1980s and early 1990s, the health insurance industry, along with health maintenance organizations, was concerned with the cost of screening. Armed with cost-benefit studies suggesting that screening made economic sense only in those communities where the incidence was high, these interests, as well as state and local associations of pediatricians, opposed calls for universal screening. But this national debate over screening was less relevant for New York City. Although CDC recommendations for universal screening carry a great deal of weight, absent federal law passed by Congress, states have the final authority on whether to mandate screening. And even with the cost-benefit studies questioning the wisdom of universal screening, New York State was one of those jurisdictions where universal screening made sense. The state mandated universal screening in 1992; but by that time the city was well on its way to a universal screening program.

New York City's lead-based paint hazard abatement policy adopted in 1982 was opposed by the real estate industry, which was instrumental in its nonenforcement by the city. City economic development interests were most involved in the fight over Local Law 101A and its regulatory approach toward building owners' responsibilities for abatement and the implications of these regulations on assessments of liability in the face of noncompliance. Critical to this discussion was that the city was the largest owner of high-risk housing and therefore bore a great deal of risk as well. Opposition from real estate interests to Local Law 101A manifested itself in two ways. First, real estate interests had a long tradition of participation in the city's electoral process through campaign contributions and electoral support.

The second way the real estate interests attacked 101A was on its merits. The essence of their argument was that the law would affect economic development in the city by stifling housing rehabilitation, since much of the housing being rehabilitated was built before 1960. Landlords as well as those who were involved in housing rehabilitation, a major piece of the city's housing industry, were concerned that expanded concepts of owner responsibility as well as shorter deadlines for action would increase their liability. This in turn would increase litigation and severely affect their ability to obtain insurance and capital (Chen 2003). Real estate and housing rehabilitation interests in the city feared the new law would decrease investment in rehabilitation projects (Hu 2004).

As the general counsel for the Rent Stabilization Association, an organization representing property owners in the city, explained, "Under the new law, however, the building is presumed to be the source of the poisoning both for the purposes of issuing a violation and for use at trial if a liability case is filed against the owner" (Romano 2004). From the perspective of the real estate industry the new law changed the "litigation dynamic" by making it "easier for lead-poisoned plaintiffs to prevail in cases against owners even if the poisoning possibly occurred elsewhere" (Romano 2004).

An official for the Community Preservation Corporation, a group that finances low-income housing, stated that as a result of the law "as many as 1,220 planned apartments could be jeopardized . . . It's going to make it easier to sue landlords . . . which is going to make it harder to funnel investment into old buildings to pay for the extensive renovations" (Hu 2004). One local newspaper editorial reported that as early as February 2004 "some developers report insurance companies are reluctant to issue policies that cover buildings for lead related liability" (*New York Daily News* 2004). An official for Phipps Houses, a nonprofit organization that owns or manages more than thirteen thousand low-income apartments in the city stated that his organization had decided not to develop some available properties because those properties had lead-based paint risks. "The costs of adequate insurance, even if available, would make ownership financially impractical" (Oser 2004).

Speaking to the part of the legislation that made landlords responsible for abating lead-contaminated dust, a representative of a group of property owners claimed that the law created an "impossible standard" (Romano 2003). He noted further, "I am sure it is obvious to most people that apartment building owners in New York City have little control over airborne dust and tracked in soil" (quoted in Romano 2003). Real estate interests were concerned that landlords might be held liable for elevated blood lead levels even if they occurred because of lead sources external to the home.

In response to these concerns, a spokesperson for the New York City Coalition to End Lead Poisoning argued that the provisions of the law were reasonable as well as practical. He noted further that under the law "landlords will not be held culpable if they can persuade a fact-finder that diligent and reasonable efforts were made to eliminate a lead-based paint hazard" (Oser 2004). Some developers agreed with this position, arguing that the insurance industry would adjust, just as it had earlier with asbestos and window guard regulations (Oser 2004).

The Bloomberg administration was equally concerned about the negative impacts of the legislation. City executive branch officials were concerned about the new law's impact not only on the private sector but also on the city's own housing rehabilitation activity. With regard to the private sector, HPD commissioner Jerilyn Perine expressed concern that the deadlines set by the new law for hazard abatement were insufficient.

A spokesperson for the mayor stated that "this misguided legislation would divert precious resources away from programs which favor reduced lead poisoning cases by 80 percent in recent years, stifle our efforts to build more affordable housing and force people into homelessness by driving up housing costs" (Chen 2003). Commissioner Perine argued that the "inspection requirements would be more costly than advocates had suggested and that the city would have to do more abatement as private owners fail to keep up with the new deadlines" (Archibold 2003).

Race and Lead-Based Paint Poisoning
Given the incidence of lead poisoning across racial groups, lead poisoning could have been a controversial issue in the city's continuing efforts to manage racial and ethnic relations. Table 2.2 displays the racial breakdown of the most severe

cases of lead poisoning, those requiring environmental intervention according to the city DOH from 2001 through 2008. Whites are consistently under-represented, although their percentage within the most severely affected group has increased over the seven-year period. Asians appear to be the most over-represented group.

Why are white children underrepresented among those who are most severely lead-poisoned? The explanation may have as much to do with class as with race. Although a large percentage of the city's housing stock was built pre-1960, through the trickle-down housing process, low-income minorities ended up living in the most dilapidated of the pre-1960 housing. That housing was the most likely to experience the type of deterioration, without rehabilitation, that produced lead-based paint hazards. In some cases, this deteriorating housing has trickled down from one low-income minority group to another. When the housing was initially built and received its first coat of lead-based paint, it was probably occupied by whites. Throughout the last three decades of the twentieth century, the housing producing the highest incidences of lead poisoning cases was concentrated in the Brooklyn and Queens minority-populated neighborhoods of Bushwick, Fort Greene, Bedford, Jamaica, Red Hook, Flatbush, and Astoria. This group of neighborhoods became known as the "lead belt" (New York Public Interest Research Group 1999). In 2008, 78 percent of children reporting an EIBLL above 15 micrograms were enrolled in Medicaid (NYC DOHMH 2009b). Poverty appears to explain a great deal of lead poisoning.

Nevertheless, given the overrepresentation of minorities among those who are lead poisoned, why has this issue not produced more controversy in the city's political system? There are several possible reasons. First, there are some cases in which the city's political system behaved in ways that could be labeled environmentally racist. But in the case of lead paint poisoning, the paint was applied long before most minority groups moved into those homes. This eliminates any proactive discriminatory intent on the part of the developers and the city. Second, although the city was not the first urban political system to take action against lead-based paint, New York City took action years before the state or the federal government. There are some areas of environmental health policy where local governments do not act until the federal government mandates that they must act. Childhood lead poisoning is not one of these cases. Minority leaders had to be somewhat satisfied with the city's initiative in tackling this issue early on, although the letter of the law frequently differed from practice and enforcement. Third, given the behavior of minority political elites, they did not appear to view the lead-based paint hazard issue as one worthy of group mobilization. The city council vote on Local Law 38 in 1999 had minorities voting on both sides of the legislation, even though advocates opposed the law and criticized it for being weak. In 2003 some advocates did accuse Speaker Gifford Miller of environmental racism given his initial reluctance to back Local Law 101A, but in the end the council voted overwhelmingly in favor (Hu 2003).

One aspect of the city's increasing diversity that has exacerbated the lead poisoning issue, and specifically the lead-based paint issue, is the increasingly diverse composition of immigrants. City health officials have begun to ask whether immigrant children are being poisoned by the housing in which they are presently living or whether they arrive in the country already poisoned. DOHMH began to report the percentage of lead-poisoned children born outside the United States in 2002. In 2002, 22 percent of those with EIBLL were born outside the United States (NYC DOHMH 2004a). The percentage of foreign-born lead-poisoned children was 17 percent in 2003 and 2007, and 21 percent in 2008 (NYC DOHMH 2004b, 2009a, 2009b). "The most frequently reported countries of birth among foreign born EIBLL children in 2002 were Haiti, Mexico, Pakistan, Dominican Republic, and Bangladesh" (NYC DOHMH 2004a). In 2008 the most frequently reported countries among foreign-born EIBLL children were Bangladesh, Pakistan, and Haiti (NYC DOHMH 2009b).

Suspicions about the source of lead poisoning among immigrant children have been strengthened by reports that a deodorant, litargirio, manufactured in the Dominican Republic, contained a high degree of lead (Johnson 2003a). The U.S. Food and Drug Administration (FDA) never banned the product because it was unaware that it existed. In 2003 DOMH issued an alert in both English and Spanish about the dangers of using litargirio (NYC DOHMH 2004b). DOHMH also attempted to convince neighborhood herbal medicine shops that catered to Hispanics to stop selling it (Perez-Pena 2003). In 2005 the city council, at the request of DOHMH, passed a law outlawing the sale of litargirio in the city (NYC DOHMH 2005b). In another instance, a folk medicine from India was reported to have produced elevated BLLs and caused the hospitalization of more than a dozen people (O'Neil 2004). Lead-glazed pottery and food has also been cited as possible sources, particularly in immigrant communities (NYC DOHMH 2005b). Of course, examples such as this feed the criticisms of Local Law 101A by real estate interests, specifically the law's presumption that the landlord is responsible for a lead-poisoned child living in landlord-owned housing. And to the extent that the sources of lead poisoning are not known because of the cultures and habits of newly arriving immigrants, lead poisoning is less preventable.

The city's diversity has also forced the DOHMH to make its Lead Poisoning Prevention Program more accessible to non-English speaking populations, some of which comprise the most at-risk communities. "The LPPP works with community and social service organizations serving immigrant communities to build partnerships and increase awareness of lead poisoning" (NYC DOHMH 2005b). Much of the LPPP literature is translated into Bengali, Urdu, Haitian

Creole, Spanish, Chinese, and French. In addition, LPPP has attempted to reach and educate non-English speaking communities through local radio stations that broadcast in the languages of the countries of origin (NYC DOHMH 2009a). LPPP has even developed an English as a second language (ESL) class for day laborers that focuses on lead-remediation safe work practices (NYC DOHMH 2005b).

Conclusion

According to DOHMH records, New York City has made great progress in reducing lead poisoning. In 2009 DOHMH reported a 92 percent decrease since 1995 in new cases of children ages six months to six years with BLLs greater than 10 micrograms. In 1995, for every 1,000 children eighteen years or younger who were tested, 49.6 had BLLs of greater than 10 micrograms. In 2008 the rate per 1,000 children tested declined to 4.5. And according to DOHMH records, in 1995 there were 82 children in the city whose BLLs tested over 45 micrograms. In 2008 there were only 7 (NYC DOHMH 2009b). Nationally, the median BLL of preschool children has declined from 15 micrograms per deciliter of blood in the late 1970s to less than 2 micrograms in 2006. In the late 1970s, more than 88 percent of preschool children had BLL over 10 micrograms. In 2006 fewer than 2 percent had BLL over 10 micrograms. There are still differences across racial, ethnic, and socioeconomic groups, but the improvement is impressive (Bellinger and Bellinger 2006).

CHAPTER THREE

MANAGING ASTHMA

New York City's policies toward childhood asthma were a response to the increase in the incidence of this condition beginning in the 1980s. Asthma's significance as a public health issue and the city's public policy in response to it were due to two different facets of the disease. First, childhood asthma was at epidemic proportions, affecting more than 10 percent of the city's children. In 2007 an estimated 300,000 children in the city suffered from asthma (Environmental Defense Fund 2007). The impact of asthma on children measured by both school absences and hospitalization rates due to the disease demanded a response from the political system. Second, asthma is a multifactorial disease. While little is known "about what causes the initial development of asthma in people previously without the disease, much is known about the triggers of existing asthma" (Das 2007). And some of the factors related to either the onset of childhood asthma or its aggravation are associated with community conditions created in part, if not entirely, by political decisions. As a result, some of the solutions to the asthma problem lay within the political system.

Asthma research has confirmed the disease's multifactorial nature but has not produced a cure for the condition. Research has, however, produced a variety of treatments that address the symptoms and allow those with asthma to manage the disease by lessening the most aggravating manifestations. The focus of public health policy addressing asthma has been to give children and their family's access to primary health care and appropriate treatments. In addition, city asthma policy has focused on educating parents and others in the community about how they can best manage their children's symptoms.

Research on the causes of asthma have also confirmed the condition's connection to economic development, particularly its by-products such as traffic and air pollution. Because the incidence of childhood asthma falls far more heavily on minority and low-income children and their communities, accusations of environmental racism and calls for environmental justice have been part of the asthma public health policy discussion.

The Science and Etiology of Asthma

"Childhood asthma is a chronic inflammatory disorder of the airways characterized by intermittent, recurrent episodes of wheezing, breathlessness, chest tightness, and cough, particularly at night or in the early morning" (Koutsavlis et al. 2001, 311). It is a "stable disease" subject to "periods of exacerbation" (Sykes and Johnston 2008, 685). Most exacerbations are due to viral infections, but the precise etiology of asthma is not known, and there are multiple triggers that result in exacerbation of the condition (Sykes and Johnston 2008; Brown et al. 1997). Asthma can develop as a response to an allergy or it can be nonallergenic. With allergenic asthma, the inhalation of an allergen produces the inflammation within the lungs that leads to hyperactivity of the airways (Institute of Medicine 2000).

Because of the variety of symptoms, there is no agreed upon clinical definition of asthma (Koutsavlis et al. 2001). As a result, identification of asthma depends on imprecise diagnoses by physicians. "Yet there is general agreement that asthma is always associated with inflammation within the lungs, and the intensity of the inflammation is related to the severity of the respiratory symptoms and the degree of bronchial hyper-responsiveness" (Institute of Medicine 2000, 23).

Asthma can affect a child's ability to play, learn, and sleep. It is responsible for numerous school absences. According to most physicians, an "asthma sufferer can live a normal, unrestricted life . . . if they get the proper medication and stick to the daily treatment and monitoring that the disease requires" (Stolberg 1999). But in low-income communities, childhood asthma sufferers often have limited access to sound primary health care. Severe cases of asthma require hospitalization, and the disease can be fatal if untreated or treated too late (Collins 1985).

As the incidence of asthma rose throughout the country and particularly in urban areas, researchers began to identify those factors they believed contributed to the disease. Asthma has both genetic and environmental roots. Genetic research as well as research of family asthma histories have "convincingly shown that the disease has a strong genetic component" (Yeatts et al. 2006, 635). A 1980 study found that "80 percent of children with asthmatic parents develop the disease compared with 40 percent of children with one asthmatic parent and 10 percent of children with no asthmatic parents" (640). Genetics, however, cannot account for the increase in asthma prevalence that occurred over the past thirty years. Changes in genetic composition that would make individuals more susceptible to asthma would take multiple generations to occur (Yeatts et al. 2006). Thus, much of the focus of asthma research and public health policy has been on the environmental factors related to the disease.

Asthma research has divided environmental factors into indoor and outdoor sources. In addition, research has established that while some factors are related to the onset or development of asthma, others are linked only to its aggravation or exacerbation. This means that for those who already have asthma, environmental factors such as air pollution, either indoor or outdoor, "may lead to disease progression such that the frequency and severity of the process along with associated morbidity are increased" (Larsen et al. 2002).

Asthma research has demonstrated stronger links between indoor air pollutants and the onset of asthma than outdoor pollutants. One of the significant links asthma research has established is between the development of asthma and secondhand smoke. This includes a connection not only between direct exposure to secondhand smoke and asthma but also between a fetus and the mother's smoking or the exposure of the pregnant mother to secondhand smoke (Gilmour et al. 2006).

Studies have established connections between indoor allergens and asthma. These allergens include cockroach, mouse, pet, house dust mites, and mold. Among the indoor factors, cockroach allergens have received the most attention. One study in Harlem found that "85% of the homes of inner city children with asthma" had detectable cockroach allergen levels (cited in Rauh et al. 2002). In 1996 a study by the National Institute of Allergy and Infectious Diseases concluded that the cockroach was a major factor in the inner-city asthma outbreak. The study concluded that childhood asthma is usually caused by "an allergic reaction to a substance called an antigen" and that of all the antigen-producing agents found in urban residences, "cockroach droppings appear to be the most powerful" (Singleton 1996). Another national study of inner-city children with asthma found that "36.8 percent were allergic to cockroach allergen, 34.9 percent to dust-mite allergen, and 22.7 percent to cat allergen" (Rosenstreich et al. 1997, 1356). The same study found that 50.2 percent of homes in the study had "high levels of cockroach allergen in dust" and that those children "who both were allergic to cockroach allergen and exposed to high levels of the allergen" had a significantly higher rate of hospitalization than other asthmatic children in the study (Rosenstreich et al. 1997). Links have also been established between mouse allergen exposure and asthma (Matsui et al. 2006).

At the same time, however, one study in inner-city Baltimore found no significant difference in the potential sources of indoor pollution in the homes of children with asthma and those without asthma. The researchers concluded that, while indoor air pollution exposure may exacerbate existing asthma, these pollutants by themselves were not linked to the development of childhood asthma. They suggest that indoor air pollutant exposure may play a "role in the development of asthma among genetically susceptible individuals" (Diette et al. 2007).

Most of the indoor allergens are linked to deteriorating housing found in low-income areas of cities. "Substandard housing is marked by poor indoor air quality, with mold, mildew, dust and cockroaches, all likely triggers for asthma attacks" (Das 2007). In 2008 the New York City Department of Health and Mental Hygiene (DOHMH) reported that at lower-income levels there was a higher prevalence of cockroaches being reported in the home as well as a higher prevalence of there being at least one smoker in the home (NYC DOHMH 2008). In fact, there are studies that confirm a positive relationship between housing deterioration and allergen levels, controlling for income and race or ethnicity. A study conducted in northern Manhattan found a significant association "between cockroach allergens and housing disrepair, independent of income" (Rauh et al. 2002).

Minority leaders in some communities affected by asthma have argued that the cockroach theory was merely an attempt by the government to "divert attention" from the broader environmental causes of asthma and blame the victims (Calderone et al., 1998a). They argued that roaches had been around for decades but the rise in the incidence of asthma was a recent phenomenon, coinciding more with increases in outdoor environmental pollutants and the siting of specific environmental hazards in low-income minority communities (Calderone et al., 1998b).

While most research has not linked outdoor air pollutants to the development or onset of childhood asthma, these pollutants have been linked to asthma aggravation, including increased bronchial hypersensitivity, inflammatory changes, increased use of medication, and hospitalization (Koenig 1999). Air quality degradation due to outdoor pollution both produces greater exposure to ozone and increases in particulate matter. Both have been linked to asthma aggravation.

Outdoor air pollution is a common occurrence in all industrialized urban areas with the primary source being vehicle emissions. Multiple studies have found associations between vehicular traffic intensity and hospitalization for asthma. One study of children in the Netherlands found that "children living near roads with high intensity truck traffic" had "lower lung function and more chronic respiratory symptoms compared to children living on roads with less truck traffic" (Brauer et al. 2002). A similar study in the Bronx found that residential proximity to major sources of air pollution was one of three factors, along with poverty status and race, that were helpful in predicting whether a child's hospitalization was due to asthma (Maantay et al. 1999). Finally, in 2007 the Environmental Defense Fund, in conjunction with Harvard's School of Public Health, conducted a study examining environmental "risk zones," those areas within five hundred feet of a heavily used roadway. Having synthesized much of the traffic-related pollution studies over the prior decade, the researchers worked under the assumption that within these zones, pollutants including particulate matter (soot) plus nitrogen oxides (smog) were sufficient to be a threat to human health and a trigger if not a cause of asthma. The study found that more than two million New Yorkers lived within these risk zones. Also located within these zones were large numbers of health facilities, schools, and playgrounds (Environmental Defense Fund 2007).

Outdoor pollutants have been the focal point of community and environmental groups' asthma studies. Citing diesel-fuel-powered buses and trucks and the continued use of coal burning furnaces in many of the city's public schools, environmental groups and their researchers argued that air pollution was a significant part of the problem as well (Kassel and Kennedy 1996). An environmental group in the Bronx cited the large number of diesel exhaust vehicles that drive through low-income communities, such as Hunts Point where an estimated sixty thousand trucks passed through in a month (Calderone et al. 1998b; Stolberg 1999). Despite the studies that linked asthma and other illnesses to outdoor pollutants, there was also evidence that, overall, air pollutants in the city, including low-income neighborhoods, had decreased, despite the citing of environmental nuisances in many low-income communities (Lobach 1996).

Another factor that environmental and community groups cited as a possible cause for increased asthma in parts of the city was the placement of waste transfer stations. In the late 1990s, there were approximately seventy-five waste transfer stations in the city, and most of them were located in low-income, minority-populated areas of the city. The Greenpoint and Williamsburg sections of Brooklyn had twenty-four waste transfer stations alone (Stewart 2000). In a small section of East Harlem there were four waste transfer stations and four bus depots, in addition to the automobile exhaust created by Tri-Borough Bridge traffic (Wakin 2001). No studies have linked waste transfer stations with asthma; however, waste transfer stations produce truck exhaust. They also create rodent and roach infestation. As a result, their disproportionate location in high-asthma neighborhoods has become a factor in public health policy discussions.

Several studies have examined the role that stress plays in modifying the impact of air pollution on the development of childhood asthma. The rationale is that low socioeconomic-status families are subject to high stress, making children more susceptible to asthma development. "Stress has pro-oxidant effects that can increase airway inflammation" and "also increase vulnerability to antigens through direct effects on the endocrine system, autonomic control of airways and immune function" (Shankardass et al. 2009, 12407). A study of asthmatic children in Southern California found that the risk of asthma due to traffic-related pollution was greater for those children whose parents reported high stress. The same study found that stress was also a factor in increasing susceptibility to asthma of children who had been exposed to tobacco smoke in utero (Shankardass et al. 2009). Another study of children in East Boston found a relationship "between traffic related pollution and asthma" only among children who were found to have elevated exposure to violence, clearly a factor that produces stress (Clougherty et al. 2007).

Obesity, a public health problem in its own right, has also been a factor related to the development of childhood asthma. Studies have confirmed that the risk of asthma increases with increasing obesity. Other research has suggested that "obesity is a strong predictor of the persistence of asthma into adolescence" (Yeatts et al. 2006, 637).

Asthma Prevalence

Measuring the prevalence of asthma and its impacts has been a challenge because of the different ways in which it has been diagnosed and the fact there have been few consistent measures of the disease's surveillance since it began to increase in prevalence in the 1980s. Some have noted that when infants are included in asthma prevalence studies, there are additional problems because it is "difficult to differentiate respiratory infections from asthma in this age group" (Gergen et al. 1988, 2). In New York City in particular, it has been reported that hospitals within the city differ in their diagnosis of infant symptoms, labeling some as asthmatic while labeling others as having bronchiolitis (Stevenson 2003).

Despite the diagnostic variability, there is little doubt that the prevalence of asthma increased in the last quarter of the twentieth century. Asthma is now the most common childhood chronic disease in the United States. For all age groups, according to National Health Interview Survey data, "the self reported prevalence of asthma increased 75% between 1980 and 1994" (Institute of Medicine 2000, 73). This increase occurred across all racial and ethnic groups, and all age groups as well. The death rate from asthma also increased. During the 1970s, asthma mortality declined more than 7 percent annually. But during the 1980s, it increased by more than 6 percent annually, "increasing faster among children ages 5–14 years than among adults 15–34 (Weiss and Wagener 1990).

Nationally, between 1980 and 1996 the prevalence of asthma for children up to age seventeen years increased from 3.6 to 6.2 percent, an average increase of approximately 4.3 percent per year. Since 1996, childhood asthma prevalence appeared to level off (Akinbami and Schoendorf 2002). In 2011, however, the U.S. Centers for Disease Control and Prevention (CDC) reported that childhood asthma (affecting those younger than eighteen) had increased to 9.6 percent (US CDC 2011). For black children, prevalence had increased from 11.4 percent in 2001 to 17 percent in 2009 (Rabin 2011).

Children living in urban areas, particularly inner-city minority children, have disproportionate rates of asthma and suffer from more severe cases of asthma as well. During the period when childhood asthma was increasing, the gap between black and white non-Hispanic children grew. In the early 1980s, black children had an asthma rate 15 percent higher than non-Hispanic white children. By 2000 black children had an asthma rate that was 44 percent higher than white non-Hispanic children. In 2000 Hispanic children had an asthma rate higher than non-Hispanic whites but lower than black children (Akinbami and Schoendorf 2002). In 2011 the CDC reported that the asthma rate among poor children was 13.5 percent and among non-Hispanic black children the rate was 17 percent. The asthma rate for all children was 9.6 percent (US CDC 2011).

New York City has engaged in only limited surveillance of childhood asthma prevalence. Using a 2003 telephone survey the NYC DOHMH reported that "17% of children ages 0–17 have been diagnosed with asthma at some time in their lives compared with 13% of children nationwide" and that nine percent "are classified as having current asthma," while the national average is 5 percent (NYC DOHMH 2008).

There is somewhat more consistency and duration of data collection on hospitalization rates for asthma than for other measures of prevalence. As a result, asthma hospitalization rates have been used by many not only as a proxy measure for asthma prevalence but also as a measure of the condition's severity. Despite the availability of hospitalization data for asthma over a much longer time period than other measures, there are still some problems with using this measure to gauge the nature of the disease. First, hospitalization for asthma may measure the failure of primary care to address asthma as much as the severity of the condition. This is particularly the case in low-income communities where primary health care may be in short supply. Asthma rates are highest in those areas of the city that are underserved by health and medical community and where higher percentages of those who lack health insurance live. More-affluent asthma sufferers with insurance see private physicians. Less-affluent sufferers, predominantly in minority communities, with Medicaid or no insurance are subject to treatment by a resource-limited public health care system and as a result are far more likely to end up hospitalized or to be seen in the emergency department of a hospital. At the same time, however, to the extent that public health policy makers can reduce hospitalization rates by providing asthma sufferers with adequate primary care or disease management capabilities, this is a significant step forward. So while hospitalization rates may not be the most accurate measures of asthma prevalence, it is still a valuable measure for public health policy makers. Since there is no cure for asthma, the most promising strategy for public health policy makers to pursue is to reduce hospitalization rates. It indicates that either severity decreased or primary care and disease management services have been provided. Reducing hospitalization places less of a burden on the child, the family, and the public purse.

Second, there are problems in interpreting asthma hospitalization rates, since some hospitals have treated children with debilitating symptoms by admitting them to the hospital, while other hospitals have treated children with similar symptoms in emergency departments. This variation was noticed even among hospitals in New York City (Stevenson 2003). Related to this, some have also suggested that over time "the threshold of attack severity for a hospital admission has likely increased" (Akinbami 2006, 6). Recent hospitalizations may represent more severe cases.

TABLE 3.1

New York City and U.S. Childhood Asthma Hospitalizations,

1990–2007 (rate per 10,000)

Year	United States (0–17 years)	New York City (0–4 years)	New York City (5–14 years)
1990	28.4	131.3	52.3
1991	30.6	140.6	55.7
1992	30.8	169.0	60.7
1993	25.4	175.4	71.8
1994	26.8	154.6	66.4
1995	32.7	171.9	65.5
1996	29.8	155.9	68.2
1997	32.4	155.0	63.3
1998	24.4	111.2	45.4
1999	28.1	138.6	53.0
2000	29.6	108.4	42.4
2001	26.2	111.7	41.5
2002	26.9	108.3	41.9
2003	31.2	116.9	49.8
2004	27.1	99.5	45.7
2005		83.5	39.2
2006		88.3	37.8
2007		79.9	35.4

Sources: Laura Akinbami. 2006. The State of Childhood Asthma, United States.
1980–2005. Advance Data From Vital Health Statistics, Centers for Disease
Control and Prevention, Number 381, December 29; New York City Department
of Health and Mental Hygiene, Asthma Initiative. 1999. Asthma Facts; New York
City Department of Health and Mental Hygiene, Asthma Initiative. 2003.
Asthma Facts (2nd edition), May; New York City Department of Health and
Mental Hygiene, Asthma Initiative. 2010. 2000–2008 Asthma Hospitalization
Tables and Figures. (Bureau of Environmental Surveillance and Policy), May.

Nationally, the asthma hospitalization rate for children up to seventeen years
of age was 21.0 per 10,000 in 1980. It increased throughout the 1980s and early
1990s and peaked at 32.7 per 10,000 in 1995 and 32.4 in 1997. Since then it has
leveled off at slightly above or below 30.0 (Akinbami 2006). Similar to prevalence, childhood asthma hospitalization rates vary by race. "In 1998–1999, the
asthma hospitalization rate among black children was 3.6 times the rate for white
children" (Akinbami and Schoendorf 2002, 318). The rate was 56.9 for black children and 15.5 for white children (Akinbami and Schoendorf 2002).

By the late 1990s, asthma was the leading cause of hospitalization among the
city's children. NYC DOHMH reports hospitalization rates for children up to
fourteen years, but in some cases they have provided rates for those up to seventeen years that can be compared with national data. In 2000 New York City's
childhood asthma hospitalization rate was 60.6 per 10,000, while the U.S. rate
for the same group was 33.6. Table 3.1 displays childhood asthma hospitalization
rates for New York City and the United States. The hospitalization rates in the

TABLE 3.2

New York City Childhood (0–14 years) Asthma Hospitalization Rates by Borough and
Selected Neighborhoods (rate per 1,000), 1995–2008

	1995	1997	2001	2004	2007–8 Average
Bronx	16.1	15.4	9.2	10.7	9.2
Kingsbridge	6.8	6.6	3.6	4.8	4.6
Hunts Point/Mott Haven	22.5	22.6	9.4	12.8	11.5
Brooklyn	9.0	8.3	5.5	6.1	4.1
Bedford-Stuyvesant/Crown Heights	15.4	14.0	10.3	10.8	7.7
Bensonhurst/Bay Ridge	2.6	2.4	1.1	1.5	1.1
Manhattan	13.4	12.3	6.9	6.3	4.0
East Harlem	36.5	29.2	16.9	13.3	11.2
Upper East Side	3.1	4.0	2.3	1.9	1.2
Queens	6.9	6.4	4.9	4.7	3.9
Bayside/Little Neck	2.7	1.4	1.5	1.9	2.3
Jamaica	10.2	9.3	7.8	7.6	6.2
Staten Island	3.8	3.7	2.8	2.6	2.0

Source: New York City Department of Health and Mental Hygiene, Asthma Initiative. 2009
Asthma Hospitalizations, New York City, by UHF Neighborhood; New York City Department of
Health and Mental Hygiene, Asthma Initiative. 2010. 2000–2008 Asthma Hospitalization Tables
and Figures (Bureau of Environmental Surveillance and Policy), May.

table, even though not entirely comparable, show that New York City childhood asthma hospitalization rates are much higher than national rates. While
national rates have fluctuated at a low level, New York City hospitalization rates
peaked in the mid-1990s and have since declined, although they are still much
higher than the national rates. These elevated rates probably indicate more severe cases of asthma as well as a lack of access to primary care on the part of
severe asthma sufferers.

Even more significant than the comparison of New York City's childhood
asthma hospitalization rates with the national rates is a comparison of hospitalization rates within the city across boroughs and neighborhoods. Table 3.2 displays hospitalization rates for children ages up to age fourteen years in the five
boroughs and selected neighborhoods from 1995 to 2008. The Bronx is consistently the borough with the highest asthma hospitalization rates, even though
these rates declined from 16.1 per 1,000 in 1995 to 9.2 in 2007–8, a decline of 38
percent. Staten Island reports the lowest rates consistently less than 4.0 per 1,000
for the ten-year period. Looking at selected within-borough neighborhood rates
indicates that the differences within boroughs are as great as, if not greater than,
the differences across boroughs. In 1995 the northwestern Bronx neighborhood
of Kingsbridge reported a 6.8 hospitalization rate, while Hunts Point-Mott
Haven in the south Bronx reported a rate of 22.5. Note, however, that by 2007–8,

the difference between the Kingsbridge and Hunts Point-Mott rates declined a great deal. For 1995, in Manhattan, the East Harlem hospitalization rate was 36.5, while the adjacent Upper East Side hospitalization rate was 3.1. Again note that by 2007–8, East Harlem's hospitalization rate was down to 11.2, while the Upper East Side was 1.2. This was the largest decrease in hospitalization rates of all neighborhoods in the city for the reported time period.

In 2002 Harlem Hospital implemented a study screening every child under thirteen years who lived or went to school in a twenty-four-square-block area of central Harlem. More than two thousand children were screened. In 2003 the hospital reported that 25 percent of its population had asthma. The results of the study suggested not only that asthma rates in low-income minority communities might be much higher than originally thought but also that there was a significant number of children suffering from asthma who were undiagnosed and therefore receiving no treatment (Perez-Pena 2003a).

New York City has not routinely published asthma hospitalization data disaggregated by race or ethnicity. Examining childhood asthma hospitalization rate differences across the city's neighborhoods can be used as a proxy for focusing on minority asthma hospitalization. In Table 3.2, neighborhoods with a high percentage of minority residents reported higher asthma hospitalization rates than neighborhoods with fewer minority residents. In the absence of disaggregated race or ethnicity data, another proxy measure that has been used in New York City is income. Corburn et al. (2006) concluded that asthma hotspots in New York City had high concentrations of minorities, individuals living below the poverty line, public housing, and deteriorating housing.

Most studies that have examined asthma hospitalization data disaggregated by race or ethnicity have not looked specifically at children. Two studies that did look at asthma hospitalization rates for the entire population disaggregated by race and ethnicity revealed significant differences among major racial and ethnic groups. Carr et al. (1992) examined asthma hospitalization data for the years 1982–86. The study found that the average asthma hospitalization rates for whites, blacks, and Hispanics in New York City for those years were 12.2, 59.9, and 62.9 per 10,000 respectively. De Palo et al. (1993) examined disaggregated hospitalization data for the years 1989–91 and found that the hospitalization rate per 10,000 population was 24.2 for whites, 81.0 for blacks, and 103.0 for Hispanics. Although there is no guarantee that the hospitalization data examined in the two studies are comparable, the data indicate that asthma hospitalizations increased for all groups. The study by Carr et al. (1992) suggests that difference among racial and ethnic groups may predate the increase that took place in the mid-1980s and early 1990s.

New York State has published data on childhood asthma prevalence for selected years disaggregated by group but not by county. For 2002–3, the state

TABLE 3.3

New York City Asthma Emergency Department Visits and Hospitalization Discharges for Children (0–17 years) by Borough (2006–8, 2008–10 averages)

	Emergency Department Visits (rate per 10,000)			Hospital Discharges (rate per 10,000)		
	2006–8	2007	2008–10	2006–8	2007	2008–10
Bronx	396.7		362.5	84.0		84.0
Brooklyn	189.2		198.5	40.9		41.0
Manhattan	290.4		286.8	41.7		38.6
Queens	164.0		169.5	36.8		33.7
Staten Island	101.2		109.0	19.0		19.1
New York State	144.4		142.4	29.3		28.8
New York City		267.0			54.0	
Rest of New York State		59.0			12.0	

Sources: New York State Department of Health Public Health Information Group Center for Community Health. 2009. New York State Asthma Surveillance Summary Report. October; New York State Department of Health, www.health.state.ny.us/statistics/ny_asthma (accessed: June 24, 2011); New York City Department of Health and Mental Hygiene. 2010. 2000–2008 Asthma Hospitalization Tables and Figures (Bureau of Environmental Surveillance), May.

reported that the asthma prevalence (self reported or reported by parent or guardian) rates for children up to seventeen years were 7.2 percent for whites, 10 percent for blacks, 10.9 percent for Hispanics, and 4.3 percent for Asians (NYS Department of Health [DOH] 2007). In 2005 the state reported little variation in asthma prevalence among its high school students with non-Hispanic white, non-Hispanic black, and Hispanic students having prevalence rates of 17.1, 18.0, and 17.5 percent respectively. These were very similar, although slightly higher than rates reported for all U.S. high school students (NYS DOH 2007). Recently the state has reported emergency department visits as well as hospital discharges for those up to seventeen years, disaggregated by county. These results appear in Table 3.3. For emergency department visits, with the exception of Staten Island, all boroughs are well above the state rate. For hospital discharges, both Staten Island and Manhattan are below the state average rate with the Bronx being more than two times the state rate. In 2007 the city's rate of childhood asthma emergency department visits was more than four times that of the rest of the state while the hospitalization rate for the same group was more than four times the rate of the rest of the state (NYS DOH 2009).

As a result of New York City's recent attempts to combat asthma, in 2008 the DOHMH began to report the numbers of those children in the city who had an Asthma Action Plan. In 2008 DOHMH reported that 41 percent of those children in households earning less than $50,000 had a plan while 54 percent of those in households earning more than $50,000 had a plan (NYC DOHMH 2008).

New York City's Asthma Policy

Table 3.4 displays policy tools implemented to combat asthma in New York City. The development of public policy toward asthma is hampered by several factors. First, at present there is no known cure for asthma. As a result there is no guarantee that addressing the known causes through public policy will eliminate or even reduce the prevalence of the disease. Second, since asthma cannot be eradicated, the goal of public policy is reduced to decreasing those symptoms of childhood asthma that are most debilitating. Controlling asthma, by either controlling the factors that trigger attacks or giving children and their families the resources to manage the disease, can reduce both the number and severity of attacks and ultimately decrease hospitalizations.

The implicit goal of New York City's policy toward childhood asthma has been to reduce the number and severity of attacks and thereby reduce hospitalizations, school absences, and any other negative manifestations of the disease. In pursuing this goal, the city has followed two broad strategies. The first strategy is to address factors that exacerbate or trigger childhood asthma or cause asthma attacks. This would include both indoor and outdoor pollutants. The second strategy involves giving families access to medical and health-related resources as well as providing them with education to allow them to manage their children's asthma in an attempt to reduce its severity. The multifactorial nature of asthma and the consequent breadth of the city's approach to dealing with it provide an example of the World Health Organization's concept of seeking "health in all policies" (World Health Organization 2010).

Much of the city's attempt to deal with pollutants that cause asthma has been focused on outdoor pollutants and, in particular, those pollutants related to vehicular emissions. The federal and state governments have been involved in addressing air pollution since the 1970s. Although federal, state, and city efforts to combat air pollution were never designed to combat asthma exclusively, any improvement in air quality should improve the health of those with asthma.

Through education and some regulation, the city has attempted to address those indoor pollutants that both cause asthma and trigger attacks. Formulating public policy, however, that speaks to indoor pollutants involves intervention, however mild, in households and family living. In addition, those indoor factors that had been identified, such as roach feces and body parts, created difficult, if not intractable, problems for policy makers. Because the target families were, in many cases, low-income minorities, the issue of government intervention became a much more sensitive undertaking. As a result, community-based organizations have played a valuable role in dealing with indoor asthma triggers. At the same time, by the 1990s there had been a several-decade history of government involvement in regulating outdoor pollution, particularly related to motor vehicles

TABLE 3.4
Public Policy Tools Addressing Asthma

MONITORING AND SCREENING
New York City
Department of Education, Board of Education: Adds questions on student medical forms asking about asthma
New York State and New York City
Collect data on asthma hospitalization and emergency department visits

EDUCATION (DISEASE MANAGEMENT TO PREVENT EMERGENCY ROOM VISITS AND HOSPITALIZATION)
New York City
Department of Health
Asthma Initiative: Educates families and school officials about asthma management, primarily through community organizations, such as East Harlem and Hunts Point Asthma Centers
Asthma Counselors (East Harlem DPHO)
Asthma Training Institute: Funds education for local physicians on the most current methods for treating asthma
Creating a Medical Home for Asthma: Provides asthma management program developed by health professionals to train health professionals
Compiles directory of asthma services in conjunction with the movement of New York City's Medicaid recipients to managed care
Public education campaign promotes awareness about asthma and management of the illness: Reduces exposure to substances that may trigger asthma attacks (via posters, billboards, ads on subways) and partners with community groups
DOHMH Asthma Action Line (telephone)
Asthma Partnership: Includes community organizations and individuals interested in furthering the city's campaign against asthma (plays an advisory role for the DOHMH)
Department of Education
Managing Asthma in Schools: Trains public school teachers to recognize asthma symptoms and help students manage the disease
Nonprofit organizations (examples)
American Lung Association Open Airways program: Trains both school health professionals as well as children with asthma to help them control their asthma
Harlem Children's Zone community workers: Teach families and children how and when to use asthma medications
Harlem Children's Zone workers: Inspect homes and educate families on possible indoor asthma triggers and how to eliminate them
Reducing Indoor Allergens and Study Team (Northern Manhattan and South Bronx): Educate families members about pest management, using laminated information sheets
Federal government
National Heart, Lung and Blood Institute: Funds a Medical Home for Asthma

TABLE 3.4 (continued)

EDUCATION (OUTDOOR POLLUTION)
New York City
    Clean Heat Program: Makes building owners aware of financing, incentives, and technical assistance in converting buildings to cleaner heating oil

REGULATIONS (OUTDOOR POLLUTANTS)
New York City Charter
    Fair share siting guidelines (not currently being enforced)
New York City laws
    Department of Citywide Administrative Services
        Regulations on city's vehicle fleet
    Department of Education
        Regulations on school buses serving the city
            Diesel fuel regulations
            School bus idling regulations
    PlaNYC
        Building/home heating oil regulations
    Taxi and Limousine Commission
        Regulations and incentives encouraging a cleaner taxi fleet
    Department of Sanitation
        Solid waste management policy (reduces waste transfer stations in areas with high asthma prevalence)
New York State
    State responsibility for achieving National Ambient Air Quality Standards pursuant to the U.S. Clean Air Act
    MTA conversion of bus fleet to hybrid buses and buses using ultralow sulfur diesel and compressed natural gas
    State attorney general's agreement with school bus companies on idling
Federal government
    Air quality regulations (subject to enforcement)
    EPA consent decree with truck and automotive engine industry regarding new diesel engines

REGULATIONS (INDOOR POLLUTANTS)
New York City
    Department of Housing Preservation and Development
        Housing code: Mandates that owners/landlords alleviate deterioration that could possibly be linked to asthma including water leaks that could produce mold and ventilation (subject to housing code enforcement)
        Safe Housing Act: Amends the Department of Housing Preservation and Development's (HPD) Alternative Enforcement Program. Several hundred buildings with the most housing code violations (asthma-related) are singled out for expedited enforcement. Landlords are given three months to correct code violations. If they fail to address the violations, HPD will do it and charge the landlords

SERVICE PROVISION
New York City
    PlaNYC, Million trees initiative: Plants more trees to combat air pollution
    Department of Health
        Asthma Resource Centers in Hunts Points (Bronx), and East Harlem: Facilitate
            coordination of efforts of physicians, community health workers, schools, and
            parents to prevent and treat the illness
        Asthma Resource Centers: Provide spacers and peak flow meters for those not eli-
            gible for Medicaid or SCHIP
New York State
    Medicaid and SCHIP: Fund the provision of spacers and peak flow meters
    Funding of regional asthma coalitions: Develop evidence-based strategies that could be
        implemented at community level to improve the delivery of asthma care
Nonprofit organizations (examples)
    Harlem Children's Zone: Builds links between health care practitioners, schools, and
        families in order to create asthma management plans
    Reducing Indoor Allergens Study Team (Northern Manhattan and South Bronx):
        Recruits families and goes into homes with carpenters, cleaners, and environmental
        researchers to combat indoor asthma triggers

FINANCIAL ASSISTANCE
Federal government
    NIH: Funds research into the causes of asthma
    Department of Housing and Urban Development Healthy Homes Initiative: Focuses
        on indoor pollution
    EPA: Funds air pollution monitoring
    Department of Transportation Asthma Free School Zones Project: Focuses on engine
        idling near schools and clean fuel technologies
    Department of Health and Human Services Preventive Health and Human Services
        Block Grant

with the federal government playing the leading role. Under federal air pollution guidelines, air quality improved significantly in New York City.

Reducing Vehicular Emissions

The local efforts to reduce vehicular emissions as a means to decrease asthma severity or prevalence was not always led by the city's elected officials. Community groups from affected parts of the city had a major role in moving the policy agenda. Most important, to the extent that efforts to reduce vehicular emissions succeeded, and not all did, there is little evidence that the efforts had any impact on reduced asthma severity or declining asthma hospitalizations. The city's attack on outdoor pollution took several forms. First, at the community level, there was an attempt to halt the placement of any additional bus depots in northern Manhattan, where asthma rates were high. Second, communities were also concerned about pollution created by diesel school buses and school bus idling. The city council and the Bloomberg administration formulated a policy to convert the city's vehicle fleet to one that produced cleaner emissions. They also attempted to do the same with the city's taxi fleet. They were assisted in this effort by U.S. Environmental Protection Agency (EPA) mandates that all diesel vehicles use cleaner fuel by 2006. The Bloomberg administration also produced a solid waste management plan designed to produce less truck traffic in the city. Finally, the Bloomberg administration hoped to reduce automobile emissions in the central business district through a congestion pricing plan. The primary tools in dealing with air pollution have been regulations.

Much of the city's efforts to attack air pollution were focused on diesel-powered vehicles. Diesel vehicles produce particulate matter that aggravates lung functioning and can exacerbate asthma. One of the targets of the city's efforts to reduce diesel fuel pollution was the city's school bus fleet, operated by private bus companies (Perez-Pena 2003b). School buses produced two related issues for the city and childhood asthma: the pollution that diesel fuel produced, and the additional pollution that school buses idling near schools produced. In 1971 the city council passed a law prohibiting cars and buses from idling for more than three minutes with fines for violations. An investigation by the council in 2004 found that bus companies frequently violated the law, factoring the fines into the cost of doing business on those few occasions when they were caught (*Gotham Gazette* 2010a). In addition, research demonstrated that children sitting inside diesel-powered buses were exposed to even more exhaust than those immediately outside the bus (NYC Council 2009).

The city council increased the fines in 2004 but enforcement of the law was not given teeth until the New York State attorney general, Eliot Spitzer, got involved that same year. An investigation by the attorney general's office found that some bus companies had routinely allowed their buses to idle for up to a half hour. This was in violation not only of the city three-minute idling law but also of a state five-minute idling law. According to the state investigation the additional idling produced 1.3 million tons of soot, including sixty tons of nitrogen oxide and twenty tons of carbon monoxide. Faced with steep fines, the bus companies agreed to retrofit many of their buses with new exhaust filters. This, combined with low sulfur fuel use, would significantly reduce harmful pollution (DePalma 2004). Spitzer was later able to get many of the school bus companies to agree to a "no idle" policy near schools (Egbert 2005).

In 2009 Mayor Bloomberg and the city council produced legislation to "retire old school buses and require filters to reduce the amount of pollution inside" those buses (Kassel 2009). In 2009 the Bloomberg administration also promulgated legislation reducing bus idling to one minute near schools and three minutes elsewhere in the city. This was done in conjunction with a "Turn

It Off" Campaign publicizing the dangers of bus idling. The law has been poorly enforced—so much so that in 2012 the city's Department of Environmental Protection announced a two-week crackdown on school bus idling in schools with high asthma rates, along with a new "Stop Idling" Campaign that would take place during Asthma Awareness Month (NYC Department of Environmental Protection 2012).

In 2000, when the Metropolitan Transit Authority (MTA) proposed using new diesel-powered buses in the city, the proposal was opposed by environmental groups as well as public health experts. They argued that medical studies had "established a direct link between diesel emissions and respiratory ailments" (Lueck 2000). With pressure from the city and community groups, the MTA slowly began to convert its bus fleet to hybrid electric buses and those using compressed natural gas. In 2003 the MTA reported that it had reduced bus emissions by 65 percent over the prior four years (NYC Council 2000). But its bus depots in northern Manhattan still housed buses burning predominantly diesel fuel.

In 2003, in an effort to minimize diesel pollution in Lower Manhattan, the city council passed legislation regulating construction vehicle fuel in Lower Manhattan. The legislation mandated that construction vehicles use low-sulfur fuel that would produce significantly less pollution. Construction vehicles using sulfur fuel can emit sulfur levels up to an unacceptable 3,400 parts per million. The city law called for fuel that would reduce sulfur emissions to 15 parts per million. The Port Authority, a major developer in Lower Manhattan, agreed to comply with the law (Lombardi 2003). In 2005 the city council passed and the mayor signed legislation mandating that the city purchase cleaner cars as it replaced its own vehicle fleet. The legislation forced the city to "buy only cars or vans that are the least polluting models available" (DePalma 2005b). Yet the city was still criticized by those arguing that it had missed an opportunity to switch to vehicles fueled by natural gas (DePalma 2005a).

The city council also passed several pieces of legislation attempting to reduce pollution from the city's taxi fleet, in addition to school buses, construction vehicles, and the city's own vehicle fleet. In 2003 the council passed and the mayor signed legislation mandating that the Taxi and Limousine Commission (TLC) achieve a taxi fleet with 9 percent of all new taxis using natural gas or electricity (*Gotham Gazette* 2010b). In 2006 legislation was passed and signed mandating that the TLC develop a plan to increase the number of clean-air taxis (*Gotham Gazette* 2010c). This was supported by legislation that lengthened the replacement cycle for clean-air taxis (*Gotham Gazette* 2010d). When litigation derailed the mayor's original plan to convert the taxi fleet, his administration produced a set of incentives that has "led to a significant increase in the number of hybrid taxis" (Kassel 2009).

Several of the city's efforts to increase air quality came out of Mayor Bloomberg's PlaNYC, announced in 2007. The plan involved more than one hundred proposals, all of which were designed to make New York a more environmentally friendly city. Several of the proposals were designed to have an impact on air quality. The most controversial of these plans was a congestion pricing proposal for the city's central business district. According to the mayor's plan, cars or trucks entering or leaving Manhattan south of 86th Street between 6 a.m. and 6 p.m. would pay a fee of $8 or $21 respectively, using an E-Z pass type technology (Kassel 2008a). The mayor argued that the plan would reduce central business district driving by almost 7 percent, reduce asthma, and raise more than $400 million for transit improvements (Kassel 2008a). But critics argued that the mayor's congestion pricing plan would increase driving precisely in those areas of the city, outside the central business district, where asthma rates are the highest (Hakim 2007). Needing state approval, the congestion pricing plan failed when it was rejected by state legislative leaders.

Another element of PlaNYC was the goal to plant one million new trees in New York City in ten years. Research conducted in the city had demonstrated that the presence of street trees was "associated with a lower prevalence of early childhood asthma" (Lovasi et al. 2008). As part of the program, in its first year the city planted more than 174,000 trees. In 2009 the city received a $2 million grant from the U. S. Department of Agriculture to create jobs in horticulture and forestry for graduates of the Million Trees NYC training program (NYC Office of the Mayor 2009a). The program was also supported by the New York Restoration Project, a group long involved in the city community garden movement.

Building Emissions

Unlike most cities, a major source of air pollution in New York is its buildings. For decades more than ten thousand buildings burned heating oil that emitted large amounts of sulfur dioxide as well as particulate matter (soot) (NYC Office of the Mayor 2013). The mayor's office estimates that for the years 2005–7, high levels of particulate matter in the city contributed to more than "3,100 deaths, over 2,000 hospitalizations for cardiovascular and respiratory disease, and 6000 emergency department visits for asthma annually" (NYC Office of the Mayor 2013). In 2011, as part of Mayor Bloomberg's PlaNYC, the city issued regulations that would ultimately phase out the use of the two most highly polluting forms of heating oil. Beginning in 2011, no new building boilers were allowed to use No. 6 or No. 4 heating oil. And all buildings were mandated to phase out No. 6 oil by the end of 2015 (New York City PlaNYC 2014). In conjunction with these regulations, the city initiated the Clean Heat Program. The program assists buildings converting to cleaner heating oil. Coordinated through

PlaNYC, the city serves as a clearinghouse for information on how buildings can finance and install cleaner oil systems, making building owners aware of incentives and technical assistance (NYC Clean Heat 2013). The incentives are provided by oil providers and energy service companies, not the city.

In September 2013 Mayor Bloomberg announced that the city had achieved the lowest levels of air pollution in fifty years, with sulfur dioxide decreasing by 69 percent since 2008 and soot pollution declining by 23 percent since 2007. Much of the decline was attributed to the more than twenty-five hundred buildings that had converted to cleaner heating oil since 2011. The Mayor also noted that another twenty-five hundred buildings were in the process of conversion (NYC Office of the Mayor 2013).

Solid Waste Management

Another way in which the city attempted to reduce air pollution, especially in some of its high-asthma areas, was a revamping of its solid waste management policy. In 2006 much of the city's solid waste sat in waste transfer stations until it could be trucked out of the city. Diesel-powered trucks would line up at these stations, with motors idling, waiting to dump their loads. Then other trucks would line up at the same stations to load the waste in order to move it out of the city. The stations were not only a source of air pollution from the trucks, but they were also a potential source of rodent and roach infestation for the entire community. Most of these stations were in the South Bronx or part of Brooklyn where asthma rates were high. In 2005 Mayor Bloomberg proposed a plan where each borough would be responsible for dealing with its own waste. In addition, to reduce truck traffic in the city and the high number of waste transfer stations in minority and low-income neighborhoods, waste transfer stations would be located along the waterfront to facilitate barges moving the waste out of the city, rather than trucks. Under the Bloomberg plan, approved by the city council in 2006, one of Manhattan's marine waste transfer stations would be located along the East River in the 90s, adjacent to some affluent white neighborhoods. At a city council hearing, when councilpersons representing the Upper East Side criticized the plan for locating a marine waste transfer station adjacent to their neighborhoods, Councilperson Charles Barron from Bedford-Stuyvesant in Brooklyn responded. "I find it interesting how now people are concerned about waste transfer stations in densely populated areas . . . Where have you been for all these years when we had 19 in Brooklyn, 15 in the Bronx and none in Manhattan? Where were all you people of conscience? . . . We've been concerned about environmental racism for decades. You have to share the burden. I don't want any child to get asthma . . . It is disingenuous now when you raise the issues because it is coming to your neighborhood but as long as it was in our communities, it was alright" (NYC Council 2006). Upper East Side groups went to court to stop the waste transfer station in their neighborhood. Recently, some of the solid waste problem has been solved through the increased use of rail and barge transport of waste out of the city, but lower-income, minority-populated communities are still the most affected.

It is difficult to assess the impact of all the regulatory efforts by the city and other levels of government in reducing air pollution and subsequently reducing asthma hospitalizations. While these regulatory efforts were probably responsible for reducing some pollution, there were other nonregulated sources of pollution in many of the high-asthma neighborhoods. For instance, many of these neighborhoods were situated near major highways, and little or nothing was done at the local level to alleviate this situation. Federal air quality regulations are at the backbone of air pollution controls and are, in large part, responsible for the improvement in New York City air quality since the 1970s.

Addressing Indoor Pollution

With little or no policy template from which to work, city efforts at attacking indoor pollution were limited. The city's housing code mandates that owners and landlords address a variety of deterioration issues that could possibly be linked to asthma, including water leaks that produce mold and ventilation issues. But the alleviation of these problems was always subject to the quality of housing code enforcement. DOHMH "published specific guidelines for how landlords could safely remediate mold problems . . . but the guidelines are not binding and therefore have not been strongly enforced by the housing courts" or the Department of Housing Preservation and Development (Das 2007). In a few cases, tenants who were being assisted by local community organizations were able to use the organization's legal services in forcing landlords to make needed repairs.

In 2010 the city council developed legislation to address indoor pollution in some of the city's most poorly maintained buildings. The legislation would force landlords to "take steps to eliminate garbage, mold, and vermin—all factors that have been linked to asthma" (Hernandez 2010). The legislation focuses on several hundred privately owned buildings "with the most violations involving garbage, insects, mold, mice and rats. Landlords would be given three months to make changes; if they failed to comply, the city would execute the work itself and charge them for it" (Hernandez 2010). In early 2011 Mayor Bloomberg signed the legislation amending the Department of Housing Preservation and Development's Alternative Enforcement Program to include those housing code violations related to indoor pollution asthma triggers (NYC Office of the Mayor 2011).

Managing Asthma: The Asthma Initiative

In order to reduce asthma hospitalizations, the key component of the city's asthma policy was to give families the information and resources to manage their child's condition to the point where hospitalization was unnecessary. This probably did more to reduce asthma hospitalizations than any other program. It required the education of families, health care providers, and school personnel, as well as the provision of medical services to families and others to allow more effective management of childhood asthma. City public health authorities conducted education, outreach, and referral to provide families or the community organizations dealing with childhood asthma with knowledge and access to the services.

For physicians and health professionals in communities where the incidence of asthma was high, the challenge was not only educating parents on how to recognize and treat the illness but also delivering care to populations and communities that lacked resources. Many of the neighborhoods reporting the highest asthma rates had the fewest health and medical resources. Low-income individuals receive substandard health care, and many were often unaware of what condition they had or the availability of inexpensive medications. As a result, asthma was often undiagnosed until an individual suffering from a severe attack went to the emergency room.

In the early 1990s, hospitals in high-incidence areas established clinics to address the increasing number of asthma cases (Sheridan 1998). Research suggested that the disease could be controlled if resources were available. High hospitalization rates in low-income communities were evidence of the failure to manage the illness on an outpatient basis (Lobach 1996). In more affluent areas of the city, where asthma rates had also increased, hospitalization rates from the illness remained low (Noble 1999).

The city did not implement a citywide policy to combat asthma until 1998. In the early 1990s, the New York City Board of Education diagnosed and treated children with asthma but was ill-equipped to respond effectively. Children with asthma have more school absences than other children, which inhibits successful school performance (Strouse 2001). Without proper training or medical devices, schools were forced to call 911 when asthma attacks became serious (Calderone et al. 1998c). It was not until September 1998 that the Department of Health, with the cooperation of the Board of Education, added questions on student medical forms asking about asthma so the schools and the Health Department could track the illness (Sugarman 1998). Treatment posed a challenge for a city school system in need of more resources. Before the fiscal crisis of the 1970s, there was a nurse in every public school in the city. By the early 1990s, there was approximately 1 nurse for every 7,000 students, and 139 nurses for 1,069 schools (Richardson 1993). Some schools in low-income areas of the city were able to maintain clinics with the help of federal, state, and private moneys. In the early 1990s the state expanded the number of school-based clinics and made services delivered at the school clinics Medicaid reimbursable. As New York State

Medicaid recipients were shifted to managed care plans in the late 1990s, the state began phasing out Medicaid reimbursement for visits to school clinics. Moreover, many of the students visiting the clinic did not qualify for Medicaid or the State Child Health Plus Program and remained uninsured (Holloway 1999).

In a few cases, with the help of local hospitals and nonprofit organizations some schools were able to address the asthma problem by holding classes to educate children with asthma and their parents on how to live with and treat the illness (Bonforte and McLeod 1995; Belluck 1996). In the mid-1990s, the Board of Education, in cooperation with the American Lung Association, implemented the Open Airways for Schools program. The program trains both school health professionals and children with asthma. The curriculum for children includes six forty-minute sessions that provides them with "information that will help them control their own asthma more effectively" together with handouts to take home to their parents (NYC DOHMH 2010a). By 2004, more than thirty thousand children and approximately fourteen hundred school health professionals had participated in the program. In 1998 an American Lung Association evaluation concluded that those children who participated in the program had two fewer absences from school than those who did not (NYC DOHMH 2010a).

In 1998 the city adopted a comprehensive approach to treat asthma in the city's high-incidence areas. Mayor Giuliani and the Department of Health implemented a multifaceted program, the Asthma Initiative. The primary goal of the program was to reduce asthma morbidity, especially in low-income minority areas of the city. Additional goals were also to reduce asthma hospitalizations, emergency department visits, and school absences (Cohen 1998; NYC DOHMH 2003). This would be achieved by educating families, school officials, health care providers, and community groups about how asthma could be managed, as well as providing these individuals and groups with information on resources and best practices.

One of the principal strategies of the initiative was to foster partnerships with community groups, health providers, and schools, many of which were already dealing with childhood asthma (NYC Childhood Asthma Initiative 2001a). The initial focus of the program was on three communities with extremely high asthma hospitalization rates: Hunts Point (Bronx), Williamsburg (Brooklyn), and East Harlem (Manhattan). The goal was to create partnerships with community groups that would serve as intermediaries between the DOH and the affected neighborhoods. They would provide the education and information to allow families to manage their children's asthma and would assist families in gaining access to services. These communities received additional resources (including community health outreach workers), support, and training for health care providers. These communities also received additional education on medical services, case management services, smoking cessation programs, and making a home asthma proof (Cohen 1998). The program was slowly expanded to other communities. At a press conference in 2000, an official from the Jamaica, Queens Center for Children and Families explained that her agency had been educating families about indoor pollutant triggers that cause or aggravate asthma, particularly secondhand smoke (NYC Office of the Mayor 2000).

The city initiated a public education campaign to promote awareness about the illness, assist children and their caregivers in managing the illness, and assist families in reducing exposure to substances that may cause asthma (NYC Office of the Mayor 1998a). At the mayoral press conference where the Asthma Initiative was formally announced, a citywide poster campaign was unveiled with posters of children stating, "I have asthma but asthma doesn't have me" (NYC Office of the Mayor 1998b).

The Department of Health established a hotline about how and where to get help for asthma (NYC Office of the Mayor 1998b). Callers to Asthma Action Line learned how to reduce exposure that could cause an attack (Calderone 1998c). The Department of Health devoted considerable funding to community outreach, distributing posters and placing ads on billboards and subways on the availability of services (NYC Childhood Asthma Initiative 2002). Since the implementation of the initiative, NYC DOHMH has published educational materials on its website, including guides for parents on how to manage their child's asthma or get schools to administer asthma medication and fact sheets for parents, physicians, and school personnel on popular asthma medications explaining what the medications are for, how they are taken, and potential side effects (NYC DOHMH 2010d).

Rabin (2010) assessed the impact of the Asthma Initiative and found that "aggressive management" of asthma "by a primary care provider can produce better outcomes while reducing costs." The two hundred African American and Hispanic children followed in the study had significant reductions in asthma severity and emergency department utilization and a (near statistically) significant reduction in hospitalization due to asthma. The average annual cost savings due to the program totaled $4,525 per patient (Grant et al. 2010). There were concerns about the city's ability to respond to the epidemic. In 1999, as the city's Medicaid population was being moved to managed care providers, the program compiled a directory of asthma services for the new health care providers (NYC Office of the Mayor 1999). But there were complaints that managed care providers were not educating patients about triggers or management, referrals to specialists, or providing spacers and peak flow meters to asthmatic children (NYC Council 1998). Some physicians in the affected communities argued that the major problem was that children did not have access to primary care physicians (Bowen 2001).

In a further attempt to use mediating structures at the community level to implement the city's asthma programs more effectively, the DOHMH established the Asthma Partnership approximately a year after the announcement of the Asthma Initiative. Although convened and funded by the city, the Asthma Partnership is an independent entity whose members include community organizations and individuals from across the city interested in furthering the city's fight against childhood asthma. Initially the partnership was designed to foster greater community involvement in the effort to combat childhood asthma. Over time, the partnership has come to play an advisory role for the DOHMH as well, giving city officials feedback and advice about asthma programs. For instance, the partnership was instrumental in getting the city to streamline the school health forms needed to get a child's asthma treated at school (reducing the three forms needed to one), to establish automated student health records, and to expand the city's asthma programming to day care centers (Davis 2010).

The Asthma Initiative also attempts to engage community health professionals. Through its Asthma Training Institute, the program funded education for local physicians on current treatment methods. The institute also offers training for nurses, social workers, community educators, and homeless shelter workers (NYC DOHMH 2010b). One of the cornerstones of the city's health care provider education efforts is the Creating a Medical Home for Asthma (CMHA) Program. Funded by a federal grant from the National Heart, Lung and Blood Institute, this asthma management program was developed in the 1990s by a team of health care practitioners and public health officials, including officials from the NYC Department of Health and the NYC Health and Hospitals Corporation. The program was designed to train health care providers to increase the quality and continuity of asthma care at health clinics in New York City to reduce asthma hospitalizations (NYC DOHMH 2010c).

To assist the schools, the Department of Health and the Board of Education cooperated on a program, Managing Asthma in Schools, to train public school teachers to recognize asthma's symptoms to "help students avoid attacks and handle emergencies" (Calderone 1998b). With the cooperation of the Board of Education, the program included several questions on school health forms that measured the prevalence of asthma among schoolchildren (NYC Office of the Mayor 1998b). It also funded a community-based asthma resource center in Hunt's Point in the Bronx, a high-asthma-incidence area, where physicians, community health workers, schools, and parents could coordinate their efforts to prevent and treat the illness (NYC Office of the Mayor 1998a). A similar project was implemented in East Harlem in 2001 in which hospitals communicated with primary care physicians, school nurses, and community outreach workers to decrease school absences and hospitalization once asthma was diagnosed (NYC Childhood Asthma

Initiative 2001b). In some communities, the program funded home visits by health workers to assist families in managing the disease (Wakin 2001).

Some of the program's funds went for the distribution of spacers and peak flow meters, two devices used in the treatment of asthma, to those who could not afford them on a regular basis or were ineligible for Medicaid (Calderone 1998a). "A spacer allows small children to get the proper dose of medicine by holding the mist-like medication in a chamber so it can be inhaled properly . . . A peak flow meter helps forecast serious asthma attacks by measuring lung capacity" (Calderone 1998a). Asthma treatments are known and inexpensive compared to other medical interventions. Although Medicaid provided reimbursement to pharmacies for spacers, the reimbursement provided was so low that some pharmacists admitted refusing to dispense spacers to Medicaid recipients. Some physicians and hospitals reported handing out spacers supplied by drug companies for free (Calderone et al., 1998a). The program also subsidized additional staff at health clinics in those parts of the city where asthma hospitalization rates were highest (Calderone 1998a).

In areas of the city where health disparities are the most glaring, the DOHMH District Public Health Offices (DPHO) were established in 2002 to coordinate department activities at the neighborhood level (NYC DOHMH 20014). These offices implement the city's Asthma Initiative in the three city communities where they were established: East and Central Harlem, the South Bronx, and Northern and Central Brooklyn. In East Harlem, the DPHO assisted in establishing the Harlem Asthma Network and the East Harlem Asthma Center of Excellence (EHACE) involving over a dozen community-based and citywide nonprofit organizations. The primary goal of the center was to reduce the rate of asthma hospitalizations. The program includes the assessment of indoor asthma triggers, pest management, mold remediation, housing repairs, and smoking cessation programs (Hayes 2014). In order to better implement the city's asthma programs, the East Harlem DPHO also established the Asthma Counselor program. Asthma counselors teach children and families how to use medication, advise families about the prevention and cessation of indoor asthma triggers, and distribute mattress covers and roach eradication products (Hayes 2014).

In 2007, furthering the efforts of the city's attack on childhood asthma, the Bloomberg administration, in conjunction with the East Harlem DPHO, opened the East Harlem Asthma Center, a storefront that would serve as the center of community outreach and education about asthma. Although asthma hospitalization rates had fallen significantly since the start of the 1998 Asthma Initiative, East Harlem childhood asthma hospitalization rates were still the highest in the city. Together with borough president Scott Stringer, the Bloomberg administration implemented a program that would concentrate on identifying children with asthma, provide follow-up care to asthmatic children who had been seen in an emergency room or who had been hospitalized, and develop self-management plans for each asthmatic child in the community (NYC Office of the Mayor 2007). In 2009 the first walk-in center was established in East Harlem where families could get information on how to manage their children's asthma, learn about reducing exposure to asthma triggers, and receive referrals for asthma related care (NYC Office of the Mayor 2009b).

The Role of Nongovernmental Groups

Working alongside of the NYC DOHMH Asthma Initiative were nonprofit organizations with roots in specific communities and, in some cases, significant amounts of private funding. Many of these organizations were members of the city's Asthma Partnership. These organizations complimented what government agencies were attempting to achieve. In some cases they employed a level of intervention, as a public health policy tool, for which city officials lacked the funding and, in some cases, the community roots to implement. Throughout the city, NYC DOHMH sought to partner with community-based organizations to take advantage of their ability to successfully conduct outreach in their respective neighborhoods, resulting in more effective implementation of programs combating asthma.

The Harlem Children's Zone (HCZ) had been running social, health, and educational program in parts of Harlem since the 1970s, so when the asthma epidemic hit Harlem in the late 1990s, HCZ had the community credibility and institutional infrastructure to mount a major campaign. With private funding and a relatively small geographic base, HCZ implemented a level of intervention beyond what the city's Asthma Initiative was able to do. Having already established programs in area schools, HCZ built links between health care practitioners, schools, and families to create asthma management plans. Without physician and parent cooperation, medication could not be administered at school, and children having asthma attacks would be sent to emergency rooms and possibly hospitalized (Jean-Louis 2003). HCZ joined the East Harlem DPHO Asthma Network soon after it was created.

Begun in 2003, by late 2004 HCZ's asthma programs had tested more than three thousand children. It found almost one thousand had asthma and had enrolled more than three hundred in its program (Santora 2005). With many of its families, HCZ was able to intervene directly in the home not only to educate families about their child's asthma but also to identify and sometimes remove indoor asthma triggers. To a great extent, HCZ was able to conduct the outreach and enroll families because of its long-standing roots in the community. HCZ community workers taught families and children how and when to use asthma medications. With family participation, HCZ workers inspected homes and educated families on possible indoor asthma triggers and how to get rid of them. This included dust, roaches, mice, and rats, in addition to household pets, carpets and bedding, plumbing and ventilation, and smoking in the house. With outside funding, HCZ supplied families with indoor air cleaners and hepa vacuum cleaners to address problems of dust. HCZ social workers acted as go-betweens for families in dealing with building owners in addressing larger indoor asthma trigger problems. And when building owners proved to be intractable, HCZ was able to draw on free legal assistance in taking landlords to court for housing code violations (Jean-Louis 2003).

In 2005 HCZ reported that, while 35 percent of its participating children reported going to the hospital in the months prior to joining the program, only 8 percent reported going to the hospital after joining. And while 8 percent reported spending at least one night in the hospital in the months prior to joining the program, there were no reported hospitalizations among this group after joining the program. HCZ officials reported that it was costing approximately $1,700 to treat each child, but a night in the hospital cost $4,500 (Santora 2005).

HCZ was not the only nonprofit program working alongside the city. In northern Manhattan and the South Bronx, the Reducing Indoor Allergens Study Team recruited families and went into homes with carpenters, cleaners, and environmental researchers for extended periods to combat indoor asthma triggers. The team hired educators from the community to work one-on-one with family members. Family members were educated about "pest management" and laminated information sheets were left in each household to reinforce the education. They noted two significant constraints on their efforts. First, given limited resources, the team targeted its efforts in each apartment rather than throughout the dwelling. Efforts were limited to the bathroom, kitchen, child's bedroom, and hall. Second, the team noted that the overall poor quality of housing "complicated the residents' ability to sustain the environmental improvements" (Kinney et al. 2002).

The contributing role of nonprofit organizations in assisting the city in combating asthma makes it difficult to assess to what extent the city's Asthma Initiative alone was responsible for lowering asthma hospitalization rates.

Not all programs or policies work as designed, especially when diverse implementation agents are involved, as was the case with the city's Asthma Initiative. A 2001 study (Snow et al. 2005) by health practitioners in the Bronx found that an extremely small percentage of teachers were "very familiar" with the Board of Education's asthma program. In fact, from the survey of school officials the researchers concluded that the Board of Education had no "formal policies for managing students' asthma during the school day" (Snow et al. 2005, 52). At the same time, another study conducted in the Bronx in 1999–2000 found that those schools with school-based health centers (SBHC) reduced asthma hospitalizations by 15 percentage points more than those schools without health centers. Interestingly the same study found that there was no difference in the asthma hospitalization rate decline for those SBHC schools that conducted an aggressive asthma intervention program (Webber et al. 2005). This may speak to the efficacy of access to primary care as a major component in combating asthma.

Economic Development and Asthma Policy

Pollution and the production of waste are two of the negative by-products of economic development. Many types of economic development create negative impacts on the environment, but some produce more pollution and waste than others do. In densely populated urban areas, the management of pollution and waste creates financial and logistical challenges for planners and politicians. Although diesel buses move people efficiently and with less harm to the environment than if the bus passengers all drove automobiles, they still create harmful air pollution, although the move to compressed natural gas and ultralow sulfur diesel fuel buses is solving this problem. And finding a place for waste disposal close to population centers reduces transportation costs but may expose populations to the harmful effects of waste disposal.

Over time, better planning for sustainability and environmentally friendly technologies may reduce if not eliminate the environmental degradation and harmful health impacts produced by economic development. The city's recent series of regulations on school buses, its own vehicle fleet, and taxis suggest that many of these improvements may not be far off if elected officials have the political will to pursue them.

But few are suggesting that economic development be curtailed as a means to reduce pollution and its negative impacts on health. The same families whose children suffer from asthma need the jobs produced by economic development; and they are some of the first individuals to suffer if economic development declines. Just as important, economic development allows the city, with a stable tax rate, to raise revenue to pay for the programs combating childhood asthma. In the aftermath of the September 11 terrorist attacks, the city suffered a decline in revenue due to the devastation of the World Trade Center site and the consequent lost jobs and economic activity. With no immediate increase in economic development in sight, the city raised property taxes 18 percent but even this was not enough to stave off significant cuts in the city's budget. Seeking to save $5 million, the Bloomberg administration proposed cutting twelve pediatric clinics administered by the Health and Hospitals Corporation, a city agency. These clinics treat children regardless of their ability to pay. For many children, the clinics were the source of primary care and "the first line of defense in treating childhood asthma" (Phua 2003).

Race and Asthma Policy

Environmental racism is as much an artifact of urban economic development as it is racial and ethnic politics. The de facto segregation of minorities and people of low socioeconomic status into residential areas "creates and compounds social and health risks, including the likelihood of living in poor indoor and outdoor environments" (Das 2007). Mayor Bloomberg's deputy mayor Daniel Doctoroff noted that, because of the scarcity of real estate, "there will always be things that nobody wants, and we have to find places to put them" (Little 2007). Those who criticize the concept of environmental racism argue that "disparate impact . . . is not evidence of intentional discrimination in the placement of polluting facilities—it's just economics" (Little 2007).

Finding the highest asthma prevalence and hospitalization rates in communities of color made the disease controversial. Unlike lead-based paint poisoning, which was also most prevalent in minority communities, the actions that caused or triggered asthma had not been halted at the time of the increase in prevalence. Unlike lead-based paint poisoning, the causes of asthma were either unknown or so diffuse as to deflect attention away from any one causal factor. As a result minority communities and their representatives could point not only to the increased suffering of their children but also to a variety of activities, still taking place, that were in some way responsible for the condition of their children. Because some of the activities were causing or triggering asthma through the degradation of the air in those communities, accusations of environmental racism were raised, with subsequent calls for environmental justice. In New York City, the impact of asthma on minority children became the primary factor in the mobilization of the environmental justice movement (Sze 2007).

Environmental racism involves the placement of facilities that produce toxic or hazardous air or water quality in communities that are heavily populated by minorities, particularly low-income minorities who lack the political power to oppose the facility or the economic ability to move (Weisskopf 1992). Environmental racism is premised on the hypothesis that environmentally hazardous sites are not equitably distributed across the city (Bowen et al. 1995, p. 641). It is as much an issue of class as it is race or ethnicity, but in urban areas race and class are frequently linked (Weisskopf 1992). Whether the siting of hazardous facilities in low-income minority areas has been a matter of public policy or merely a function of diffuse but systemic values regarding race and class is a subject of debate among those who study the concept (Bowen et al. 1995, 658; Maher 1998, 360). The environmental justice movement has it roots in the late 1980s. The United Church of Christ Commission on Racial Justice published a report concluding that "people of color bear a disproportionate burden of environmental pollution across the United States" (Sustainable Cleveland

Partnership 2010). "In 1998, EPA issued new guidelines regarding Title VI of the 1964 Civil Rights Act. The guidelines stated that EPA could withhold federal funds from state and local agencies' projects if those projects were found to be harming minority communities" (Sustainable Cleveland Partnership 2010).

Despite the multifactorial nature of asthma, the environmental justice movement focused on those factors related to outdoor air pollution, neglecting those less controllable indoor sources. In addressing the significance of outdoor pollution and its links to asthma, the environmental justice movement cited the "precautionary principle" (Sze 2007, 94). Leaders argued that the "science of risk assessment was inadequate to deal with the cumulative exposure that their residents faced" (94). As a result, in those communities that had already been burdened by a large number of polluting facilities, "special protective precautions" were appropriate (94). In the late 1990s, when research linking asthma and indoor pollutants such as dust mites and cockroaches began to appear, the environmental justice movement responded that roaches, dust, and those factors emanating from low-quality housing had been around for decades, long before asthma increased. They worked to deflect the innuendo that minority children got asthma because their parents were bad housekeepers (Sze 2007). At the same time, however, the Harlem Children's Zone, the Reducing Indoor Allergens Study Team, and others were working with community residents to clean up their dwellings.

In dealing with outdoor air pollution in those New York City communities with high rates of asthma, the environmental justice movement, composed primarily of residents from affected neighborhoods, was at the forefront of the battle against bus depots, diesel buses, and other polluting facilities. They were joined by the city council in those efforts to decrease air pollution in the city, particularly council members from those communities of color where asthma rates are the highest. And in many of their efforts, they were also supported by the Bloomberg administration. Since the MTA, the primary target of the environmental justice movement, was a state agency, the Bloomberg administration was not constrained in its criticism of the MTA or its support of environmental justice issues.

In 2000 WE ACT, an environment group in West Harlem, filed a complaint against the MTA with the U.S. Department of Transportation. The complaint accused the MTA of discrimination, violating Title VI of the Civil Rights Act. The complaint was based on the MTA's placement of diesel bus depots. At that point, six of the eight bus depots in Manhattan were north of 96th Street in minority neighborhoods (Shipp 2000). The complaint stated that the MTA's actions "had the effect of discriminating against residents of northern Manhattan on the basis of race and exposing them to disproportionately high health risks from diesel exhaust" (Shipp 2000). Analysis conducted by WE ACT found that a disproportionately higher number of minorities and a disproportionately lower number of whites lived within a quarter mile of a bus depot, compared to a racially neutral location of depots (WE ACT 2006a).

In 2003 the MTA proposed to reopen a bus depot in East Harlem, closing one on 16th Street in southern Manhattan (Kugel 2003). With support from U.S. senators Hillary Clinton and Charles Schumer, the community organized to protest the bus depot (Gonen 2003). With the opening of the new depot, all but one of the depots in Manhattan would have been located north of 96th Street. Some of the depots have been in the same locations for almost a century, formerly serving as trolley barns. The MTA argued that it was too costly to move the depots and that it was trying to decrease the pollution the depots produce (Jones 2006).

In 2004 the U. S. Department of Transportation ruled that the MTA was not in violation of Title VI of the Civil Rights Act. It did state, however, that the MTA would have to comply with federal rules, including conducting environmental analyses prior to the reconstruction or rehabilitation of its bus depots, planning to ensure "equal, non-discriminatory distribution of service facilities," curtailing the practice of idling buses, providing greater opportunities for community participation in MTA planning, and incorporating "principles of environmental justice into their siting decisions" (WE ACT 2006b). Later in 2004, WE ACT and the Natural Resources Defense Council entered into discussions with representatives of the MTA in an attempt to settle the dispute over MTA activities in northern Manhattan. The discussions broke down in 2005 when the MTA decided that it was not going to convert one of its northern Manhattan bus depots to compressed natural gas but instead was going to use diesel hybrid-electric at that depot (WE ACT 2006b). In 2009, more than a decade after WE ACT began its campaign to make the MTA more environmentally accountable, the MTA agreed to rebuild one of its bus depots according to green principles and with input from WE ACT and the community (WE ACT 2009).

Another one of the major political skirmishes where there were charges of environmental racism took place in the South Bronx where a coalition of community groups joined with regional as well as national environmental groups. They campaigned to close a medical waste incinerator that was constructed in the early 1990s. When it was built in the early 1990s, the incinerator was equipped with the most up to date pollution scrubbing equipment. The incinerator served not only its host, Bronx Lebanon Hospital, but also several other hospitals that had been disposing of their medical waste using "outmoded and much dirtier incinerators" (Dao 1997). Community and environmental groups formed the South Bronx Clean Air Coalition but had been unable to stop the incinerator from opening in 1992 (Frankel 1992). In 1997 the private company running the incinerator closed under threat of litigation by New York State governor George Pataki and the attorney general Dennis Vacco (Feinberg 2001). The incinerator had "routinely violated state pollution standards" in its six years of existence. Some of the violations involved the release of carbon monoxide, a pollutant that had been linked to respiratory problems, in excess of permitted levels (Dao 1997).

In 2000 Brooklyn congresswoman Nydia Velazquez, citing the large number of waste transfer stations in the Greenpoint, Williamsburg, and Red Hook sections of Brooklyn, proposed federal legislation, the Community Environmental Equity Act. The legislation, which never passed, would have required state and local governments to perform impact assessments before siting residential or industrial waste facilities in communities. The legislation would have also imposed a fair-share concept on local governments, "limiting how many facilities can be placed in any one community" (Liff 2000).

The City Charter includes a fair-share siting concept, which has been applied more to social services, such as homeless shelters and drug rehabilitation centers, than to facilities that produce environmental harm. The Charter mandates that the city create guidelines for the siting of public facilities. The guidelines produced by the city council required that if a community had more than its fare share of a certain facility, then any new facility must meet certain criteria. These criteria included that the new project respond to a critical need, that it would last for two years or less, or that the community is the only feasible alternative for siting (Collin et al. 1995, 371). The city has been criticized for never fully enforcing or implementing the fair-share concept (NYC Department of City Planning 1995).

Because of asthma's prevalence among racial and ethnic minorities, it is critical that the NYC DOHMH develops and disseminates materials in ways that are both multilingual and culturally sensitive. This is particularly important if public policy is going to address the indoor pollutant causes and triggers of asthma, those factors that may be part of housekeeping and family life. As with many public health issues, New York City public health policy makers have to address "linguistic isolation" of those immigrant populations in order to prevent the adoption of unhealthy behaviors and risk factors (Bernstein 2004). Just as important, "children in immigrant homes are less likely than those in native families to have health insurance" (Bernstein 2004).

DOHMH has attempted to address the diversity of the childhood asthma population in two ways. First, and most importantly, they have worked through community organizations, those groups with connections in high-asthma-impact neighborhoods. These groups, such as the Harlem Children's Zone, employ community residents as points of contact with families. As a result, they can engage in outreach more successfully and can provide feedback to asthma policy officials on what is successful. In a related manner, DOHMH has attempted to work through the schools, which also have roots in the community. Second, DOHMH has translated all its materials into Spanish.

The Federal and State Governments and Asthma Policy

The federal government has had a significant impact on asthma in New York City primarily through its air quality regulations. Under the Clean Air Act, the EPA sets air quality standards for various pollutants, including ground-level ozone, carbon monoxide, sulfur oxides, and nitrogen oxides. Standards are set according to EPA's understanding of the impact of these pollutants on human health. The standards become federal mandates that states are supposed to meet. The Clean Air Act gives the states considerable flexibility in achieving the federal standards. States that fail to meet EPA standards are required to submit a plan to EPA, accompanied by a timetable. There are sanctions for not adhering to these regulations (Kassel 2008b). Owing to federal ambient air quality standards, and state and city efforts to meet these standards, air quality in New York City has improved significantly, although the levels of fine particulate matter and ozone in the city do not yet meet federal standards (NYC DOHMH 2009).

New York City's and New York State's efforts at cutting diesel pollution to meet federal standards has been assisted to a great extent by federal policy. Because of a 1998 consent decree between EPA and the truck and automotive engine industry, new diesel engines in 2002 emitted 40 percent less pollution (Kassel 2008b). And the EPA has issued new regulations mandating cleaner fuels and engines in diesel trucks and buses (*New York Times* 2006). The additional diesel engine standards, which must be met by 2007, were supposed to reduce diesel fuel emissions by 90 percent (DePalma 2005a). New York State's program of converting the MTA fleet has also been successful. One report suggested that between 1995 and 2008 the MTA fleet has experienced a 97 percent reduction in "particulate soot pollution" (Kassel 2008b). With all of the reduction in diesel pollution, in 2008 the state Department of Environmental Conservation "predicted that the downstate region of New York State (including all of the city, plus Long Island and the lower Hudson Valley) soon will meet the federal annual standard for soot (a.k.a. fine particulate matter) for the first time ever" (Kassel 2008b). As of fall 2009, however, the city still failed to meet the federal standard for ground-level ozone, otherwise known as smog, or particulate matter (soot) (Kassel 2009).

Despite the impact of federal air quality regulations and activities, federal laws at times have been subject to lax enforcement as well as regulatory standards rollback. During the George W. Bush administration, many air quality pollution standards were modified (Braiker 2003). In some cases states were allowed to delay implementing policies to achieve emission standards (Leonnig 2005). In 2005 EPA issued a ruling allowing states to delay "stricter smog controls," effectively reducing air quality in many urban areas, including New York City (Leonnig 2005). Although the Obama administration backed off strengthening ozone regulations in 2011, in 2012 the EPA announced new regulations for fine particle soot, a recognized trigger of asthma aggravation. The new regulations would reduce fine particle emissions from 15 to 12 micrograms per cubic foot, a move that was supported by public health officials and the American Lung Association (Kaufman 2012).

Another element of federal involvement in treating asthma is through the establishment of treatment protocols. The National Institutes of Health (NIH) together with the National Asthma Education and Prevention Program have established protocols for those with asthma to aid in the home-based management of asthma. These protocols include advice on identifying symptoms of the disease, when to seek medical intervention, how to recognize asthma aggravation triggers, and using medication correctly (NYC Council 1998).

The other major way in which the federal government participates in the city's asthma policy is through funding. The primary mechanism of federal funding is Medicaid, the federal health insurance program for many low-income families and children. In addition, since the late 1990s, the federal government has funded the State Child Health Insurance Program (SCHIP) for children whose families fall slightly above Medicaid eligibility criteria. Both Medicaid and SCHIP are matching programs so the state must match federal funds. For New York the federal-state matching ratio is approximately 50–50, while for SCHIP the federal contribution is 65 percent. In the case of Medicaid, counties in New York State, including New York City's five boroughs must pay for approximately half the state's matching share. This places quite a fiscal burden on the city.

As previously noted, for those who were Medicaid or SCHIP eligible, Medicaid and SCHIP paid for primary care for children with asthma, spacers, peak flow meters, and other medication, as well as emergency room visits and hospitalization. Health officials certainly hoped that those children with access to primary care, through Medicaid or SCHIP, would not need emergency room care or hospitalization. Low-income children in New York State enrolled in Medicaid or SCHIP are one and a half times more likely to see a physician more regularly than children who are uninsured (Marks 2003).

Another response by the federal government to the increase in asthma rates among children was to allocate greater funding to research. Two schools in New York City, Columbia University's School of Public Health and Mt. Sinai School of Medicine received grants from the federal government in 1998 (Kiely 1998). Because of the lack of knowledge about asthma, much of the federally funded research focused on the causes of the illness more than the cure.

The federal government operates several small categorical grant programs, administered by a variety of federal agencies including the Department of Transportation (DOT), Housing and Urban Development (HUD), EPA, and the

CDC in the Department of Health and Human Services (HHS). These programs, however, account for a small amount of federal funding, especially when compared to Medicaid and SCHIP funds. In 2000 the U. S. Department of Housing and Urban Development implemented the Healthy Homes Initiative. The program provided grants for the renovation of "dilapidated homes with damp or musty conditions that promote asthma" (Hsu 2000). New York City was one of five cities to receive funding from the federal government under this grant (Hsu 2000). In 2003 the East Harlem Working Group, administered out of Mt. Sinai Hospital's School of Medicine was receiving funding from both EPA and HUD (Ellin 2003). EPA also funded air pollution monitoring surveys in several low-income neighborhoods (Fernandez 2006).

Through a Congestion Mitigation and Air Quality grant, the U.S. Department of Transportation funds the Asthma Free School Zone project. This nonprofit organization, formed in 2003, has worked to reduce engine idling near schools, increase clean fuel technologies on school buses, and eliminate coal-burning heating systems. It has also participated in community education programs as well as measured air quality near schools in all five boroughs (Asthma Free School Zones 2010; Das 2007).

Some federal funds are funneled to the city through the state. The CDC gives funds to New York State that are used to support asthma programming in the city (Heigel 2010). The federal Preventive Health and Health Services Block Grant gives states discretionary funds to use for a wide range of health-related activities including emerging health threats as well as monitoring and education activities in the area of preventive health (Catalog of Federal Domestic Assistance 2010).

The federal courts also became involved in the asthma issue in 2000 when the Legal Aid Society sued the city and state for "failing to screen, diagnose and treat children with asthma in the city's shelter system," as federal Medicaid law required (Sengupta 2000). The Legal Aid Society accused the city of placing children with asthma in apartments or city shelters with many of the conditions that aggravated their conditions. Homeless children in the city were already known to suffer extremely high rates of asthma (Sengupta 2000). A study (McLean et al. 2004) conducted in the late 1990s but not published until 2004 concluded that approximately 40 percent of children entering the shelter system had asthma, six times the national rate. In the study's sample, 26.9 percent entered the shelter system with a physicians' diagnosis of asthma, and another 12.9 percent reported symptoms "consistent with moderate to severe asthma" (244).

The suit alleged that approximately 90 percent of homeless children in the city were not being adequately treated for their conditions. The suit was a cause of some tension between the city and the state as each argued that the other level was responsible for the implementation of this aspect of Medicaid. They also argued that since Medicaid legislation did not refer to asthma or the homeless, they were not responsible for treating children in homeless shelters. The suit was settled in 2003 when a federal judge ruled that homeless children are entitled to health care under Medicaid. The city agreed not only to make asthma treatment available to homeless children but also to disseminate information inside shelters so that homeless families would be aware of the services available to them. In addition, as the city had done in the public schools earlier, the city agreed to train the staff of homeless shelters to "recognize and treat asthma" (Pear 2003). During the three years in which the case was being decided, the population of children in New York City's homeless shelters increased by almost 90 percent (Pear 2003).

The state has also had a significant role in the city's fight against childhood asthma. Similar to the federal government, a primary contribution of the state to the city is its funding and administration of the Medicaid and SCHIP programs. The New York State Department of Health administers Medicaid through its county offices. In New York City, the program is administered through the Human Resources Administration, not the Department of Health and Mental Hygiene. Medicaid and SCHIP not only provide low-income New Yorkers with health insurance but are also a major source of funding support for city hospitals and clinics in less affluent parts of the city where health care providers and institutions receive much of their reimbursement from these programs.

The state is responsible for achieving the National Ambient Air Quality Standards under the federal Clean Air Act. In accordance with this mandate, the State Department of Environmental Conservation (NYS DEC), along with other state agencies, enforces emission limits on motor vehicles, as well as encourages car pooling and the use of public transportation. NYS DEC also monitors air quality across the state, including the city. "NYS DEC monitors provide continuous data on hourly and daily fluctuations in air quality, that are related to changes in weather, meteorological conditions and emissions" (NYC DOHMH 2009, 11). As part of the implementation of PlaNYC, city officials concluded that the state's pollution monitoring, conducted with a few fixed monitors mostly on rooftops, was not designed to measure neighborhood air quality variations. As a result, in 2007 the city carried out its first Community Air Survey using portable air monitors mounted on lights poles near the street level (NYC DOHMH 2009).

In 2006 the state began funding regional asthma coalitions across the state. The purpose of the coalitions was to combat childhood asthma through the development of evidenced-based strategies that could be implemented at the community level. The overall goal was to improve the delivery of asthma care in those communities that had been overburdened by the disease so as to decrease asthma mortality, hospitalization, emergency room visits, and school absences (NYS

DOH 2005). Eleven coalitions statewide were awarded funding after a competitive application process. Three coalitions, in the South Bronx, Northern Brooklyn, and Northern Manhattan, were funded by the program. Funding included state funds plus federal funds being passed through the state (Heigel 2010). State officials also participate in the city's Asthma Partnership. In one example, state funds paid for a van that traveled through parts of the Bronx, screening children for asthma and other diseases (Davis 2010).

As noted previously, State Attorney General Spitzer was involved with the city, in getting school bus companies to comply with state and city laws on bus idling (DePalma 2004). Ultimately it was Spitzer who was successful in getting the companies to stop. In late 1999, State Attorney General Vacco sued power-generating companies in the Ohio Valley, arguing that coal-fired power plants were contributing to increasing asthma rates in New York City (Edwards 1999).

Asthma Policy Success Story

Since medical research has not yet produced a cure for asthma, the goal of public health policy has been to reduce the number and severity of asthma attacks. Public health policy has apparently succeeded in doing so. Compared to the mid-1990s, childhood asthma hospitalizations have declined significantly; so too, have emergency department visits, school absences, and deaths due to asthma. Despite these gains, asthma remains the leading cause of childhood hospitalization in the city. Moreover, the declining rate of hospitalization and emergency room visits says nothing about the prevalence of the illness but only how it is being treated or managed.

Asthma is a multifactorial disease with multiple causes and multiple known triggers. In response to this, public health policy to combat asthma developed a multifactorial strategy. Yet it is difficult, if not impossible, to assess which of the asthma policies or programs have been the most instrumental in reducing the severity of attacks. In dealing with the possible environmental causes and triggers of asthma, policies have focused on both the indoor and the outdoor environment. Those regulatory efforts targeted at the outdoor environment can be further disaggregated into those promulgated at the national and state levels and those targeted by the city and state at high-asthma communities, recognizing the overlap among the two sets of policies.

Beyond the comprehensive environmental regulatory effort in which all three levels of government were involved, the city and a myriad of community organizations attacked childhood asthma at the neighborhood level. The city and these organizations conducted education and outreach, training parents, school personnel, and providers in managing childhood asthma. They focused on the reduction of asthma triggers inside the home and at the most local of levels, the neighborhood. And they facilitated access to primary care in order to give children the health care that would keep them out of the emergency room and the hospital. In this effort, they received assistance from the state and federal levels through Medicaid as well as the state's implementation of its Child Health Insurance Program in the mid-1990s and the federal SCHIP program in the late-1990s.

The problem of childhood asthma demonstrates the need for multiple tools to solve complex public health problems.

CHAPTER FOUR

LIVING WITH HIV/AIDS

As a public health issue, AIDS appeared suddenly and with little warning. At its outset, it appeared to be spreading rapidly. Public health authorities had no prior information or data about the etiology or emergence of the disease, which added to the initial public fears. Also, unlike other recent public health threats, the AIDS death rate was high.

Much has been written about HIV/AIDS in New York City, particularly its early years (Chambre 2006; Joseph 1992; Perrow and Guillen 1990; Shilts 1987). While this chapter summarizes the tools employed early in the fight against HIV/AIDS, it does not provide another history of this period. The focus instead is on the more recent period where AIDS does not constitute an automatic death sentence and where people are capable of living long lives with a chronic debilitating condition. Public health authorities today face different challenges from those faced in the 1980s. There still is no cure for the disease, but public health education has slowed its spread, and the development of drugs has allowed those with AIDS to live a longer life. In addition, in 2010–11, there were several potential pharmacological breakthroughs in the fight against HIV/AIDS. One clinical trial demonstrated that gay men taking a combination of drugs daily in one pill could significantly reduce their chances of being infected with HIV (McNeil 2010b). Another study in 2010 showed that women using a microbicidal gel could also increase their protection against contracting HIV (McNeil 2010a). Finally, in 2011, a study concluded that "people infected with the virus that causes AIDS are far less likely to infect their sexual partners if they are put on treatment immediately instead of waiting until their immune systems begin to deteriorate (McNeil 2011a).

The history of HIV/AIDS suggests that, compared to other public health crises, it created much more of a challenge to the public health establishment. This was due not only to the incidence and virulence of the disease itself but also to the various ways in which the disease was contracted and the connection of the disease to lifestyles that were out of the mainstream. Two different but both marginalized populations fell victim to AIDS. Gay males in the 1980s were as much a minority group as intravenous drug users. And although these communities' responses to the AIDS crisis were quite different, they represented minority groups' responses to government action or inaction, in many cases fostered by discrimination. Most importantly, unlike childhood asthma or lead-based paint poisoning, AIDS was self-inflicted due to the at-risk behavior of the individual. In some ways, this should have made it easier to eradicate. But the behaviors that resulted in AIDS were so ingrained in their respective populations that public health officials could only hope to moderate the behavior to lower the risk. In part, if not entirely, the at-risk behaviors that led to AIDS, unprotected anal or vaginal intercourse and intravenous drug use, defined the marginalized groups in the eyes of the public. This made persons with AIDS far less sympathetic and increased the challenge of the public health infrastructure to obtain the needed resources to respond (Perrow and Guillen 1990).

New York City was and continues to be one of the epicenters of the AIDS crisis. Yet the city's response to AIDS is as interesting for the public health tools not used as it is for those employed to combat the disease. While opposition to the employment of public health policy tools is not unusual, in the case of HIV/AIDS some of the resistance came from those most vulnerable to the disease and those in their communities. Aside from the advent of powerful drugs, education programs became the centerpiece of public health AIDS prevention tools. Mandatory testing and contact tracing were never adopted. Needle exchanges to combat the spread of HIV among intravenous drug users were only adopted years after knowledge about how the diseases transmission was known.

Once the city's AIDS infrastructure was in place, it was forced to adjust both the implementation and the target of its attack on AIDS as the incidence of the disease slowly changed from homosexual males to minority intravenous drug users and their contacts. In addressing AIDS in the gay community, the city was assisted to a great extent by community-based volunteer organizations, some of whose efforts in fighting AIDS predate the city's involvement. As the locus of AIDS changed to minority IV drug users, their sexual partners and children, city resources were stretched as was the entire health care delivery system. And in many ways this challenge was typical in dealing with health issues among the "most vulnerable, alienated, and impoverished subgroups of the population who typically lack education, social resources, and group structures to develop self help initiatives" that existed in the gay community (Mechanic and Aiken 1989, 17).

Critics have argued that the response to AIDS on all governmental levels was delayed and never enough. According to these critics, to the extent that the response was in any way effective was due to the pressure that the emerging gay community was able to place on the political system. Despite its marginalization, the gay community that organized the initial demands for a public response to HIV/AIDS was middle class and educated. Unlike IV drug users, they were not wholly without resources to launch a successful advocacy campaign.

The Etiology of HIV/AIDS

Acquired immunodeficiency syndrome (AIDS) is the final stage of the human immunodeficiency virus (HIV). HIV attacks the immune system, the part of the human body that fights infections. HIV harms the immune system by destroying white blood cells (T cells or CD4 cells), central to the body's ability to fight disease (U.S. Centers for Disease Control and Prevention [CDC] 2010a). "It can take years for a person with HIV, even without treatment" to be diagnosed with AIDS (US CDC 2010a). And "most people have few, if any, symptoms for several years after they are infected" (Gay Men's Health Crisis [GMHC] 2010). "Having AIDS means that the virus has weakened the immune system to the point at which the body has a difficult time fighting infection" (US CDC 2010a).

HIV is a fragile virus that can be killed with alcohol, bleach, or a simple detergent (Batchelor 1988). As a result, HIV can be transmitted only from an infected human to another usually through the blood, semen, or vaginal fluid. It can also be transmitted from an infected pregnant woman to her fetus before or during birth, or from a breastfeeding mother to her infant through breast milk (US CDC 2010a). HIV can also be transmitted through blood transfusions with infected blood, although today this is vary rare since all blood is now tested for HIV before its use in transfusions (US CDC 2010a).

HIV was first identified in the United States in 1981. In May 1982, the *New York Times* reported that the federal Centers for Disease Control was tracking "a serious disorder of the immune system" that was affecting male homosexuals. Of the more than three hundred people known to be afflicted with the condition, approximately half lived in New York City. At that time, the condition was labeled GRID, for gay-related immunodeficiency (Altman 1982). Two years later, there were approximately a thousand reported cases of AIDS in New York City. It was not until the mid-1980s that researchers had developed a conclusive test to identify HIV or understood how the disease was transmitted (US CDC 2010a).

In 1996 drugs became available that allowed individuals to live with the disease. Triple therapy, the combination of three antiretroviral drugs essentially transformed AIDS from a "fatal infection to one resembling a chronic disease" (Bertozzi et al. 2009, 1581). In 2008 the CDC estimated that there were more than a million people in the United States living with HIV or AIDS but that more than 200,000 of these were not aware that they had the disease (US CDC 2010a).

Incidence

Table 4.1 displays AIDS incidence statistics for New York from 1981 through 2011, the most recent year for which data are available. The definition of AIDS has evolved over the years with the federal CDC changing the definition of the

TABLE 4.1
New York City HIV/AIDS Cases, 1981–2011

Year	AIDS Cases Diagnosed	HIV Cases Diagnosed	Persons Living with AIDS	Deaths Due to AIDS
1981	162		140	591
1982	541		480	201
1983	1,097		985	592
1984	1,841		1,720	1,106
1985	2,869		2,765	1,824
1986	4,227		4,273	2,719
1987	5,221		6,151	3,342
1988	6,437		8,290	4,301
1989	6,877		9,817	5,351
1990	7,780		11,881	5,717
1991	9,096		14,514	6,469
1992	10,910		18,461	6,977
1993	12,699		23,733	7,412
1994	12,656		28,046	8,340
1995	11,360		31,096	8,308
1996	9,375		34,407	6,067
1997	7,411		38,394	3,421
1998	5,659		41,269	2,785
1999	5,385		43,863	2,790
2000	6,179		47,349	2,692
2001	5,608	5,684	85,903	2,869
2002	4,730	5,091	90,063	2,878
2003	5,331	4,570	93,141	2,843
2004	4,402	4,186	96,287	2,728
2005	4,179	4,315	98,704	2,545
2006	3,802	4,157	102,153	2,419
2007	3,582	4,208	105,271	2,327
2008	3,336	4,186	107,506	2,303
2009	3,022	3,868	109,475	2,202
2010	2,571	3,532	111,461	1,711
2011	2,208	3,404	113,319	1,690

Source: New York City Department of Health HIV Epidemiology and Field Services Program (1981 through 2011). New York City HIV/AIDS Annual Surveillance Statistics.

disease as more was learned about it and as emerging groups of disease victims displayed symptoms not previously seen. For instance, in 1992 the CDC added three diseases, "pulmonary tuberculosis, recurrent bacterial pneumonia, and invasive cancer of the cervix to the list of diseases used to classify an HIV infected person as having AIDS" (Navarro 1993b). Before this, the CDC had been criticized by health advocates because its definition of AIDS did not include "many conditions seen most often in HIV infected woman and intravenous drug users" (Navarro 1991a).

In 2001 the New York City Department of Health and Mental Hygiene (DOHMH) shifted its reporting requirements from persons living with AIDS to persons living with HIV or AIDS, which explains the significant increase from 2000 to 2001 reported on table 4.1. Diagnosed AIDS cases and deaths due to AIDS peaked in the mid-1990s. In 1996 the New York City Department of Health and Mental Hygiene (DOHMH) reported that for the first time in the twentieth century, the life expectancy of males born in the city declined by half a year, primarily due to AIDS (Firestone 1996). According to the CDC, by the mid-1990s AIDS was the leading cause of death for Americans between the ages of twenty-five and forty-four (Collins 1997).

Because of the availability of drugs, in 2011 there were more than 100,000 individuals in the city living with HIV or AIDS. In addition, according to the DOHMH, "an estimated 1 in 4 New Yorkers living with HIV do not know that they are infected" (NYC DOHMH 2005, 4). As a result, not only must the city's health care system deal with the medical needs of a growing population of persons with AIDS or HIV, but this increasing critical mass of disease carriers forces the city's public health system to maintain vigilance in combating the spread of the disease.

For AIDS diagnoses in each given year, table 4.2 displays the percentage of those diagnosed cases that were due to homosexual sexual contact or intravenous drug use, as well as the percentage of diagnoses in any given year comprised of blacks or Hispanics. In some minority communities there are males who, while not identifying themselves as gay, have stated that they do have sexual relations with other men—men who have sex with men (MSM).

The data in table 4.2 display two types of transitions. First, there have been shifts among the types of causal groups who have been diagnosed with AIDS. Early in the reporting of the disease, gay men composed a majority of diagnosed AIDS cases. Early on, though, IV drug users composed more than a third of diagnosed AIDS cases, which is frequently overlooked. Given the level of organization within the gay community relative to the IV drug user community, as well as the gay community's superior access to physicians, it is entirely possible that IV drug users with AIDS were being missed at the outset of the AIDS crisis. By 1988, however, IV drug users surpassed gay men as the predominant group of new AIDS cases, composing more than half of new cases until the mid-1990s and the most prevalent group until early in the new century. The shift in the AIDS population from gay males to IV drug users is also significant because "addicts with AIDS suffer a higher rate of acute opportunistic infections than do homosexuals and thus require more intensive medical intervention" (Drucker 1986, 168). Moreover, very few IV drug users have health insurance.

In the early 2000s, as the total number of new AIDS cases began to decline, the percentage of cases attributable to IV drug use also declined, as drug users began "changing their behavior to reduce exposure to AIDS" and older, infected addicts were dying off or quitting (Foreman 1989). But the percentage attributable

TABLE 4.2

AIDS Incidence by Selected Group by Year, 1981–2011 (% of total cases)

Year	Gay Men / Men Who Have Sex with Men	IV Drug Users	Heterosexuals	Blacks	Hispanics
1981	65.4	25.9	1.9	27.8	23.5
1982	55.5	34.9	3.0	33.5	21.1
1983	54.1	35.9	2.6	31.4	24.2
1984	55.7	34.4	2.8	32.8	22.1
1985	52.7	37.6	3.3	34.1	24.1
1986	51.7	38.4	3.5	31.6	26.2
1987	46.0	42.1	4.9	34.3	28.2
1988	40.3	47.1	5.0	36.4	29.4
1989	38.4	47.8	5.8	37.3	29.4
1990	34.2	51.2	6.4	39.7	31.2
1991	31.6	52.8	7.1	40.7	31.5
1992	29.6	53.2	8.3	41.7	32.2
1993	28.2	52.4	10.5	42.6	33.9
1994	28.5	47.5	12.0	41.2	35.1
1995	24.7	43.5	14.0	43.0	34.6
1996	22.0	39.9	16.0	46.2	35.2
1997	20.4	37.6	18.2	47.5	35.0
1998	20.5	35.0	19.4	49.3	35.1
1999	21.7	33.6	19.1	49.8	34.6
2000	21.4	29.0	18.6	50.3	32.7
2001	21.7	23.6	19.6	51.7	32.1
2002	22.7	19.7	20.7	53.0	30.1
2003	25.1	18.8	18.7	50.5	31.1
2004	27.2	19.4	19.2	51.0	31.5
2005	28.6	16.7	20.5	51.3	31.4
2006	30.7	15.3	23.4	48.1	32.5
2007	30.5	15.7	24.8	49.4	33.1
2008	32.4	13.7	22.5	51.0	32.5
2009	31.6	12.6	25.3	50.3	32.4
2010	34.4	11.6	24.3	52.3	31.3
2011	36.4	11.8	23.9	53.2	31.9

Source: New York City Department of Health. HIV Epidemiology and Field Services Program (1981 through 2011). New York City HIV/AIDS Annual Surveillance Statistics.

to homosexual relations began to increase. This increase corresponds with survey information collected by the NYC DOHMH in the late 1990s reporting an increase in unprotected sex among young gay males (Richardson 1999). In addition, in 2006 some evidence began to appear that a small group of new HIV cases was the result of straight men having sex with other men, what became known as "down-low" behavior, producing the MSM category (Fallik 2006). As displayed in table 4.2, the combined percentage of new AIDS cases attributable to IV drug users or homosexual relations composed less than half of all cases after 2000. Several new groups began to appear in greater numbers on DOHMH AIDS surveillance reports (NYC DOHMH HIV Epidemiology and Field Services Program 2009). The first of these groups were heterosexuals who represented approximately one fifth or more of new AIDS cases beginning in 2001. Although the number of newly diagnosed AIDS cases attributable to IV drug use declined, the population of IV drug users "is by and large heterosexual and in an age range in which most are sexually active" (Drucker 1986, 171). So even though AIDS was not being spread by dirty needles, it may still have been spread by sexually active IV drug users with HIV.

Also among heterosexuals, in the early 2000s the rate of teen HIV infection and women with HIV began to climb, particularly after 2004 (Boyle 2008). A third group, not appearing on table 4.2, is those new AIDS cases reported by DOHMH for which the cause of AIDS is unknown. Thus the challenge for public health policy is not only the shift in groups being reported with new cases of AIDS but the increasing number of new cases of unknown origin.

The second shift was the racial and ethnic composition of the AIDS population. In the early 1980s when AIDS was first being reported, blacks and Hispanics made up half of those reported with AIDS. The percentage of Hispanics increased slowly over time, and this group represented a little less than a third of annually reported cases in 2011 and for most of the previous decade. Blacks with AIDS, however, increased at a greater rate and composed more than half of newly diagnosed cases beginning in 2000. In 2012 DOHMH reported that although deaths to due AIDS among blacks had declined by 41 percent between 2001 and 2010, black men still composed 43 percent of newly diagnosed cases among men, and black women 64 percent of newly diagnosed cases among women (NYC DOHMH 2012).

The data in table 4.2 addressing at-risk groups and newly diagnosed AIDS cases in the city correspond to similar national percentages for at-risk groups produced by the CDC (McNeil 2011b). Despite the decline in AIDS cases in the early 2000s in the city, the CDC reported that by 2006 HIV cases were increasing in New York City at three times the national rate (Chan 2006a). With regard to race and ethnicity, the CDC estimates suggested that whites in New York were "infected at four times the national rate, Hispanics at three times the national rate, and blacks at almost twice the national rate" (Chan 2006a).

The City's Response to AIDS

Because of the complexity of the disease and its varied impacts on the public, the city's response to HIV/AIDS was multidimensional. A multidimensional public health policy toward AIDS was necessary because of the direct impact it had on various groups in the city as well as the indirect impact it had on the broader public. Table 4.3 displays the extensive array of tools used to combat AIDS. Although all agreed that the most pressing goal was to prevent the transmission

TABLE 4.3
Public Policy Tools Addressing HIV/AIDS

MONITORING AND SCREENING

New York State (and City)

Department of Health: Opens storefront clinics offering HIV testing and counseling (1986). City expanded testing availability throughout 1980s, 1990s, and 2000s; testing is at first anonymous, later confidential

New York State

Requires pretest counseling regarding the nature of the illness, information about discrimination problems that disclosure of the test could cause, and legal protections against discrimination—protocol is shortened in 2010

Screens all newborn infants (mid-1990s)

Requires reporting of HIV-positive cases to the state (2000)

Provides opt-in screening program for pregnant women (late 1990s)

Federal government

CDC: Monitors and tracks AIDS

CDC: Establishes testing protocols

CDC: Decides which groups are at risk (e.g., Haitians)

EDUCATION (PUBLIC)

New York City

Mayor's office (Koch): Meets with experts and then issues statement to quell public concern with the spread of HIV/AIDS

Department of Health: Issues public information pamphlet to address concerns about AIDS

Federal government

Surgeon General's office: Distributes AIDS brochure, "Understanding AIDS," to American households

EDUCATION (PREVENTION)

New York City

Human Resources Administration: AIDS Helpline (1985)

Department of Health, Education Unit: Issues pamphlets, brochures, public presentations, wallet-sized cards urging safe sex, condom use. Disaggregated by victim group type:

Heterosexuals/homosexuals—campaign via television, radio, newspapers on safe sex / condom use

IV drug users (presence of risk, how to reduce risk)

Outreach workers

Pamphlets

Board of Education

Sex education: AIDS prevention education (via contracted nonprofit groups) (discontinued)

HIV/AIDS Curriculum Guide (with state) (2005)

New York State

AIDS Institute: Funds prevention programs targeted at women and adolescents

HIV/AIDS Materials Initiative: Produces materials promoting prevention and service availability, including video and audio presentations, computer software

Department of Health: Produces and distributes public-service announcements pro-
moting safe sex (ran on television stations)
Department of Education HIV/AIDS Prevention Curriculum Guide (with city) (2005)
Federal government
CDC: Funds some of DOH's educational materials
CDC: Develops education and prevention programs targeted toward minority groups
Nonprofit groups (examples)
Gay Men's Health Crisis (GMHC)
Provides educational services to the gay community
Provides newsletters, brochures, informational forums, announcements in gay com-
munity publications
Telephone hotline
Contracted by the city to provide educational services to the gay community in 1985
GMHC: Targets specific minority victim groups (2006)
Peer street outreach by community groups in minority communities
Project WAVE: Raises AIDS awareness in minority communities through radio stations
Community groups: Offer AIDS prevention education to NYC high school students
outside of school and trains peer educators

EDUCATION (MEDICAL AND SOCIAL SERVICE PROFESSIONALS)
Nonprofit groups (examples)
GMHC: Provides social service and training in hospitals (under contract to the city)
Minority Task Force on AIDS
New York City
Department of Health, AIDS Education Unit
Issues pamphlets, brochures, public presentations
Conducts outreach conferences with professionals and community groups
Issues special report on dealing with children with AIDS
New York State
AIDS Institute, clearinghouse for information: Produces AIDS prevention materials
for hospitals and clinics
State HIV Clinical Education Initiative
State HIV Care Networks (funding via federal Ryan White funds): Local associations
of health care providers and community-based organizations
AIDS Advisory Council (formed by state) comprising representatives of medical insti-
tutions, state and local health departments, and nonprofit organizations
Federal government
CDC, National AIDS Clearinghouse
CDC, National AIDS Information Line: Disseminates information to medical and
social service professionals
CDC: Sponsors conferences dealing with AIDS in minority communities

REGULATIONS (DISEASE DEFINITION)
Federal government
CDC: Establishes what symptoms constitute AIDS

TABLE 4.3 (continued)

REGULATIONS (PREVENTION—CONTACT/PARTNER TRACING)

New York City

Department of Health in cooperation with physicians and community groups: Voluntary partner counseling and notification assistance

New York State

Defers responsibility of partner notification to those with HIV (1990).

Requires doctors, through new state law, to discuss with their HIV infected patients those whom they may have exposed to HIV infection. If patients offered names of partners, physicians could either notify the partners themselves or contact the city Department of Health to make contact. Patient's name would be kept confidential (2000).

Gives physicians legal permission to notify patient's partners or refer names to DOH (1989), but infected individuals were not legally obligated to give names of partners

Federal government

CDC: Makes partner notification programs a condition for the receipt of HIV Prevention Program funds, but New York's program was viewed as acceptable to the CDC

REGULATIONS (PREVENTION—CHILDREN WITH AIDS)

New York City

Board of Education: Establishes a panel of physicians and experts on AIDS to determine whether a child with AIDS should be allowed to go to school

New York State

Screens all newborn infants for HIV (mid-1990s)

Informs mothers of test results (1997)

REGULATIONS (PREVENTION—BLOOD SUPPLY)

Nonprofit groups (examples)

New York City Blood Centers: Require donors to use coded stickers to indicate whether their blood should be used or not (prior to the availability of blood test for AIDS)

Blood banks: Screen blood for AIDS/HIV

Federal government

FDA: Develops questionnaire to given to those donating blood to be used in determining whether donor blood should be used (1983)

FDA: Bans blood donations from any man who has had sexual intercourse with another man

REGULATIONS (DRUGS AND PROPOSED CURES FOR AIDS)

Federal government

Food and Drug Administration: Provides routine drug approval protocol (including fast track) and regulation

REGULATIONS (PREVENTION—NEEDLE EXCHANGE PROGRAMS)

New York State

Department of Health: Provides waivers to allow for clean needle exchanges (overrides law dealing with drug paraphernalia)

REGULATIONS (PREVENTION—GAY BATHHOUSES, BARS, AND MOVIE THEATERS)
New York State
> Issues regulations banning certain sexual behaviors from any venue that allows sexual activity to take place; state health and sanitation code amended (1986)

New York City
> Department of Health: Provides enforcement power of state regulations (some bathhouses are closed for violating regulations)

REGULATIONS (HOSPITALS)
New York State
> Issues new regulations making it easier for hospitals to shift from intensive inpatient care to more appropriate levels of outpatient care
> Adjusts Certificate of Need regulations to allow for expansion of hospital bed space

REGULATIONS (FEDERAL OVERSIGHT AND REGULATION OF STATE/CITY ACTIVITIES)
CDC: Funds HIV/AIDS prevention with requirement for HIV prevention planning
Federal judge: Places Division of AIDS Services under federal oversight (2000), as a result of Housing Works lawsuit

SERVICE PROVISION
New York City (assisted by the state)
> Department of Health
>> Changes testing centers to counseling centers over time to provide testing, case management, and coordination
>> Provides condom distribution through STD clinics and other venues
>> Provides housing (contracts with nonprofit groups)
>> Provides rent subsidies through city and state Supportive Housing Agreement (2005)
>> Field Service Unit: Contacts those who have tested positive for AIDS, linking them to appropriate care (2008)
> Human Resources Administration (later Division of AIDS Services, later still HIV/AIDS Services Administration)
>> Assists AIDS patients in dealing with city agencies offering benefits, including hospitalization, case management, housing/home care, nutrition, transportation, Medicaid eligibility, food stamps, employment and vocational assistance, counseling for clients and families, guardianships, and permanency planning
>> Provides food stamps and meal subsidies provided for indigent
> Health and Hospitals Corporation: Provides care for insured and uninsured
> Department of Homeless Services: Provides shelters dedicated to AIDS patients
> Board of Education, Department of Education: Distributes condoms in NYC High Schools (1991), with parental opt-out
Nonprofit groups (examples)
> GMHC
>> Publishes lists of physicians familiar with AIDS management
>> Offers therapy sessions for AIDS patients, partners, and families

TABLE 4.3 (continued)

Cleans apartments, does laundry, provides transportation, and serves as intermediaries with social service providers

Offers medical services center (in cooperation with NY-Cornell Hospital)

AIDS Resource Center: Provides housing

Housing Works: Provides housing

Churches in minority communities: Sponsor housing for those with AIDS

Life Force in Brooklyn: Provides services to minority women

Nursing homes: Accept AIDS patients

Clean needle exchange programs

New York State

HIV Care Networks (funded in part by federal Ryan White funding): Create local associations of health care providers, community-based organizations, and individuals with AIDS, identify persons at risk, and provide a comprehensive array of services

Drug rehabilitation services

Medicaid: Modifies program to address needs of AIDS patients (e.g., hospital reimbursement modification for AIDS Designated Care Centers)

Enrolls Medicaid patients in HIV Special Needs Plans

AIDS Institute: Funds community-based activities, including prevention programs, services for children and families, home and family-centered care, and peer-delivered education programs

AIDS Institute: Funds grants to find homes for foster children and creates pool of state funds for those AIDS patients who have no insurance or with private insurance running out

Harm Reduction Initiative: Provides services to substance abusers, their families, and communities

Federal government

Medicaid

Ryan White funding: Subsidizes the provision of emergency services to those with AIDS

Ryan White funding: Subsidizes state drug treatment as well as mental health service for substance abusers

Minority AIDS Initiative Fund

FINANCIAL ASSISTANCE

Federal government

Ryan White Comprehensive AIDS Resource Emergency Care Act (1990):

Emergency money to cities for AIDS-related services

Funding to assist persons with AIDS to maintain insurance or purchase drugs

Funding for case management services

Grants for prevention projects

Funding for AIDS Education and Training Centers to provide training for health care professionals (1996)

Funding for some gaps not addressed by Medicaid

Medicaid

CDC grants: Assist state and local governments with screening and surveillance

CDC grants: Focus on state and local government prevention efforts

CDC grants: Assist with education and training of health care professionals
CDC: Funds local prevention efforts and AIDS education demonstration programs in selected cities
Department of Health and Human Service grants: Address prevention in selected at-risk groups (e.g., women and minorities—Minority AIDS Initiative Fund)
Social Security Administration: Reduces waiting period so those with AIDS can receive Supplemental Security Income payments
Federal housing assistance
New York State
Supports funding of programs by AIDS Institute
Medicaid
New York City
Medicaid

---

of HIV/AIDS to additional individuals, this goal was complicated by a variety of factors. First, in some cases, protecting the civil rights and privacy of those with the disease took precedence over prevention (Joseph 1992). As a result, some public health tools used previously for dealing with contagious or infectious health threats were not used in the fight against AIDS. Second, nongovernmental organizations in the homosexual community were the first groups to address the presence of AIDS, not the city government. As late as the mid-1980s, in the absence of a comprehensive city, state, or federal program on AIDS, one commentator noted that "the homosexual community has shouldered the primary responsibility for crucial counseling, public information and support services" (Whitmore 1985).

The first public health problem created by HIV/AIDS was ignorance and the fear produced by that ignorance (Herman 1982). In the gay community, organizations arose almost immediately to address the needs of those members of the community with AIDS as well as the broader concerns within the entire homosexual community. In the early years, Gay Men's Health Crisis reached the gay community using "brochures, announcements in gay publications, and informational forums" (Chambre 2006, 16). In examining the response of the general public toward AIDS in the early to mid-1980s, it is difficult to distinguish where fear of AIDS ended and where bias and discriminatory behavior toward homosexuals began. The fact that gay men and intravenous (IV) drug users were the primary victims of AIDS reinforced existing stereotypes. Mayor Koch attempted to quell public fears, and the New York City Department of Health issued pamphlets answering basic questions about AIDS (NYC Office of the Mayor 1983; NYC DOH 1985). Ultimately, the city and its public health officials had to walk a fine line. On the one hand, they had to convince the public that AIDS was not transmitted through the air or by everyday contact. On the other hand, they had to convey a vigilance that AIDS was potentially everyone's problem (Fineberg 1988).

Despite pronouncements by national and city political and health officials about the limited way in which AIDS was transmitted, concerns were voiced. Parents, for example, questioned whether children with AIDS should be allowed to attend school, forcing the school system to establish a panel of physicians and experts who decided who could attend school on a case-by-case basis (Adler 1985). By the mid-1980s there were also a few reported cases of individuals who had contracted AIDS through blood transfusions (Clark 1985). Since there was no test to screen for HIV until 1985, there was some risk involved in any blood transfusion (Clark 1985). Ultimately, many blood centers, including those in New York, dealt with this issue by "requiring donors to indicate by coded stickers, which can only be read by computer, whether their blood should be transfused or not" (Eisenman 1985). Once developed, the HIV antibody test was used to screen the blood supply.

Screening blood, however, did not end the issue of blood safety. Once someone is infected with HIV, antibodies detectable in blood may not be produced for months or even longer. If an infected person donates blood during this period, HIV will not be detected at the time. As a result, the federal Food and Drug Administration (FDA) developed a questionnaire to be given to all those donating blood and in 1983 began to recommend the exclusion of some groups on the basis of answers to those questions. Among the groups designated for exclusion by the questionnaire were men who had sexual relations with other men, anyone who ever had sexual relations for money, IV drug users, "and the sexual partners of anyone in these groups" (Lambert 1990b).

As of 2011, the FDA ban on blood donation for any male who has had sex with another male remained in place. In 2010 the federal "Health and Human Services Advisory Committee on Blood Safety and Availability voted against changing the policy" (Paul 2010). The panel noted that "current research did not yet justify the lifting of the ban" (Paul 2010). Because the ban stigmatizes all gay males, advocates from the gay community have argued that the multiple tests used by blood banks to test the blood, plus the questions posed to all prospective donors, makes it virtually impossible for HIV blood to be undetected (Paul 2010).

Testing and Reporting

Early in the epidemic, AIDS was monitored as patients were hospitalized or died. A test for the virus that caused AIDS was not publicly available until 1985. In March 1985 the FDA "approved the first of five applications from pharmaceutical companies to market a blood test kit to detect" the HIV virus (Levine and Bayer 1985, 8). While initially in 1985 the test was available from only private physicians and a few hospital clinics, in 1986, in a program funded by the state, the city and state opened storefront clinics offering free HIV testing and counseling. According to a state health official, the privacy of the individuals being tested would be protected by giving each person a number. "No one knows the result but the individual and the counselor" (quoted in McQuiston 1986). Throughout the 1980s and into the 1990s, the city added new clinics where testing and counseling were offered.

Once the test became available, however, it was not immediately embraced by AIDS advocates and leadership in the gay community. Since there was no cure or treatment for AIDS at that point, knowledge of having the virus, while certainly valuable to some, was seen as little more than a death sentence to many. Opponents of testing programs argued that a positive test for HIV or AIDS was "a de facto marker for homosexuality" and would subject the individual to additional stigma and discrimination (Burr 1997). Groups emphasizing civil liberties and fearful that those with HIV would be the victims of discrimination argued that testing should be voluntary and anonymous. If the individual wants to be tested or know the outcome of a test, that is fine, but no one else should know (Burr 1997).

On the other side of the debate were those who wanted to employ the entire range of public health tools in fighting the spread of HIV/AIDS. This group noted that there were examples of routine testing for infection, often without patient consent, as well as the reporting of names to local public health authorities. They argued that with sexually transmitted diseases, there were laws or regulations requiring reporting to state departments of health and that these agencies had an excellent record of keeping this information confidential. This group, primarily from the field of public health, argued that AIDS was being made an exception by the abandonment of traditional public health practices. They argued that voluntary testing would "miss populations that disproportionately need to be reached" (Burr 1997). How could public health policy makers understand "the pattern of HIV infection" and respond appropriately unless an accurate sample of the population was tested (Joseph 1992, 131)? Voluntary testing, as well as persons at risk being discouraged from getting tested, inhibited the city's ability to gauge the size and diversity of the epidemic.

By the mid-1990s, a slight majority of all states had regulations requiring the reporting of positive HIV tests to public authorities. New York did not (Burr 1997). New York State law, positioned on the civil liberties side of the debate, required that those who voluntarily decide to be tested must "give written consent and that they receive counseling before and after the test" (Navarro 1993c). In 1985 the state and city established the Anonymous HIV Counseling and Testing (ACT) Program. The program provided "free, anonymous, HIV counseling and testing to individuals at risk for HIV infection" (NYS Department of Health [DOH] AIDS Institute 2009, 6). The city established sites where anonymous testing would take place. In addition, the state had no law requiring the reporting of HIV positive cases to the state until 2000. Up until 2000, New York

City reported AIDS cases to the state without reporting any personal identification information. State law passed in the late 1980s mandated that information on HIV testing and records remain confidential except in a few exceptional cases (Joseph 1992). Both gay advocacy groups and many public health officials opposed reporting because of not only concerns about privacy and confidentiality but also beliefs that reporting "might leave people less willing to seek voluntary HIV testing and counseling" (Bayer 1991, 89). Over time, the anonymous testing program encouraged those who tested positive to change their status from anonymous to confidential (NYS DOH AIDS Institute 2009).

In 1990 the NYC Health and Hospitals Corporation announced that it would encourage all adult patients to be tested for HIV (Lambert 1990d). The same year, the state commissioner of health, David Axelrod, initiated a public promotion campaign urging sexually active individuals or anyone who had used illicit drugs to get tested (Lambert 1990e). But in 1995 the NYC DOH announced that it would "no longer carry out free and anonymous HIV tests for patients who have private insurance or Medicaid" (Mooney 1995). In the late 1980s and 1990s, with the availability of drugs such as AZT that might prolong life, major gay organizations changed their position on testing. But while urging individuals to get tested, they still maintained the position that all testing should be voluntary (Lambert 1989e). A few advocacy groups called for HIV positive cases to be reported to the state (Richardson 1998).

In 2005 the NYC Department of Health and Mental Hygiene (DOHMH) reported that "an estimated 1 in 4 New Yorkers living with HIV do not know that they are infected" (NYC DOHMH 2005, 4). The study noted further that in 2004 more than a thousand New Yorkers did not find out that they had HIV until they were diagnosed with AIDS (NYC DOHMH 2005). In 2006 the city commissioner of health, Thomas Frieden, called for a more aggressive HIV testing protocol in New York. Frieden's recommendations were based not only on the availability of drugs that could effectively treat an HIV infection but also on reports that by 2005 the number of people dying from AIDS had not declined since 1998 (Frieden et al. 2005). Frieden termed the current approach to HIV screening "outdated," stating that the current policy fails "to identify infected patients promptly" allowing the epidemic to continue to spread (Frieden et al. 2005, 2398). He cited that in 2004 the CDC estimated "that more than half of new HIV infections are spread by HIV-positive people who are unaware that they are infected" (2399). In 2002, 1,429, of the city's new HIV cases (26%) learned that they were HIV positive on the same day they learned they had AIDS (Altman 2004).

Frieden wanted the elimination of the written consent form required by state law before an HIV test. The law had been in place since 1988. He also wanted to "do away with the requirement that physicians detail the reasons a patient may not want to be tested for HIV," part of the pretest counseling required by state law (Santora 2006a). He believed that the written consent form and the pretest counseling discouraged individuals from getting tested (*New York Times* 2006). Even though the state had reduced the amount of pretest counseling time required, according to the law before the written consent form is signed, the physician or clinician ordering the test "must provide an explanation of the nature of AIDS and HIV related illness, information about discrimination problems that disclosure of the test could cause and legal protections against such discrimination" (Perez-Pena 2006a; 2006b). Some physicians noted that the test protocol was a "barrier in emergency rooms, where doctors often feel it interferes with more immediate needs" (Hartocollis 2008). While Frieden referred to the state law as being too rigid, AIDS advocacy groups called it "patient centered" (Welsh 2006). Although "thirty-eight states do not require patients to sign separate consent forms for HIV testing," the New York State legislature, supported by AIDS advocacy and civil liberties groups, did not change the law as proposed by Commissioner Frieden and supported by the CDC (Chan 2006b).

Attempting to bend the state law as much as possible, the city increased its HIV testing at city hospitals and clinics in 2006. Commissioner Frieden noted that the city was attempting to see what it could "do within the confines of existing state law" (Perez-Pena 2006b). In 2008, still under the constraints of the state law, the city launched a campaign to get every adult in the Bronx tested. At that point, the Bronx was the borough most affected by AIDS. Under the Bronx initiative, the NYC DOH was able to get hospital administrators in the Bronx to agree to conduct HIV tests in emergency rooms "while still following state law" (Hartocollis 2008). The director of an AIDS program at a Bronx hospital stated that "she had carefully constructed a script for doctors that follows state law but squeezes what is typically a 20-minute counseling and consent process into five minutes" (Hartocollis 2008). She noted that a skilled physician could do it in three minutes. The city campaign included public-service announcements encouraging residents of the Bronx to get tested and informing them where tests were being given (Hartocollis 2008). The city also partnered with more than sixty community groups in the Bronx to help get the word out (Jaccarino 2009).

Finally in 2010 Governor David Patterson signed into law regulations that eased the HIV testing protocol. The new protocol allowed "patients to agree to HIV testing as part of a general signed consent to medical care that remains in effect until it is revoked or expires" (NYS Office of the Governor 2010). Opt-out language for HIV testing is included in the new consent protocol as opposed to the prior opt-in language (NYS DOH AIDS Institute 2012). And the new regulations also allow oral consent for a rapid HIV test. Under the new law, HIV tests must be "offered to every individual between the ages of 13 and 64 years of age receiving health services" (NYS Office of the Governor 2010).

Although testing has remained voluntary for all but a few designated groups, the city and state have done a great deal to make HIV testing a routine part of health care. In the 2000s, testing is available in every emergency room, all public clinics, and even at health fairs. And the availability of a rapid AIDS test means that individuals can get results in an hour (NYC Council 2007). In 2012 the FDA announced the availability of a home HIV test, although the initial price of the home test, forty dollars, would probably be prohibitive for many (McNeil 2012). While certainly increasing privacy, the availability of a home test could confound public health policy makers who use testing results for epidemiological purposes.

The policy on the testing of infants and informing the parents followed a different path from others. In the late 1980s, the city hospitals began to test babies for HIV without seeking the consent of the parent. But the program was anonymous, so while the state knew how many infants tested positive for HIV, it did not know whom, nor was the information reported to parents. It was not until the mid-1990s that the state implemented mandatory infant screening for HIV. Newborns were already screened for a variety of genetic disorders. For some this created a conflict between the rights of the child and the privacy rights of the mother, especially once medication became available to prolong the life of child born with the virus. Since there was no mandate that pregnant women take the test, some women would find out that they were HIV positive at the same time they found out that they transmitted the virus to their infant. And "some women refused to take the test even when reached by HIV counselors" (Navarro 1993c). In some cases women feared discrimination, or even loss of their child, if they tested positive (Navarro 1993c).

In 1994 research funded by the federal government concluded that it was possible to prevent most cases of AIDS in babies (Kolata 1994). The study strengthened the argument for mandatory testing of pregnant women. On one side of the debate were bioethicists arguing that, "if you can prevent a young child from being infected, it would seem . . . that you are under an obligation to take the necessary steps necessary to prevent that harm" (quoted in Kolata 1994). But other ethicists stated their opposition to "requiring pregnant women to do anything" (quoted in Kolata 1994). They argued that "mandatory testing or attempts at mandatory treatment 'reinforces concern for the fetus or child to . . . the possible detriment of the pregnant woman'" (quoted in Kolata 1994).

In 1997 a new state law mandated that the hospitals inform mothers of their infants' test results without seeking their consent (Sontag 1997). This was done primarily by passing the information to the "patient's doctor, so that the mother could get treatment" (Santora 2005). The new state policy raised several issues. First, there were women who were unaware that they had HIV as well as being unaware that the disease could be given to a fetus through perinatal transmission. Second, since hospitals would not receive the test results for as few as two or as many as six weeks, they would have to track down the mothers in a timely manner, especially since "breastfeeding increases the chances that H.I.V. positive mothers will pass the virus to their babies" (Sontag 1997).

In the late 1990s, the New York State also began a program targeted specifically at pregnant women urging them to get tested (Staley 2006). But the state maintained its opt-in policy of HIV screening for pregnant women, as opposed to those states that have an opt-out policy that assumes screening will take place unless the pregnant women actively declines the test (Kaiser Family Foundation 2008). In 1994 a drug was developed that could reduce the "vertical transmission" of HIV by two-thirds. In the years following, major medical organizations called for mandatory testing, routine testing with a right of refusal, and universal opt-out screening (Bayer and Fairchild 2006).

With the mandatory testing of infants, the program urging pregnant women to get tested, and the advent of new drugs, the city was able to reduce the number of newborns with HIV dramatically. In 1990 there were 321 newborns with HIV. In 2003and 2004, there were five babies born with HIV each year (Santora 2005; Lite 2006a).

Contact Tracing and Partner Notification

Another part of the debate revolved around the practice of contact tracing or partner notification. Since the virus was passed primarily through sexual intercourse or needle sharing, public health authorities wanted to treat HIV similar to venereal diseases. "Contact tracing for a venereal disease starts with a diagnosis reported confidentially by a physician, hospital or clinic. A health department worker then asks the patient to identify any sexual partners. Without revealing the patient's name, the worker privately informs those partners that they may be infected and urges testing" (Lambert 1987). AIDS was never identified, categorized, or treated as a venereal disease in New York State so contact-tracing laws that apply to those diseases or tuberculosis did not apply to AIDS (Sullivan 1987b). But even within the city public health establishment there was debate over the value of AIDS virus contact tracing. One member of the City Board of Health argued that contact tracing can "destroy peoples' lives in the process" (quoted in Lambert 1987). And an AIDS specialist for the American Civil Liberties Union stated: "We oppose contact tracing. The state should not maintain any list of names. You're worried about losing your job and your insurance" (quoted in Lambert 1987). The proponents of contact tracing argued that the privacy rights of the individual carrying the virus should not be given priority over the carrier's sexual or intravenous-needle-sharing partner's right to know (Hentoff 1987). In 1987 the NYC Department of Health reported that more than a thousand women had contracted AIDS and many of them did not know their spouses or partners were infected (Sullivan 1987b).

From the outset of testing, public health authorities in New York wanted to engage in partner notification for those who tested positive. But with anonymous testing they realized that this type of program was going to be voluntary at best (Sullivan 1987a). By the late 1990s, all states had some regulations that could pass as partner notification or contact tracing, but the differences among the states were significant. A majority of states had laws that allowed "doctors or public health officials to notify the sex or needle-sharing partners of those with AIDS or infected with HIV," but only four states required it (Burr 1997). New York State relied on "patient referral, deferring the responsibility of notification" to those infected with HIV (Burr 1997). In 1989 New York State gave physicians legal permission, by state law, "to notify their patients' partners or to refer their names to the health department," but there was no requirement that this be done (Lambert 1990d). AIDS counselors encouraged but did not require those who tested HIV positive to alert their partners, offering DOH's help in doing so (Lambert 1990d). Strict rules on patient confidentiality made partner notification programs impossible (Bayer 1991).

In 2000 New York State strengthened its reporting and partner notification law somewhat. The law required "doctors to discuss with their HIV-infected patients those whom they may have exposed to HIV infection through sex or needle sharing" (NYC DOHMH 2010b). If patients offer names of partners, physicians can either notify the partners themselves or contact the DOH who will do the contacting. Partners would be advised to get tested and counseled, but the partner would not be informed by whom he was identified. The original patient's name would be kept confidential. Under the law, however, infected individuals were not legally obligated to reveal the names of partners who might be at risk. Individuals were still being counseled to inform their partners directly or to seek help from a physician or AIDS counselor. Also, the state and city still operated sites where individuals could be tested anonymously, frustrating any effort at contact tracing (NYC DOHMH 2010b).

In 2006 DOHMH established eight HIV Field Services Units (FSU) "to assist HIV medical providers and patients diagnosed with HIV infection with partner services and linkage to medical care" (NYC DOHMH 2011). The FSU reported that in 2010 "543 partners were notified, 378 were tested for HIV infection and 46 were newly diagnosed with HIV" (NYC DOHMH 2011). These numbers are small but more than double the number for all categories in the FSU's second year (2007) of operation (NYC DOHMH 2011).

Public Education and Condom Distribution

In addition to testing and reporting, public education was at the center of the city's attempts at prevention. The challenge for the city in mounting an educational campaign geared to disease prevention was addressing the highly diverse publics, which included gay males, IV drug users, the medical community, the minority communities, sexually active teens, and heterosexuals in general. The gay community organized and initiated its own prevention campaigns well before the city got involved in any organized way. As a result, the city was able to enlist and borrow from the gay community's tactics and information in its own prevention efforts. Because of the political system's legacy of discrimination against homosexuals, many in the gay community viewed the government with suspicion, if not hostility. As a result, the fact that initial prevention efforts were run by organizations within the gay community and not governmental institutions enhanced the credibility of those programs (Perrow and Guillen 1990).

In the case of AIDS education there were a number of challenges for public health policy makers. The desired behavioral changes involved "biologically based, socially complex behaviors," including sexual practices and drug use (Fineberg 1988, 593). Realizing that the abolition of these behaviors was not within the realm of public policy, public health authorities sought to make them safer in order to lessen, if not eliminate, the risk of the individual getting HIV/AIDS as a result of the behavior. But seeking to make the behavior safer, many outside the public health policy arena viewed the actions of public health officials as sanctioning, if not enabling, the behavior. To some, safe sex education, and the provision of condoms, was tantamount to approval of homosexual and premarital heterosexual intercourse. Teaching IV drug users to clean their needles with bleach was supporting IV drug use (Fineberg 1988).

Early city efforts included telephone hotlines, resource guides, and pamphlets distributed throughout the city (NYC Office of the Mayor 1985). The DOH established an AIDS Education Unit that made public presentations and distributed brochures. The DOH produced a nine-page pamphlet on AIDS that was being widely distributed to city employees (NYC Office of the Mayor 1985). DOH also distributed wallet-sized cards that included the AIDS Hotline number as well as a brief description of the disease, information about who was most at risk, and information addressing what one could do if he was at risk or believed that he had AIDS (NYC DOH 1986). Finally, the city also contracted with GMHC to produce a series of pamphlets targeted to specific at-risk populations and to hold a series of public forums on AIDS throughout the city (NYC Office of the Mayor 1985). In addition to the publication and distribution of brochures, pamphlets, and print media, in 1987 the city's AIDS Education Unit conducted numerous outreach conferences with professional and community groups. In 1988 alone, the unit participated in seventy-one conferences (Lambert 1989e).

As the city began to disaggregate its education campaigns to different at-risk populations in the 1990s and 2000s, it relied heavily on community groups and groups with experience in dealing with HIV/AIDS. A 2006 campaign targeting low-income women in Brooklyn was run by GMHC, now more adept at dealing with AIDS in minority communities. The campaign included posters in subway stations and the distribution of "5000 promotional postcards at beauty salons and health fairs" (Grace 2006). In 2009 DOHMH assistant health commissioner Monica Sweeney reported that DOHMH had recruited "porn stars" and sex workers as "peer connectors" to help educate hard-to-reach groups. In addition the department rented a van that would go into neighborhoods where isolated groups were located. The vans would offer both testing and counseling (Sweeney 2009).

In some cases, public health officials were stymied by a lack of knowledge about how to reach certain at-risk populations. At a city council hearing addressing the growing incidence of AIDS among men of color, one witness noted that there is little known about men who have sex with men and how to make them safe. Addressing the problem of younger homeless men, another witness stated that it comes down to "where am I going to sleep and what will I have to do to find a place to sleep" (NYC Council 2008).

In attempting to reach the diverse at-risk populations in the city, public health officials and those assisting them became aware that the means by which information was delivered was as important as the message itself. "Information must be provided in a culturally appropriate manner, and channels of dissemination must be used that will reach the target groups" (Peterson and Marin 1988, 875). This meant that medium and vocabulary as well as the level of sophistication of the message had to be gauged properly. Most importantly, differing cultural norms among at-risk groups had to be understood. For some populations, verbal communication by peers was far more effective than written communication. Street outreach campaigns, such as street fairs, employing knowledgeable minority men proved to be far more effective in minority communities than distributing brochures in public places (Peterson and Marin 1988).

Intravenous drug users composed more than a quarter of the diagnosed AIDS cases in New York City in 1982 and had surpassed gay males in diagnosed AIDS cases by 1988. They posed the greatest challenge for AIDS prevention education efforts. IV drug users were a hard-to-reach population whose addiction behavior was difficult to modify. Clearly the most effective means of reducing the incidence of AIDS among IV drug users would have been to enroll them in drug treatment programs that would have attempted to cure their addiction. But amid the many drug treatment programs in the city, there were only enough slots at any point in time to accommodate no more than 20 percent of those in need (Drucker 1986). Because of the shortage of treatment slots, AIDS prevention education targeted toward IV drug users did not so much concentrate on attempting to eliminate drug use as it did attempt to take some of the risk out of drug use. In 1987 the NYC DOH AIDS prevention effort produced pamphlets targeted toward IV drug users. While the pamphlets counseled individuals not to inject drugs, they urged users to protect themselves from AIDS by not sharing needles or by cleaning needles with bleach, ethyl alcohol, or boiling water before sharing (NYC DOH 1987a; 1987b).

Delivering the prevention message to IV drug users was as problematic as the content. According to a state program, city outreach workers were supposed to persuade addicts to take a blood test and then arrange transportation for the addict to a nearby center. At the center the addict would take a blood test and then meet with a counselor who would describe safe sex techniques as well as methods of sterilizing syringes. If possible, the counselors would also seek spaces in drug treatment programs. In 1987 the city's commissioner of health, Stephen Joseph, noted the limited success of this type of program in reaching drug users (Freedman 1987).

Much of the city's AIDS preventive education campaign revolved around the concept of safe sex. Beginning in the mid-1980s, DOH pamphlets urged condom use (NYC DOH 1985a). By 1987 the DOH safe sex message had more clarity. The city's pamphlet, "AIDS, The Straight Facts" stated, "About having sex . . . Always use a rubber and practice safer sex, so body fluids (especially semen) are not passed between you," and "Avoid any practice where blood could be passed between you" (NYC DOH 1987b). In the late 1980s, in order to reach a larger public, DOH began running a comic strip that appeared on thousands of subway cars. Entitled "Decision" and appearing in both English and Spanish, the story line included a soap-opera-type romance along with AIDS prevention education (Barron 1993). The comic strip was paid for, in part, by a grant from the federal CDC (Barron 1993). DOH also embarked on an advertising campaign including "television, radio, and newspaper messages directed primarily at heterosexuals" (Gross 1987a). The advertising campaign by the NYC DOH, in conjunction with an advertising agency, was designed to convince sexually active persons between the ages of eighteen and thirty-four to use condoms as a means of lowering the risk of contracting HIV (Fineberg 1988). One of the ads included the message "Don't go out without your rubbers" (Gross 1987a). Another ad had a scene of a couple entangled amid bed sheets with the caption, "Bang, you're dead" (Gross 1987a). Critics argued that the ads were in bad taste, or even promoted promiscuity. In response, Commissioner of Health Stephen Joseph stated, "The Department of Health is not the guardian of public morality. We are the guardian of public health" (Gross 1987a).

Once drugs made it possible to live longer with HIV, the city's education program was forced to shift focus. On the one hand, educational messages could no longer push the message that HIV was a "death sentence" (Hartocollis 2011). On the other hand, public health officials in DOHMH wanted to convey the message that living one's life on anti-HIV drugs did not "guarantee good health" (Hartocollis 2011).

The city is supported in its efforts to produce educational materials by the New York State HIV/AIDS Materials Initiative. The initiative produces materials not only promoting prevention but also about service availability. The materials include video as well as audio presentations and computer software. The materials are produced in various languages. Most the materials can be accessed from the state's website (NYS DOH AIDS Initiative 2009).

The New York State Department of Health also produced and distributed public-service announcements promoting safe sex, which ran on several television stations in the city. The announcements included two gay men talking about condom use at a gym as well as a "man returning home to his wife and family after his male date refused to use a condom" (Davis 1993). All of these announcements concluded with: "Use a condom. Take charge. Take care" (David 1993). The federal government ran radio and television ads as well, some of which involved celebrities urging young people to take steps to avoid HIV (Navarro 1994a). Among some segments of the population, the efforts at education appeared to be working. In 1999, DOH reported a sharp drop in infected gay men attributable to an increased use of condoms and safer sex (Altman 1999b).

The distribution of condoms by the city became a major element of the AIDS prevention program. The city's DOH had been distributing condoms since the 1970s, initially through sexually transmitted disease (STD) clinics. In the 1980s, distribution was expanded to those organizations that were dealing with IV drug users and other HIV/AIDS service delivery groups (NYC DOHMH 2010a). In 1987 teams from DOH distributed free condoms at "singles bars, pornographic movie theaters, massage parlors and sex clubs throughout the city" (Sullivan 1987a). In the 1990s DOH began distributing the female condom as well. In 2005 DOHMH initiated a condom website where organizations could order condoms online. "Average monthly condom distribution increased from 250,000 to 1.5 million" (NYC DOHMH 2010a). In 1999 a study by GMHC in cooperation with DOH found that gay males had in fact "reduced their levels of risky sexual behavior," contributing to the decline in gay males contracting HIV throughout the 1990s (Altman 1999a).

But in 2005 Commissioner of Health Frieden complained that condoms "are not widely available, nor is their use strongly promoted, and they are still used infrequently in high risk sexual encounters" (Frieden et al. 2005, 2399). That same year the NYC Commission on HIV/AIDS recommended making condoms available at as many public places as possible (Meyer and Colangelo 2005). In 2006 the NYC DOH reported that they were distributing more than a million free condoms a month. Finally, in 2007 the city, in cooperation with Lifestyles condom launched its own NYC Condom, increasing condom awareness as well. Since then the city has also designed NYC Condom dispensers and placed them in bars, restaurants, community service agencies, and STD clinics (NYC

DOHMH 2010a). This included the creation of a Facebook page devoted to condom use promotion (Chan 2009).

Some public health experts were concerned that campaigns to promote the use of condoms to decrease HIV infection would create a "false sense of security" among those who engaged in at-risk behavior (Gruson 1987). Although condoms reduced the risk of HIV, experts were not sure how effective they were. U. S. surgeon general, C. Everett Koop, warned against any sexual contact with those who had HIV. According to the surgeon general, "if you use a condom for protection against AIDS the way you use them for birth control, then you are in danger" (Gruson 1987). Concerns about decreased condom usage increased in the late 1990s once new life-saving drugs became available. Some public health experts sensed that among younger gay males who had grown up during the AIDS crisis, there was a greater willingness to take risks and not use condoms (Stolberg 1997).

When it came to educating children about AIDS, a number of issues arose. First, although there was agreement that AIDS education should attempt to reach children before they became sexually active, there was the question at what age or grade level should AIDS education begin? Because a significant number of New York City schoolchildren were aware of people dying from AIDS, there were those who wanted to begin the AIDS discussion in the early elementary grades. The second issue, more controversial than the first, was how to educate preteens and teens about AIDS as they approached the age of potential sexual activity. While some wanted to bring safe sex education into the classroom complete with condom demonstrations, more conservative elements pushed for an abstinence-only AIDS education program. In the early 1990s, the tension surrounding this debate was exacerbated by an additional debate over whether and how the city's public schools should include gays and lesbians in instruction about tolerance for different groups.

Until the second year of the Bloomberg administration, health education in the city's public schools was controlled by the quasi-independent Board of Education, not the DOH. The board had seven members, two appointed by the mayor, and one by each of the borough presidents. The seven-member board was responsible for hiring a chancellor who administered the school system. Administration of the city's school system was also decentralized, so that the fifty-one elected community school boards had some control over policy especially at the elementary and middle schools levels. This all changed in 2002–3 when the state gave the mayor control over the school system, and the Board of Education and the elected community school boards were abolished.

From 1985 through 2002, the city's school system was headed by eight chancellors. This only added to the lack of continuity in school policy on AIDS education. Early on, the school system relied on outside groups to develop and implement AIDS education courses. This approach produced considerable controversy as outside groups, on an approved list, had different approaches for educating students about AIDS prevention (Berger 1990). In the 1990s, the city school board became more convinced that the promotion of abstinence was the proper method of AIDS education. Many groups stopped working with the schools because of the new policy (Dao 1993). Some of the groups, such as Montefiore Hospital's Adolescent AIDS Program ran weekend workshops training students to be peer educators in HIV/AIDS prevention (*New York Times* 1999). In the mid-1990s, Chancellor Raymond Cortines "revised the curriculum to emphasize abstinence" and gave "parents the right to keep their children out" of those discussions where safe sex was the focus of prevention (Sengupta 1997).

In the early 1990s, the New York City school system became the first to distribute condoms in its high schools (Marks 1993). With pressure applied by Mayor Dinkins, the Board of Education voted in 1991 to not allow parents to take their children out of the condom distribution program (Berger 1991). But in the mid-1990s at the insistence of the Board of Education, Chancellor Rudy Crew scaled back the city's high school AIDS prevention education program by "calling for an end to condom demonstrations in the classroom and requiring every high school to establish a resource room staffed by volunteer teachers where students" can request a condom demonstration as well as pick up free condoms (Sengupta 1997). In the school's health education curriculum, abstinence was promoted as the primary means to avoid contracting AIDS (Newman 1995).

Under Mayor Bloomberg's control, the schools last updated their AIDS curriculum in 2005. Although the program does educate junior high and high school students about condom use to reduce the risk of HIV infection, the program still stresses abstinence (NYC Department of Education 2006). In addition, rather than relying on outside groups to provide HIV/AIDS prevention education in the schools, the state and city produced HIV/AIDS prevention curriculum guides for each grade from kindergarten through the twelfth grade. The seventh grade curriculum guide note to teachers states: "Abstinence from sexual intercourse is discussed and emphasized throughout the curriculum. It is also important for students to know the facts about condoms so that they can make informed choices that help lead to a healthier life" (NYC Department of Education 2005a, 112). The twelfth-grade curriculum guide emphasizes that condom use reduces but does not eliminate the risk of becoming infected from HIV, while abstinence does eliminate the risk. At the same time, the twelfth-grade guide gives explicit instructions on how to use both male and female condoms (NYC Department of Education 2005b).

The schools send a letter to parents explaining the city's AIDS curriculum: "State Regulations require that all students attend lessons on the nature of the disease and methods of transmission. However, parents or legal guardians have the right to ask that their child not participate in the lessons dealing with prevention" (NYC Department of Education 2010). The letter explains that parents who wish to have their child excused from prevention instruction must "assure that the pupil will receive such instruction at home" (NYC Department of Education 2010). In 2009 a spokesperson for Gay Men's Health Crisis reported to the city council that HIV/AIDS prevention education differed from school to school and was implemented at the discretion of the principal (NYC Council 2009).

Parents of high school students in the city also have the option to take their children out of the Condom Availability Program run by the city school system. Under this program, every city high school must make condoms available to students through its health resources room. This room must be opened at least ten periods a week and must be staffed by both male and female staff. Students must be made aware of the program's existence. And new students must receive information along with a letter to the parents giving them the ability to opt out of the program (NYC Department of Education 2009). Despite these regulations, significant variations have been reported in how individual high schools handle condom distribution in the city. Some high schools have posters advertising the program and aggressively make sure that each student receives the mandated six lessons. Other schools' programs exist on paper only (Richardson 1997c).

Needle Exchanges

Just as critics had opposed condom distribution, believing that it would promote increased sexual activity, there were many who argued that the political system should not be supporting drug use in any way. Some argued further that the distribution of clean needles to drug addicts was in violation of the law. Minority group representatives were vocal in their opposition to needle exchange programs. Since the majority of IV drug users in the city were minorities, leaders from the minority communities viewed needle exchanges as giving up on drug treatment and writing-off minority drug users (Anderson 1991).

Advocates of needle exchanges agreed that although needle distribution or exchanges were controversial, such methods were effective at "harm reduction" (Anderson 1991). Because harm reduction strategies accept the reality that many will continue to engage in at-risk behaviors even once informed of the danger in doing so, these strategies have not been "universally accepted in the United States, despite evidence that they have been effective in other countries" (NYC Commission on HIV/AIDS 2005). Opponents of harm reduction strategies believed this approach legitimized, if not encouraged, the at-risk behavior. Congress voted to withhold money from needle exchange programs in 1988, and this was not reversed until 2009 (*New York Times* 2010). Responding to the critics, the head of the American Foundation for AIDS Research (amFAR) stated:

"I never heard of anybody starting drugs because needles were available or stopping because they couldn't find a clean one" (quoted in Anderson 1991, 1510).

Although needle exchange programs were already being employed in other countries, New York State law would not allow such a program, and the administration of Mayor Ed Koch refused to initiate one (Nix 1985). The state commissioner of health has the ability to "define who may legally possess needles and syringes" (Joseph 1992, 194). Mayor Koch's own commissioner of health, David Sencer "proposed that needles be sold over the counter to encourage addicts not to share needles" (Nix 1985). In 1985 public health officials in New York City reported that some IV drug users were beginning to take precautions to avoid AIDS by purchasing illegal, but clean, needles from street sellers (Altman 1985). Mathilde Krim, cofounder of the amFAR, stated: "Giving needles to addicts 'is not something we like to do, but if we don't, people are going to die for lack of a stupid needle" (quoted in Lambert 1991). In January 1988 a Brooklyn community drug treatment group, the Association for Drug Abuse Prevention and Treatment (ADAPT) announced that it was distributing free needles and syringes to addicts in exchange for dirty ones, in defiance of state law (Anderson 1991).

In 1988 Governor Cuomo allowed the city to run a limited pilot project where clean needles would be given to addicts entering drug treatment programs (Kerr 1988). For those participating in the needle exchange program, the HIV infection rate was cut by 80 percent (*New York Times* 2010). But Mayor Dinkins abandoned the project responding to opposition by the Black Leadership Commission on AIDS (Lambert 1990c). Lobbied by the public health community, Dinkins approved privately run needle exchange programs later in his term (Navarro 1991c; 1991d). By 1994 there were several needle exchange programs operating in the city with at least two each in Manhattan, Brooklyn, and the Bronx with more than twenty-five thousand participants. All operated with "waivers from the State Department of Health because New York" was still one of a few states making it a "crime to possess or use syringe needles without a prescription" (Lee 1994). The programs received funding from the State Department of Health and amFAR (Lee 1994).

An evaluation of New York's needle exchange programs in 1994 found that program participants had a lower rate of HIV infection than those drug users who did not participate (Lee 1994). In 1998 studies conducted by the NYC DOH in conjunction with the Chemical Dependency Unit at New York's Beth Israel Medical Center found that the spread of AIDS among the city's IV-drug-using population had leveled off, in part due to the proliferation of needle exchange programs. The studies also documented a significant decline in needle sharing (Knox 1998).

Despite the documented effectiveness of needle exchange programs, the controversy surrounding them remained. The Clinton administration refused to fund needle exchange programs (Moynihan 1999). In 2004 Commissioner of Health Tom Frieden skirmished with a community board in Queens over the need for a needle exchange program in that borough. NYC DOH had found that there were several Queens neighborhoods with high rates of HIV due to IV drug use, and Commissioner Frieden wanted to place a mobile needle exchange van in that borough to service those neighborhoods. But even in 2004 needle exchange programs still needed a waiver from the State Department of Health; and the state agency demanded local support before granting the waiver (O'Grady 2004).

In 2010 Governor Paterson signed into law an amendment to the state penal code stating "that a person does not act unlawfully by possessing a hypodermic needle or syringe if he or she participates in a needle exchange or syringe access program authorized under the Public Health Law" (NYS Office of the Governor 2010). In addition the new law stated that a "residual amount of a controlled substance on a needle or syringe does not constitute a criminal act" (NYS Office of the Governor 2010). On the federal level, in 2009 President Obama "repealed the 21-year old ban on federal financing for programs that give drug users access to clean needles" (*New York Times* 2010). But there was a delay in the U.S. Department of Health and Human Services issuing regulations for states or local governments seeking to use federal money to start new needle exchange programs or expand existing programs (*New York Times* 2010).

Closing Bathhouses and Theaters

Early in the campaign against AIDS one of the tactics the city used in attempting to curtail the transmission of HIV was to target those places where transmission was likely to take place. For the gay community, bathhouses, clubs, and movie theaters served as venues where gay males engaged in sexual relations. The gay community was divided over whether these establishments should remain open or be closed down. While many of these venues were viewed as places where gay males engaged in unsafe sex, many in the public health and gay communities saw them as useful places to educate individuals about AIDS prevention. Some gay organizations in the city had attempted to change behavior at the bathhouses by issuing guidelines to be followed by owners and attempting to educate patrons, but even they admitted that no one was in complete compliance (Gross 1985). Opponents of bathhouse regulations and closure argued that this type of governmental activity infringed on the fundamental right to privacy of consenting adults and deprived individuals of the constitutionally protected right to gather and socialize (Connelly 1985).

San Francisco had closed its bathhouses in 1984 after determining that an ordinance prohibiting unsafe sexual practices in the bathhouses could not be enforced (Lindsey 1985). In 1985 the Cuomo administration amended the state health code giving local officials the power to close those establishments allowing unhealthy sexual practices as public nuisances for sixty days (Roberts 1985). In early December 1985, a little more than a month after the state regulations were issued, the city closed a bathhouse in which city inspectors reported seeing multiple acts of unsafe sex (Purnick 1985b). Other closings followed. All of the bathhouses were not closed immediately, but in 1987 State Commissioner of Health David Axelrod said he was confident that in those bathhouses that remained open, safe sex was taking place (Bronstein 1987). Some bathhouse owners sued the city, but the court ruled in the city's favor arguing that the state "nuisance laws allow public authorities to abate essentially anything that may be injurious to the health of the public, including dangerous activities, goods and premises" (US CDC 2010b).

Concerned about possible raids from undercover city inspectors, some clubs put up signs warning patrons that sexual relations were forbidden. Other clubs and bars closed off backrooms where sexual activity formerly took place. And still others hired and trained monitors to prevent patrons from engaging in high-risk sex (Blumenthal 1985). Late in 1985, Commissioner of Health Axelrod announced that regulations that had been applied to bars, movie theaters, and clubs would also be extended to hotels that are found to be supporting unsafe sexual activity (*New York Times* 1985).

In 1993 the city began to experience a resurgence of sex-related businesses catering to gay males (Navarro 1993a). In 1994 and 1995 the city closed several gay bars, movie theaters, and clubs, once again exercising the power given to it by the state (Myers 1994; Dunlap 1995a). Those establishments sued the city, but a State Supreme Court judge ruled that, "because city officials sent warning letters before moving to close" the theater, "they had properly tried to limit high risk sexual activity there without curtailing the exhibition of movies" (Dunlap 1995b).

Direct Provision of Services

Public health's emphasis on prevention normally results in the utilization of policy tools such as education and regulation. In the case of AIDS, the public health enterprise has also employed the direct provision of health services. While AIDS is not the only instance of public health authorities involving themselves in the direct provision of health services, it is certainly an important example of the porous boundary between public health and the provision of social, health, and medical services. The provision of services by public health authorities can be divided into two types. First there are those types of services delivered to the entire public or at-risk groups to enhance prevention. In the case of AIDS, the establishment of free testing sites, the distribution of condoms, and the establishment of needle exchanges fall into this category and have already been discussed. The second category of provided services, which occurs less frequently, includes those delivered directly to those afflicted with the disease.

With HIV/AIDS, the direct provision of health services or the coordination of their provision was necessary for several reasons. First, because of the way in which AIDS is transmitted, providing services to those infected was one way of controlling the infected population and attempting to stem the spread of the disease. That is, the services furthered the goal of prevention. A second reason why public health authorities have gotten involved in the delivery of health services is that public health crises frequently fall disproportionately on low-income individuals and families, and those who lack access to the health care system. Those who do not get treated remain a threat to the health of the community. In the case of AIDS, many of the groups that were affected by the disease were precisely those groups who lacked access to the health care system and who, if left isolated, would have continued to spread the disease.

Third, because of the fatal and later debilitating nature of HIV/AIDS, a range of services was needed by persons with AIDS that went well beyond what the medical and health communities were used to providing. These included housing and social services such as nutrition and job training. While the medical community had its own understanding of what case management entailed, AIDS demanded an expanded and more comprehensive definition.

The city's public health infrastructure got a slow start with regard to the delivery of AIDS services. As a result, organizations formed to address the crisis in the gay community got a head start and in many ways set the agenda for the delivery of services to those with AIDS and later HIV. By 1983 GMHC already had a paid staff of twelve and approximately five hundred volunteers (Dowd 1983). The group ran "therapy groups for AIDS patients," partners, and families (Dowd 1983). In addition, volunteers cleaned apartments, did laundry, paid bills, picked up prescriptions, and transported patients to doctors appointments, while also "serving as intermediaries with the city's social service agencies" (Dowd 1983). In 1997 GMHC entered into an agreement with New York Hospital–Cornell Medical Center to open a medical services center on the first floor of GMHC's headquarters in Chelsea (Richardson 1997d). Over time, GMHC was joined by other advocacy groups and nonprofit organizations.

The city's program of AIDS services included assessment centers where people were sent for medical evaluation after testing positive for HIV; care at city hospitals; case management and coordination, both inpatient and outpatient; and housing. When necessary, the city also provided food stamps and meal subsidies (Lambert 1989b). For those persons with AIDS eligible for Medicaid, the federal-state-city-financed health insurance program for low-income families, the city began paying for services almost immediately. Many who were not eligible for Medicaid but could not afford care ended up in city hospitals. The city also distributed subsistence stipends of as little as five dollars a day to those who were waiting for their applications for federal or state benefits to be approved (Siegel 1995). Throughout the history of the crisis, the extent of the city's provision of services to persons with HIV/AIDS was a function of annual budget considerations. The city never appropriated sufficient funds to deliver services to all who were eligible.

Another major impediment to the effective delivery of services to persons with HIV/AIDS was, and still is, the fact that testing remains voluntary, even though the burdensome testing protocol was eased in 2010. As a result, it is difficult to reach those with HIV/AIDS when many do not know themselves that they have the disease. Because of privacy concerns regarding testing results, it was not until 2008 that DOHMH through its field services units began to link testing and surveillance data with the provision of care. DOHMH staff members, some of whom are "embedded" in city health facilities, now review and identify surveillance records (Sweeny et al. 2013, 565). They then contact individuals who have tested positive, offering to connect them with appropriate care and offer transportation (Sweeny et al. 2013).

The impact of AIDS patients on the city hospital system was much more than just a demand for bed space. In the New York City public hospital system, the typical AIDS patient was an IV drug user who entered the hospital with a variety of medical issues in addition to AIDS. The array of conditions required an intense and expensive medical response, including "chest X-rays, CAT scans, and spinal taps" (Navarro 1991e). In the late 1970s and early 1980s, in part due to the city's fiscal crisis, several public hospitals were closed and others decreased available bed space. As a result, there was never sufficient inpatient space available for AIDS victims (Lambert 1988a).

As drug development allowed persons with HIV/AIDS to live a longer and healthier life, services offered by the city changed slowly to address this new condition. Offering persons with HIV/AIDS the goal of independent living and self-sufficiency adequate to ensure that they could continue to receive the needed medical care became the new goal (NYC Human Resources Administration 2013). Attempts were made to locate service providers in communities populated by persons with AIDS. And the DOHMH AIDS hotline was revamped not only to help individuals assess their level of risk and get tested but now also to provide referrals for services (Hansell 2000).

In late 1997 Mayor Giuliani signed legislation creating the HIV/AIDS Services Administration (HASA), a permanent agency within the city's Human Resources Administration (HRA). In the same legislation, the city council expanded the benefits that could be provided by the division to include both transportation and nutrition subsidies. The bill also established a bill of rights for AIDS patients, listing the services to which they were entitled. This list included hospitalization, case management, appropriate housing or home care, nutrition, and transportation, in addition to Medicaid and food stamps (*New York Times* 1997). Over time the agency added employment and vocational assistance, "counseling for clients and their families on daily living skills and available support systems," "guardianship and permanency planning for families with children," and burial assistance (NYC HRA 2010a).

During the late 1990s and 2000s, there were several controversies surrounding HASA's delivery of services to persons with AIDS. HASA was frequently accused by activists, and occasionally the city council, of being overly punitive in its administration of services (NYC Council 2012). In the late 1990s, the Giuliani administration implemented an Eligibility Verification Review (EVR) process that appeared to subject HASA clients to greater eligibility scrutiny than all others receiving assistance from the city (NYC Council 1999). Despite a city law that mandated the least-burdensome eligibility process for those with AIDS, the Giuliani administration did not eliminate EVR until ordered to do so by the state courts. For those HASA clients who were drug abusers, cash assistance was tied to compliance with drug rehabilitation, but this was partly in response to a state mandate (Dudley 2012).

One of the most significant services that the city found itself delivering to HIV/AIDS victims was housing. Studies demonstrated that "housing insecurity is a major barrier to obtaining and maintaining medical care for HIV and AIDS patients over time" (Ruiz 2005b). Research showed that those with a stable housing situation were far more likely to receive medical care on a regular basis and far less likely to engage in at-risk behaviors (Aidala et al. 2005). In the mid-1980s, the city began to locate and rehabilitate housing for AIDS patients (Rangel 1985). In 1987, the nonprofit AIDS Resource Center, under contract with the city, opened Bailey House, a group residence for individuals with AIDS in Greenwich Village (Dunlap 1987). Since a significant number of AIDS patients were homeless, by the late 1980s the city had established homeless shelters, or sections of homeless shelters dedicated to AIDS, as well as scattered-site housing and hotel rooms when necessary. Rent subsidies were also provided when necessary (Lambert 1989b). Over time various housing options were developed for persons with AIDS, from emergency to transitional to long term (Dudley 2012). City legislation passed in 1997 required that clients of the city's HIV/AIDS Services Administration live in housing that was "medically appropriate" (Ruiz 2005b).

But even with federal and state assistance, the city and the nonprofit groups providing housing were never able to meet demand. In 1997 Mayor Giuliani's coordinator of AIDS services noted that while there were more than five thousand clients in need of housing, there were fewer than three thousand available units (Dunlap 1997). Some persons with AIDS spent nights in homeless shelters or hotels instead of medically appropriate housing (NYC Council 2000b). As more persons with HIV/AIDS survived the illness, housing needs became more long term (Richardson 1997a).

In 2010 Governor Paterson vetoed legislation that would have offered rent relief to more than ten thousand New Yorkers with HIV or AIDS. In vetoing the bill, Governor Paterson expressed his unwillingness to impose unfunded mandates on local governments in the state at a time when they did not have the revenue to fund them. Mayor Bloomberg had urged the governor to veto the legislation (Cardwell 2010). Nonprofit groups administering housing informed the city council that city housing payments to landlords were so late that they were forced to put up their own money, or the landlord would cease renting to persons with AIDS, further exacerbating the housing shortage (NYC Council 2002). There were also concerns that since HASA clients were not protected by state housing assistance regulations, many were paying more than 30 percent of their income for rent (NYC Council 2009).

While the city's relations with most of the nonprofit housing provider groups were cordial and businesslike, there was conflict on occasion. Housing Works was founded in 1990 by many of the officials who had been involved in ACT UP, one of the more militant AIDS grass-roots advocacy groups. Housing Works officials had been vocal critics of city AIDS policies, particularly whenever the Giuliani administration considered budgetary reductions in AIDS services funding (Allon 1998). The group was involved in much of the litigation on the city's efforts in delivering services to those with HIV and AIDS. In 1999 the New York State Court of Appeals ruled that the Giuliani administration "had created illegal obstacles for people with HIV or AIDS to obtain public assistance" (Hernandez 1999). At issue was the city's Eligibility Verification Review procedures whereby city investigators would conduct background checks to verify whether an individual with AIDS qualified for city benefits.

In 2000, in response to a 1995 class-action lawsuit filed by Housing Works, a federal judge found that the city had violated the Americans with Disabilities Act and ordered the city's Division of AIDS Services be placed under federal oversight for three years (*Washington Post* 2000). The judge found that the city had "chronically and systematically delayed or stopped subsistence benefits, including emergency housing, rent assistance, food stamps, Medicaid and other services" for thousands of individuals who have HIV or AIDS (Richardson 2000). Under the ruling, individuals with complaints about the Division of AIDS Services would be able to go directly to an appointed federal magistrate to lodge their complaints (Mansnerus 2000).

With court-mandated services, by 2009 the city HIV/AIDS Services Administration was delivering services to more than thirty thousand cases of HIV/

AIDS, including forty-five hundred families. This included more than seven thousand housing placements in city-administered housing and rental assistance for almost twenty thousand additional cases (NYC HRA 2010b).

New York City's Response to AIDS and Economic Development

Unlike some public health problems, HIV/AIDS was neither caused nor exacerbated by economic development issues. The city's response to the AIDS epidemic, however, provides an example of the impact of economic forces on the city's ability to respond to a public health threat. The city's fiscal problems of the early 1980s may have delayed a comprehensive response by the city. AIDS struck the city as it was emerging from the fiscal crisis of the 1970s. In addition, the impact of AIDS on New York City was exacerbated by the concurrence of homelessness and drug abuse, issues that also strained a financially weakened public health system (Bayer 1991).

Declining city and state revenues, as a result of a depressed economy, forced the city and the state to make difficult choices among programs. In 1989 an ambulatory care program at city hospitals and an AIDS prevention education program were cut (Lambert 1988a). Faced with budget shortfalls in 1995, the Giuliani administration announced that the Health Department would no longer administer free HIV tests for patients who had private insurance or Medicaid (Mooney 1995). In addition, in 1995, the city stopped giving individuals with AIDS the small daily cash stipend, less than ten dollars, while they were waiting for more comprehensive benefits to be approved (Siegel 1995).

More recently, as a result of the recession beginning in 2008, New York City's AIDS budget has encountered the stress that all city services have experienced. In 2010 the Bloomberg administration proposed cutting $10 million from the city's AIDS budget, which would have resulted in the elimination of 248 caseworkers. Threatened with a lawsuit in federal court by Housing Works, the Bloomberg administration withdrew the proposed cuts. The suit by Housing Works argued that the proposed budget cuts violated the city's own legally established ratio of AIDS caseworkers to clients (Markey 2010). But cuts were being threatened again in 2011. This time the cuts focused less on case management and more on nonprofit groups who provide a range of AIDS services (Hamilton 2011).

Just as cities in the 1980s and 1990s understood that high crime rates inhibit economic development by making a city less attractive, New York City political elites surely understood that an unabated AIDS crisis would have similarly made the city less attractive to economic development interests. As such economic development concerns probably hastened the city's response to AIDS, despite the critics' complaints about a delayed response.

New York City's Response to AIDS
and the Minority Community

Race and ethnicity have played a major role in the utilization of public policy tools in the fight against HIV/AIDS. Minorities (African American and Hispanics) have made up a majority of those diagnosed with AIDS since the outset of the crisis (table 4.2). During the first decade of the disease, while the gay community initiated a response to AIDS, many minority group leaders either were in denial or refused to believe that dealing with HIV/AIDS was their responsibility (Quimby and Friedman 1989). And from 1996 going forward, more than 80 percent of those diagnosed with AIDS were either African American or Hispanic (Chiasson 2000). Racial and ethnic disparities were even greater among women, where Latinas and black women composed 90 percent of the female AIDS cases (Ferraro 1998a). In 2008 young black and Latina females accounted for almost 30 percent of newly reported HIV cases in the city, mostly through heterosexual intercourse (Gardner 2008). And more than 100,000 minority children were orphaned by AIDS (Ferraro 1998b).

While the legacy of racism and discrimination provides part of the explanation for the delayed response of New York State and New York City to the outbreak of AIDS, the complacency of minority groups and leadership was also present. The gay community mobilized rapidly to address HIV/AIDS, but there was no equivalent mobilization in minority communities (Peterson and Marin 1988). In 1987 Manhattan Borough president David Dinkins commented: "I wish I knew why more people aren't outraged, full of fear, and speaking out on this subject . . . But I do know that in minority communities, there are so many areas of concern, so many damn problems" (quoted in *New York Times* 1987). To some extent, Mayor Dinkins was articulating the views of many of the mainstream civil rights groups in the 1980s, which saw "AIDS in the context of broader problems of poverty, drug addiction, inadequate education and unemployment" (Quimby and Friedman 1989, 405).

There was concern in minority communities that AIDS would be closely associated with minorities and become another "rationale for racism" (Freedman 1987). When the city instituted its program of giving free clean needles to intravenous drug users, some black leaders termed the program "genocide," believing that the program would expand illegal drug use in the inner city (Lambert 1988c). The plan was denounced by the black and Hispanic caucus of the city council as well as black members of Congress from the city (Bayer 1995, 141). Minority leaders wanted a comprehensive governmental response to drug abuse in the inner city, not just a response to AIDS. In many cases, black elected officials were merely representing the views of their constituents, who had strong moral views regarding homosexuality and drug abuse (Quimby and Friedman 1989).

Churches were the center of black political life in New York as well as major distributors of social services, but there was reluctance on the part of the minority religious community to embrace AIDS as a cause. Fundamentalists within the black community, as elsewhere, viewed AIDS as a sort of retribution from God on the gay and drug-using communities. In addition, the minority social agenda was already quite full with poverty, racism, and drugs (Goldman 1987). One prominent Brooklyn pastor held a forum on AIDS in 1987, but only twenty-five people attended (Quimby and Friedman 1989). There was even greater resistance by religious leaders in the Hispanic and Asian communities (Link 2005). It was not until 1989 that the black clergy mounted a coordinated effort to speak out about the threat of AIDS to minority communities (Lambert 1989c). And it was not until late in 1991 that the black religious community began delivering services to those with AIDS when church-sponsored housing for individuals with AIDS was contracted (Navarro 1991b). As late as 1996, churches in minority communities were still resistant to get involved in fighting AIDS. An AIDS forum sponsored by a Hispanic organization in East Harlem was attended by only eight of twenty-four churches invited to attend (Jacobs 1996).

The Minority Task Force on AIDS, a Harlem-based organization of social service providers, was formed in 1985. This was probably the first organized response by the minority community to the outbreak of AIDS. This group believed that the African American leadership in New York City had failed to acknowledge the extent to which AIDS was affecting the black community (Quimby and Friedman 1989). Ten years later the head of the organization, Linda Stewart Campbell, voiced concern that the minority community had still not made a sufficient commitment to dealing with AIDS. Commenting on the inability of the organization to obtain significant donations from the black community, Campbell noted: "We're still at war with ourselves about AIDS . . . What we see in the epidemic—like the drug use—reminds us of all the evils that have torn us apart" (quoted in Lee 1995).

But by the mid-1990s most minority group leaders had reached the conclusion that HIV/AIDS was their problem and that action needed to be taken to prevent the further spread of the disease in their respective communities. As late as 2000, Councilperson Una Clarke stated that "she was pleased to see that people of color are coming forward and admitting that there is a crisis in the community" (NYC Council 2000a). At that point, however, some minority leaders became critical of the gay community, controlled predominantly by upper-middle-class white males, for monopolizing much of the funding and resources.

Other minority-based groups eventually formed to deal with the AIDS problem. Some of them were religiously based, such as the Balm in Gilead, a New York–based educational group that met with minority church communities across the country to raise AIDS awareness and construct AIDS prevention programs (Blake 1999). Others were focused on a specific segment of the HIV/ AIDS demographic such as Life Force in Brooklyn, an agency that used federal funding to reach out to minority women (Gonzalez 2007).

Even once there was consensus in minority communities to address AIDS, education and prevention were complicated. In some minority communities, bisexual men having sexual relations with other men did not consider themselves gay and ignored prevention and education programs pitched to the gay community as a result (Cooper 2000; Sweeny 2009). Some health officials suggested that black and Latino men and women would "rather die than risk having family or friends find out they are sick" (Santora 2006b). In 1995, when the CDC reported that AIDS incidence rates for whites had dropped while they had increased for blacks and Hispanics, the CDC concluded that, while prevention efforts targeting the white community had succeeded, those directed at the minority community had failed (Nicholson 1995). In 2001 the Bronx Lesbian and Gay Health Resource Consortium, as part of a campaign to reach minority gay males, placed ads on bus shelters throughout the Bronx displaying "two men, one with his arm around the other" with the caption, "I'm not gay, but sometimes I have sex with other guys" (Kennedy 2001). The company that placed the ads on the shelters began receiving complaints due to the ads' reference to sex. The company removed the ads (Kennedy 2001). As services were targeted more toward minority communities, there was a demand for cultural competence if the services were going to be effective. Because of cultural differences as well as prejudice, minority men were isolated from the sources of information that were available to, and being produced by, white gay men. Gay newspapers and brochures being distributed in gay bars and clubs were simply not available to minority men. But there were also questions as to whether the messages within these newspapers and brochures would have been accepted by minority men, given varying community norms (Peterson and Marin 1988).

In a city with many ethnic enclaves and recent immigrants, cultural and linguistic isolation were common. Some cultures viewed women as second-class citizens who could not demand that their sexual partners use protection. In some traditional Latin cultures, the decision over condom usage lay with the husband (Mays and Cochran 1988). This was in direct contradiction to mainstream cultural norms where women had taken control of contraception (Mays and Cochrane 1988). At times the subordinate status of women was exacerbated by "emotional and economic dependence upon their male partners," as well as the threat of physical violence (Peterson and Marin 1988, 874). These cultural mores and practices would have to be addressed by any AIDS prevention education program targeted at minority communities. Cultural sensitivity was particularly problematic in presenting frank discussions of sexuality (Ports 2000). One witness told a city council hearing "you just can't throw a pamphlet at someone"

(NYC Council 2000a). As it developed, new media and the internet were used to reach young people at risk, as well as offer young people at risk a "space" where they could get information anonymously (NYC Council 2009).

In defense of the minority community's response to the AIDS epidemic, some argued that the New York State Division of Substance Abuse, which was aware of the potential impact of AIDS on the minority community early in the development of the disease and could have alerted and mobilized minority leaders, simply ignored the problem for several years (Perrow and Guillen 1990, 75). In addition, some have noted that organizational fragmentation among the city and state health agencies also inhibited the governmental response to AIDS among intravenous drug users. The Department of Health, the agency primarily responsible for the city's response to AIDS, dealt directly with neither low-income populations nor drug abusers. Although the Department of Health began contracting with community-based organizations for the creation and delivery of AIDS education and prevention projects in 1985, community-based organizations in minority neighborhoods were not included until 1988 (NYC Mayor's Office of Operations 1988, 390).

In the late 1980s and early 1990s, as the demographics of AIDS in the city changed from white to minority and from gay to drug user, there was tension over which groups should receive funding priority in the fight against HIV/AIDS. In 1992 a dispute arose over the appointment of the chair of the City Council Committee on Health, Enoch Williams. Gay groups opposed Williams, a black councilman from Brooklyn, as chair because of his opposition to the distribution of condoms in schools and the distribution of clean needles to addicts. Williams argued that gay opposition to his position was due, in part, to his statements that too much AIDS funding had gone to gay groups rather than the black and Hispanic communities (*New York Times* 1992). In 1996 several minority members of the Gay Men's Health Crisis Board resigned, claiming that the group had not adequately responded to AIDS in minority communities (Dunlap 1996). In 2008 one member of the city council argued that if the epidemic were affecting white men the way it was affecting men of color, there would be much more action by the political system (NYC Council 2008).

In 2001 a study by Housing Works analyzed New York State contracts awarded for AIDS prevention and service delivery. The study concluded that although 80 percent of New Yorkers with AIDS were black or Hispanic, 70 percent of AIDS funds spent by the state went to organizations run by non-Hispanic whites (Perez-Pena 2001). State officials claimed that the discrepancy was not due to discrimination but to the history of AIDS and inertia created when white gay male groups first lobbied and applied for the funding. A spokesperson for the Gay Men's Health Crisis stated that more money needed to be spent by the state on AIDS services in order to better serve minority communities (Perez-Pena

2001). In 2006 Comptroller William Thompson complained to DOHMH commissioner Tom Frieden that minority communities in the city had been shortchanged in the distribution of federal AIDS funding (Hays 2006).

In 2007 there was similar controversy in the city on the distribution of HIV/AIDS service contracts between the city and nongovernmental organizations using federal Ryan White funding. A study conducted by the Community Preventive Health Institute found that between 2006 and 2007 there was a maldistribution of contracts among the five boroughs with Manhattan receiving 60 percent of the funds although it had only 30 percent of the city's residents living with AIDS. Using the boroughs as surrogates for minority representation, the study attempted to link the funding preference being given to Manhattan with higher AIDS death rates among minorities in the outer boroughs (Norwood 2007). Lost on the researchers was the fact that funding given to nonprofits in Manhattan for the delivery of AIDS services was not necessarily going to be spent in Manhattan. Nor did the study ever explain how the federal funding, only a small portion of total HIV/AIDS services funding, could determine deaths due to AIDS.

Possibly the most important difference between the delivery of services to minority HIV/AIDS victims and to their white counterparts were socioeconomic status and subsequent access to adequate health care that class differences produced. Upper-middle-class HIV/AIDS victims could access a private, nonprofit health care system, while low-income minorities at best had access to an overcrowded public health care system. This difference frequently meant not being tested and diagnosed early and not having access to the proper drugs once a diagnosis was obtained. For those who could not speak English, there were additional language barriers in communicating with the health care system (Ruiz 2005a). A study by Columbia University's School of Public Health in 1997 found a variance among races in treatment. It documented that whites were much more likely than blacks or Hispanics to have access to new drug regimens that were lowering AIDS death rates (Richardson 1997b). The NYC DOH reported that in 2004 Chelsea, a Manhattan neighborhood, continued to have the highest rate of newly diagnosed cases of the AIDS virus, with Central Harlem "close behind" (Santora 2006b). Yet those diagnosed in Chelsea were half as likely to die from AIDS as those in Central Harlem (Santora 2006b).

New York State Government's Response to HIV/AIDS

That New York State influenced the city's choice of public health tools to combat HIV/AIDS in different areas is not surprising, given the state's legal responsibility for the city, its role in financing city activities, and the exercise of state police powers. In many cases, the laws, relevant to disease prevention and education that the city's Department of Health was implementing, were state laws;

and regulations on testing and laws dealing with needle exchanges were exclusively under the jurisdiction of state elected officials and health authorities.

As AIDS treatment and prevention programs began to focus on issues of individual behavior, lifestyle, and privacy, the state frequently attempted to influence the city's implementation of state law in these areas, for example, in the case of bathhouse closings and needle exchanges, where the state amended its health code or waived parts of the criminal code giving the city the ability to act. But despite its power over the city, the state had no desire to become the level of government primarily responsible for the campaign against HIV/AIDS (Lambert 1989a).

In some cases, the state and city simply differed on which tools should be used. Much of this difference can be explained by the fact that city officials were much more responsive to constituencies at the local level and therefore felt somewhat more constrained to use every available tactic. The state pushed the city to regulate or close those commercial establishments, such as bathhouses, bars, and clubs, where at-risk sexual activity was taking place. The city was initially solicitous of the gay community's reluctance to shutdown these establishments, believing that they could be used at outlets to educate gay males about safe sex practices. Similarly, state officials were willing to give the city permission to experiment with needle exchange programs, since these programs required state authorization. City officials, however, in response to concerns from minority communities, were reluctant to exercise this authority until evidence of the efficacy of needle exchange programs from other countries and cities became so overwhelming that much of the opposition disappeared.

In 1983 Governor Cuomo and the New York State legislature established the AIDS Institute within the state's Department of Health. Over time the institute became the clearinghouse for most of the state's initiatives on HIV/AIDS, overseeing research as well as programming to combat AIDS through education and the delivery of health services (Sullivan 1983b). The institute was involved in the modification of the state's Medicaid program to address AIDS and funded activities in the city, such as the production of AIDS prevention materials by hospitals and clinics and funding grants to find homes for foster children with AIDS (Nix 1985; Gross 1987b). Over time the institute was also involved in initiating and funding community-based activities, including prevention programs targeting adolescents and women, services for children and families, home- and family-centered care, and peer-delivered education programs (NYS DOH AIDS Institute 2009).

In 1983 the state also created the New York State AIDS Advisory Council, which comprised representatives from state medical institutions, local health departments, and nonprofit organizations on the front lines in the fight against HIV/AIDS. The purpose of the council was to advise the state commissioner of health as well as the AIDS Institute. The council was at the forefront of the syringe access program (NYS DOH AIDS Institute 2009). The New York State Interagency Task Force, formed by Governor Pataki in 1997, coordinated AIDS services across approximately twenty state offices and agencies and attempted to decrease the duplication of services (NYS DOH AIDS Institute 2009).

The state exercised considerable influence over the city's delivery of services to AIDS victims through its Medicaid program, the jointly funded federal-state health insurance program for low-income families, elderly, and disabled. New York City's interest in Medicaid was not only because it funded many of the services being delivered to AIDS victims in the city but also because the state required the city, and all local governments in the state, to share in the cost of Medicaid. Since the city shared in the cost of Medicaid, any expansion in Medicaid services created additional funding requirements for the city, even though it was state officials who were making the expansion decisions.

As previously discussed, early in the AIDS crisis it became apparent to city and state officials that city hospital resources were going to be strained by the number of AIDS victims entering both the public and the not-for-profit hospitals. By 1985, AIDS was the most common diagnosis at Bellevue Hospital in Manhattan, the city's largest public hospital (Sullivan 1985). Since there was no cure, no long-term care alternative, and no specialized housing for AIDS patients, individuals with serious AIDS symptoms would enter the hospital and stay until they died. In 1987 the city's public hospitals reported that "AIDS victims cost 25% more per day to keep in the hospital, require 40% more nursing care, need twice as expensive drug treatment, and stay two weeks longer than the average patient" (*Economist* 1987).

The city, with the initiative of the NYS AIDS Institute, attempted to solve the problem by offering hospitals increased Medicaid reimbursement in exchange for being named AIDS Designated Care Centers. Hospitals would receive 20 percent more than the customary Medicaid per diem reimbursement rate in exchange for developing coordinated care plans for AIDS patients (Steinhauer 2001; Sullivan 1985). The state also issued new regulations making it easier for hospitals "to shift from intensive inpatient care to more appropriate levels of outpatient care," potentially decreasing the cost of care per AIDS patient (Sullivan 1985). Each participating hospital was also required to provide hospice care for dying patients either on site or elsewhere. By the mid-1990s, there were twenty-seven Designated AIDS Centers statewide with most being in the city (Navarro 1994b).

The state and city also attempted to solve the hospital costs problem by moving AIDS patients into managed care as they were doing with the bulk of the state's Medicaid population. But the move required approval of the federal Department of Health and Human Services. Advocates for AIDS victims in the city moved to block the proposal (Fein 1995). Studies on the limited experience of AIDS patients in managed care plans had found that many patients were unable to find a physician knowledgeable about AIDS, the drug coverage was inadequate, and waiting times for appointments were too long (Rosenthal 1996). In 1997 the federal government approved the state plan to move its Medicaid recipients into managed care. Federal officials ruled, however, that AIDS patients would not be "required to join for at least two years," while the federal government evaluated how the program would work for AIDS patients who enrolled in managed care voluntarily (Ferraro and Sorenson 1997). HIV/AIDS patients were never required to enroll in a Medicaid managed care plan. The state did create HIV Special Needs Plans in an attempt to carve out a lower-cost option for HIV/AIDS patients on Medicaid. But this remained optional for HIV/AIDS patients, as is managed care (NYS DOH AIDS Institute 2010).

Since only two-thirds of hospitalized AIDS patients qualified for Medicaid, the state also created a special pool of funds for those AIDS patients who were not eligible for Medicaid (Sullivan 1985; *Economist* 1987). For those AIDS patients who had private insurance that was running out, the state continued to pay the insurance premiums for these individuals calculating that this was less expensive than moving them to Medicaid (Sack 1991).

The state assisted the city in the delivery of services to AIDS patients through its regulatory controls over health facilities. As nonprofit groups responded to the need for long-term care facilities and housing for AIDS patients, the state had the authority to assess the need and to approve the opening of these facilities (Lambert 1988b). In the late 1980s, as the city's available hospital beds were filling up with AIDS patients, the state adjusted certificate of need regulations to allow for expansion of hospital bed space in the city (Lambert 1989d). Similar to state control over health facilities, the state also plays the leading role in training clinicians and medical personnel (NYS DOH AIDS Institute 2009).

In 1986, as a blood test to detect the AIDS virus became more reliable, the city and state cooperatively open several sites around the city where individuals could receive free AIDS testing. The state had already opened similar testing centers in other cities in the state. The state paid for the centers, but the city tested the blood samples (McQuiston 1986). Up to that point, the test was available in the city only through private physicians and at certain hospital clinics (Gross 1985).

One area of conflict between the state and the city was drug treatment. Mayor Koch was critical of Governor Cuomo for the state's failure to increase the number of drug treatment programs in the city to help reduce the spread of AIDS among intravenous drug users (Barbanel 1985b). In 1988, as intravenous drug use was becoming the primary road to AIDS infection, the city commissioner of health, Stephen Joseph, complained that although the city was making space available to the state to run substance abuse programs, the state was not allocating sufficient space to those with AIDS or at risk for AIDS (Marriott 1988).

Similar to the city, some of what the state does is funded by the federal government. The state's Harm Reduction Initiative is a program designed to "provide an array of services to substance abusers, their families and communities," primarily through contracts with service providers at the community level (NYS DOH AIDS Institute 2009, 12). CDC funds as well as federal Ryan White funding subsidizes drug treatment and mental health services for substance abusers (NYS DOH AIDS Institute 2009). In exchange for CDC funding, the state and city are required to engage in HIV prevention planning. This is done through the NYS Prevention Planning Group, comprising officials from across the state that provide the AIDS Institute with assessment and feedback on those programs that are effective (NYS DOH AIDS Institute 2009).

New York City's Response to HIV/AIDS and the Federal Government

With the exception of the Centers for Disease Control, the federal response to the AIDS crisis was too delayed and too weak for it to have a significant impact on the city's utilization of public health policy tools. Federal funding of Medicaid all along and the Ryan White Comprehensive AIDS Resource Emergency (CARE) Act in 1990 did enable the city and nonprofit groups to deliver more services to those with AIDS. But the Ryan White CARE Act, as well as Medicaid funding had little influence over the choice of services (Arno and Feiden 1986).

While there were clearly areas of federal expertise, such as medical research and national disease tracking, where the federal government could contribute to the fight against AIDS, the federal government's delay in acting prevented it from playing a leadership role for quite some time. The most important tool the federal government could, and eventually did, provide to the fight against HIV/AIDS was funding for research and the delivery of services to those with HIV/AIDS.

The first federal agency to make contact with the city was the Centers for Disease Control. Performing its legislatively mandated function, the CDC got involved in the AIDS policy in mid-1981 long before the rest of the federal government. The CDC formed a task force to investigate the outbreak and its causes. The CDC first reported the existence of AIDS symptoms in its Morbidity and Mortality Weekly Report in July 1981. Of the 116 cases reported, half were from New York City (Henig 1983). Not only did the CDC perform its mandated function of leading the nation in tracking the disease and its health impacts, but over time the agency also defined and redefined the disease as research clarified the symptoms and conditions directly related to HIV/AIDS.

The CDC also played a leading role in establishing HIV/AIDS testing protocols once a test was available in the mid-1980s. In 1986 the CDC issued recommendations for the expanded use of the HIV antibody test. These recommendations called for "confidential and anonymous HIV-antibody testing of persons at high risk in combination with risk reduction counseling, and for HIV-seropositive persons, referral of sex and needle-sharing partners for medical evaluation and testing" (US CDC 2006, 598). More recently, the CDC has issued recommendations to make HIV-antibody testing more accessible, better integrated into routine medical care, and more accommodating to "the diverse needs and preferences of persons seeking testing" (598).

The other half of the CDC's mission is education and prevention. In 1983 the CDC established the National AIDS Information Line for the purposes of disseminating the most up-to-date information on the disease and to assuage public concern (US CDC 2006). But it was not until 1987 that the CDC established a National AIDS Clearinghouse and initiated its America Responds to AIDS Campaign (US CDC 2006). As part of this campaign in 1987, the CDC initiated its National AIDS Information Campaign where it distributed public-service announcements "to broadcast media throughout the country" (Sisk et al. 1988). It also began funding prevention education demonstration projects in selected cities across the country, including New York, geared to increasing condom use. In the late 1980s, the CDC also began funding programs to train school administrators and school health personnel about addressing the AIDS crisis among school-aged youth (Sisk et al. 1988).

In 1988, under the leadership of Surgeon General C. Everett Koop, the CDC distributed a brochure about AIDS to every U.S. household (Sisk et al. 1988). The brochure, "Understanding AIDS," was a frank, if not blunt, presentation of AIDS and how it is transmitted (Levitt and Rosenthal 1999). In the introduction to the brochure, Koop noted: "Some of the issues involved in this brochure may not be things you are used to discussing openly. I can easily understand that. But now you must discuss them" (US CDC 1988, 1).

More recently the CDC has taken a leading role in responding to the increased incidence of HIV/AIDS among young minority males by developing and supporting prevention programs that target these groups. In 2007, CDC established a Hispanic/Latino Executive Committee. They have also developed prevention and education programs to respond to those minority males who, while not identifying themselves as gay or bisexual, place themselves at risk by having sexual relations with other minority males. The CDC has also implemented "social marketing campaigns designed to increase knowledge of HIV status and promote HIV risk reduction" among minority women (US CDC 2008).

The one significant disagreement that the city had with the CDC concerned the treatment of Haitians. In July 1983 the city commissioner of health, David Sencer, announced that he was removing Haitians from the city's list of groups at risk for AIDS. Sencer noted that the small number of Haitians with AIDS no longer warranted their being on the list, a status that had stigmatized the Haitian community (Sullivan 1983a; Altman 1983). In addition, Sencer noted that among the Haitians reported with AIDS, many were associated with other at-risk AIDS groups, homosexuals or intravenous drug users. Haitians claimed that their placement on the list of at-risk groups had resulted in discrimination (Altman 1983). The CDC declined to remove Haitians from its list of at-risk groups (Sullivan 1983a). Epidemiologists from the CDC noted that Haitians were ten times more likely to have AIDS than other Americans (Altman 1983). In 1990 the Haitian link to AIDS was raised again when the federal Food and Drug Administration recommended that certain Haitians be excluded from blood donations as a safeguard against contaminating the blood supply with the AIDS virus (Lambert 1990a). Haitian groups claimed that policy was irrational and discriminatory because Haitians had fewer cases of AIDS than many other groups (Hilts 1990). In New York City, Haitian groups protested this ruling and marched in Manhattan to protest the FDA's actions. Mayor Dinkins spoke at the demonstration publicly criticizing the FDA (*Washington Post* 1990). The FDA abandoned the policy later that year (Hilts 1990).

The primary contribution of the federal government to the fight against HIV/AIDS is funding. Throughout the 1980s, the federal government increased its funding for AIDS research. By 1990, "federal investment in AIDS research exceeded the level of funds invested in heart disease research" (Joseph 1992, 64). The federal government's primary financial contribution to the delivery of AIDS services was through Medicaid. As previously discussed, the federal government pays for approximately half of the cost of Medicaid with the state and New York City each paying a quarter. So although the city welcomed federal involvement in AIDS treatment through Medicaid, the AIDS epidemic put an additional fiscal burden on the city because of its share of Medicaid costs.

Other than Medicaid however, the federal government was slow to move on the financing of AIDS programs. By the mid-1990s, however, there were fewer than a dozen project grants administered by a variety of federal agencies designed to assist state and local governments in their anti-HIV/AIDS efforts. Most of the early grants were CDC funded programs targeted to state and local departments of health, schools, and nongovernmental organizations dealing with prevention. CDC grants also assisted state and local government with HIV/AIDS surveillance, the development of public information and education programs, and the education and training of health care professionals dealing with HIV/AIDS victims. As an example, the CDC funded Bronx Lebanon Hospital's Prenatal Care Initiative, which focused on HIV prevention and care for pregnant women (NYC Council 2007). The Department of Health and Human Services administered grant programs increasing the capacity of minority communities to deal with HIV/AIDS. Other federal project grants supported state and local government attempts to meet the long-term housing needs of those with AIDS and programs to address HIV/AIDS in the military (U.S. Catalog of Federal Domestic Assistance 2010).

Early on, Mayor Koch sought to include AIDS patients under the federal Supplemental Security Income (SSI) program for those who were disabled. The problem with the SSI program was that it required a two-year waiting period after the diagnosis before one could become eligible for benefits. Koch sought to have the two-year waiting period for eligibility waived, using the rationale that many AIDS patients did not live two years after the initial diagnosis (Barbanel 1985a). In the mid-1980s, the Social Security Administration reduced the waiting for people with AIDS to a few weeks allowing them to become eligible for presumptive disability payments (Arno and Feiden 1986).

It was not until 1990 with the passage of the Ryan White Comprehensive AIDS Resources Emergency Act (CARE) that the federal government committed itself to funding AIDS treatment on a significant level. The act provided funding for a variety of activities. First, it provided emergency money to cities for AIDS-related services. Most of this money was given to metropolitan areas according to a formula gauging the incidence of the AIDS outbreak (U.S. Department of Health and Human Services 1998). Second, the act provided funding to states that could be used to assist persons with AIDS to maintain their insurance or purchase drugs. A major part of this program was the AIDS drug assistance program whose funding became more critical as drugs began to play an increasing role in keeping AIDS victims alive and prevent the transmission of HIV. These funds could also be used for the provision of case management and counseling services for those individuals with AIDS, as well as mental and oral health. Third, the act provided grants for AIDS prevention projects, including pediatric AIDS (Smith 1996, 316–17; AIDS United 2011). The act prohibited the use of federal funds to pay for clean needles for intravenous drug users (Donovan 1996, 78). President Obama changed this regulation in 2009, allowing for federal funds to be used for needle exchange programs.

Federal funding for the act in the first year of the program, 1991, was more than $220 million. In 1999 New York City received $109 million in Ryan White funding, compared to $16.5 million from the CDC (Cohen 2000). In 1996 funding was added for the establishment of AIDS Education and Training Centers to provide training for health care professionals in the prevention and treatment of AIDS (U.S. Department of Health and Human Services 1998). In fiscal year 2002, total funding for the program was almost $2 billion (U.S. Department of Health and Human Services 2002). As a result of the 2008 recession and increased pressure on Congress to reduce the deficit, Ryan White funding did level off in the 2000s. In 2010, total funding was only a little more than $2 billion, of which New York State received $342 million (Kaiser State Health Facts 2012).

For New York City, the most relevant aspect of the Ryan White Act was Title I, which made emergency funding available to metropolitan areas with more than two thousand cases of HIV infection for the most recent five years (NYC DOHMH 2001). In 1991 the federal government distributed almost $88 million in Title I funding. In 2002 more than $600 million was distributed (U.S. Department of Health and Human Services 2002). In the early years of the Ryan White Act, the city received approximately 40 percent of Title I funds (NYC Mayor's Office of Operations 1992, 305). By 2001, as more metropolitan areas had established the need and infrastructure to deliver AIDS services, the city was receiving a little more than 20 percent of Title I funding, and this dropped to 17 percent in 2006 (U.S. Department of Health and Human Services 2001; Lite 2006b). On occasion both Senators Schumer and Clinton became embroiled in the reauthorization of Ryan White funding to make sure that New York did not lose its share (Lite 2006b). In fiscal year 2006, the city received almost $500 million in federal funding for AIDS services (Hays 2006).

Some of the Ryan White funding received by the city comes through the state. Under the 2006 revision and reauthorization of the Ryan White Act, the state received funds to establish HIV Care Networks across the state. These networks are "local associations of health care providers, community based organizations, community leaders and persons both infected and affected by HIV/AIDS," as well as city and state government representatives (NYS DOH AIDS Institute 2009, 57). These networks are mandated to identify populations at risk as well as to plan and provide necessary services. New York State established eleven networks, five of which are located in the city at the borough level (NYS DOH AIDS Institute 2009).

In 2001 the city Department of Health reported that, although Ryan White funds provided for only a small percentage of AIDS-related services for the city, the funding had helped to "establish and maintain" a safety net of services across the city. Ryan White Title I funding received by the city helped to fill gaps created by Medicaid. For those who were not eligible for Medicaid, the funding paid for home care and drugs. In the late 1990s, when the rate of AIDS-related deaths began to drop, many credited Ryan White Title I funding as being responsible for funding many individuals' drug regimens (Altman 1997). The funding also supported services not provided for by Medicaid, including "mental health services, housing placement, adult day care, transportation and nutrition" (NYC DOHMH 2001).

In the late 1990s, the Congressional Black Caucus and the Congressional Hispanic Caucus initiated legislation, signed by President Clinton, establishing the Minority AIDS Initiative Fund. The goal of the fund was to improve "HIV related outcomes for racial and ethnic minority communities disproportionately affected by HIV/AIDS" (Valdiserri 2011). The funds are distributed by agencies in the Department of Health and Human Services, including the CDC, the Substance Abuse and Mental Health Services Administration, and the Office of Women's Health (Valdiserri 2011).

Another federal agency involved in funding New York City's response to AIDS is the U.S. Department of Housing and Urban Development (HUD). HUD funds the Housing Opportunities for Persons with AIDS Program (HOPWA) that supports a range of housing activities from construction and rehabilitation to rental assistance. The program also funds some social services. In 2010 New York State received $1.1 million in HOPWA funds (Supportive Housing Network of New York 2013).

For almost two decades the activities of the CDC, Medicaid, and Ryan White constituted the bulk of the federal response to HIV/AIDS. In 2010 the Obama administration unveiled a national AIDS strategy. The goals of the strategy were "to reduce the number of new HIV infections, increase access to care and improve health outcomes for people living with HIV, and reduce HIV related health disparities" (White House Office of National AIDS Strategy 2011). Hampered by a recession and a Republican Congress's concerns with the federal deficit, the Obama strategy was not able to call on vast federal resources to fund new initiatives. Instead, the strategy called on those relevant federal agencies to better coordinate and direct the efforts with existing resources. As previously noted, there was a small increase in federal funding for the AIDS Drug Assistance Program, and New York City did receive some of these moneys (White House Office of National AIDS Strategy 2011). In 2010 New York State received almost a half billion dollars in federal funding for AIDS programs, not including Medicaid; and most of this funding went to the city. In addition to Ryan White, the primary sources of these funds were CDC prevention grants and HOPWA (AIDS United 2011).

Once experimental AIDS drugs became available, the federal Food and Drug Administration placed many of these drugs on the fast track, allowing them to be used before comprehensive testing. To the extent that the drugs were efficacious, this saved the city millions of dollars in treatment costs (Lambert 1989e). The AIDS Coalition to Unleash Power (ACT-UP), a group of AIDS activists who split from the GMHC in the 1980s, was instrumental in getting the FDA to move as fast as it did. ACT-UP was also involved in pushing the National Institutes of Health research agenda toward HIV/AIDS research.

Conclusion

The AIDS crisis is not over. As table 4.1 illustrates, the numbers of new cases and deaths may be declining, but the impact of AIDS on the health of the city is still significant. In 2011 there were more than three thousand new cases of HIV/AIDS diagnosed and slightly fewer than two thousand deaths attributed to

AIDS. There were 105,633 persons with HIV/AIDS living in the city. Not only is the number of persons with AIDS living in the city increasing, but also the number reported in table 4.1 represents only known cases of HIV/AIDS. Thus the spread of AIDS remains a major problem for city public health officials as well as dealing with a large population of individuals in need of medical treatment, education, and monitoring.

Because of the advent of drugs that limit the spread of AIDS among certain populations and allow persons with AIDS to live and longer and healthier lives, there is much less public fear about the disease, especially among those at-risk populations. Public health policy will have to address this new condition to prevent an increase in the spread of AIDS.

In 2005 a commission appointed by Mayor Bloomberg studied the challenges the city would face in its continued efforts to combat and deal with HIV/AIDS and made recommendations on the policy shifts needed to deal with the continuing but shifting crisis. The commission addressed two major themes in its recommendations: how to stop the continuing spread of HIV/AIDS, and how can the city adjust policies and resources to meet the needs of the growing number of New Yorkers who would live a long life with HIV (NYC Commission on HIV/AIDS 2005).

Because of the large number of individuals currently living in the city with HIV/AIDS, the provision of services has become a major piece of the public health effort against AIDS. The direct delivery of services to individuals with disease has normally not been a significant function of the public health establishment. This is normally left to private, nonprofit, or public medical providers. Many persons with HIV/AIDS lacked the economic wherewithal to demand these services on their own, and public health officials have acted as advocates in an attempt to stabilize the living situations of those with the disease. The passage of the Affordable Care Act may address some of this need. The 2005 mayoral commission also focused on the need to provide each HIV/AIDS patient with adequate case management services so that each victim has access to and receives a comprehensive continuum of care, including housing and mental health services (NYC Commission on HIV/AIDS 2005). Finally, public health officials needed to maintain contact with those persons living with HIV/AIDS as a means of continuing to educate them about remaining vigilant in not engaging in at-risk behaviors that would transmit the disease to others.

Throughout the crisis, however, prevention through education remains the primary public health tool in the fight against HIV/AIDS. Despite complaints by some public health officials who advocate the use of tools exercising more public control of individual behavior, public health officials continue to use the least invasive technique to educate individuals about risky behavior that could transmit the disease.

The 2005 mayoral commission noted that many members of at-risk communities were suffering from safe sex education "fatigue" as well as "treatment optimism," believing that, because current drug regimens could address HIV/AIDS, there was less of a need to avoid risky behaviors (NYC Commission on HIV/AIDS 2005, 18). In response to this emerging problem, the commission made several recommendations. First, the commission suggested that prevention education should be more effectively incorporated into the provision of medical care by clinicians who treat HIV/AIDS victims. Second, the commission recommended that public health officials utilize HIV-positive spokespersons in their education campaigns, similar to the CDC's "HIV Stops With Me" campaign (19). It did note, however, that federal guidelines governing CDC funding of education campaigns have inhibited, if not prohibited, the "social marketing of HIV prevention messages that would be the most effective in reaching the highest risk individuals and groups" (21). With regard to social marketing targeted to non-English speaking communities, the commission recommended that campaigns should involve "community leaders and stakeholders to maximize support, and should be culturally sensitive and not merely translations of English language campaigns" (21).

The 2005 mayoral commission also concluded that, in order to make education more effective, HIV/AIDS victims and those at risk would have to be given greater access to appropriate resources. In this regard they recommended making condoms more available through distribution at more venues frequented by those at risk. They also recommended the expansion of harm reduction programs as well the expansion of drug treatment programs to assist individuals in ending their addiction (NYC Commission on HIV/AIDS 2005).

The mayoral commission realized that in order for prevention to be effective, more individuals would have to be tested. The commission found that "most new HIV infections are transmitted by people who are infected but unaware of their status" (NYC Commission on HIV/AIDS 2005, 4). It estimated that approximately 25 percent of New Yorkers with HIV/AIDS did not know that they were infected. While the commission did not advocate for mandatory HIV testing, it did recommend that HIV testing be better integrated in normal medical care as well as increasing the availability of testing citywide (NYC Commission on HIV/AIDS 2005). It hoped that this would reduce the stigma of testing and encourage more to be tested. Also, linking testing to treatment would enhance the ability of public health officials to maintain contact with those who have HIV/AIDS and to continue efforts to prevent transmission to others (NYC Commission on HIV/AIDS 2005).

As part of the effort to test more at-risk individuals, the commission also recommended enhanced partner (contact) notification programs. Citing the innovative programs employed in Los Angeles and San Francisco that utilize the internet and email, the commission noted that "partner notification is more effective when conducted by public health officials than by the infected person or by the patient's physician" (NYC Commission on HIV/AIDS 2005, 19).

Minority politics and relations between the political system and the city's diverse groups have had a significant impact on public health policy on HIV/AIDS. In the early 1980s homosexuals were as much a minority group in the city as any racial or ethnic group. They were isolated within the city's social structure and were the victims of discrimination, even in a city with as liberal a reputation as New York. Their increasing political visibility and clout had a great deal to do with the city's response to AIDS, however delayed it was. At the same time the eventual response from all levels of government was based on the assumption, and later knowledge, that many other groups were at risk. There are those who argue that the slow response to the AIDS crisis occurred because the perceived initial and primary victim group comprised homosexuals (Shilts 1987).

In addition to its emerging political activism and power, one of the factors that served the gay community well in its response to AIDS was the community's ability to forge an organizational infrastructure to deal with the disease. The African American community, and to a lesser extent the Latino community, already had an organizational infrastructure, churches, but these institutions viewed AIDS with great antipathy. Since many of the African American and Latino HIV/AIDS patients were intravenous drug users or gay, they suffered from a double stigma. They were at a disadvantage as members of minority groups who suffered discrimination in society at large, but they were also stigmatized by their own communities.

In conjunction with the impact that the city's diversity has had on the development of policy tools to address the HIV/AIDS epidemic, the 2005 mayoral commission expressed concern about the continued stigma attached to those persons with HIV/AIDS. Although recognizing that "progress has been made in reducing HIV-related stigma," the commission recognized that prejudicial attitudes toward homosexuals as well as drug users remain (NYC Commission on HIV/AIDS 2005, 12). This prejudice manifests itself in the "loss of social support, persecution, isolation, job loss, and problems accessing health services," all of which inhibit those with HIV/AIDS from being tested and disclosing their status (12).

In 2012 the *New England Journal of Medicine* reported: "We are at a moment of extraordinary optimism in the response to the human immunodeficiency virus. A series of scientific breakthroughs including several trials showing the partial efficacy of oral and topical chemoprophylaxis and the first evidence of efficacy for an HIV vaccine candidate have the potential to markedly expand the available preventive tools" (Havlir and Breyer 2012, 1). Depending on its cost and availability, an HIV/AIDS vaccine will have significant impact on some of the behaviors that the public health community has been attempting to eradicate for decades. Will the presence of a vaccine cause the political system to defund many of the preventive tools as well the services being provided to those living with AIDS? Will the vaccine reach all of those at risk? And when the mode of prevention shifts from a complex set of educational and regulatory tools to a single injection or pill, what roles will the public health and medical communities play?

CHAPTER FIVE

HELPING A CITY LOSE WEIGHT

Obesity became a public health issue for several reasons. First, in the 1990s government health agencies at all levels, and especially the federal Centers for Disease Control and Prevention (CDC), reported an increased prevalence of obesity. This was true for both adults and children. By 2003 the CDC was reporting that more than a third of Americans were overweight and more than a quarter were obese (Kolata 2003). In the same year, the CDC also reported that there were "twice as many overweight children and almost three times as many overweight adolescents as there were in 1980" (Connelly 2003). Second, during the same time period, medical- and health-related research began establishing multiple links between obesity and negative health outcomes, including diabetes, heart disease, and several types of cancer. Third, given the preceding two facts, public health officials decided to make obesity an issue worthy of political system attention. In 2002 Surgeon General David Satcher stated that "obesity would soon succeed tobacco as the leading cause of preventable deaths" in the United States (Kolata 2002). To date, New York City has enacted possibly the most comprehensive set of policies to combat obesity of any jurisdiction in the United States.

New York City's, and the nation's, obesity problem is complex. The increased prevalence of obesity is due to various factors including poverty, poor access to nutritious foods, a decline in the number of citizens who engage in physical exercise of any type, and a significant shift in the way many Americans, and New Yorkers, eat. For New York the obesity problem is exacerbated by the fact the many New Yorkers suffer from hunger or, at the very least, food insecurity.

From a public health policy perspective, there is no consensus around a single policy tool or set of tools to assist the obese. There is opposition not only to the use of some potential tools, such as taxes, but also to any type of governmental intervention to address obesity. The opposition is based on a general antipathy toward government intervention in individual lifestyle choices, a belief that the science behind the links between obesity and negative health outcomes is still fuzzy, and a belief that many of the public health policy tools being employed in battle against obesity lack efficacy.

Obesity Defined

Being overweight and obese is due to an imbalance "between how much a particular body needs to maintain a certain weight and how much it is fed" (Henig 2006). The food we eat is digested and converted into fat, sugar, and protein. The fat and sugar that does not go to the liver to be used for bodily functions is stored in fat cells. Protein may also be converted into fat cells through excess amino acids. Weight gain occurs when there is an imbalance between the fat and sugar produced by eating and the fat and sugar needed for bodily functions. When individuals expend more energy than they consume in necessary fat, sugar, and protein, "enzymes start breaking stored fat into its component parts, which the body then burns for energy (Bor 2010). According to neurologist Barry Levin, genetics plays a major role in obesity because it governs how and how much fat, sugar, and protein are converted into energy and signals that individuals need to eat (Larkin 2007).

According to the CDC, "overweight and obesity are both labels for ranges of weight that are greater than what is generally considered healthy for a given height" (US CDC 2010a). In the mid-1990s, the World Health Organization (WHO) recommended using body mass index (BMI) as a means of establishing "graded classifications of overweight and obesity" that would permit "comparisons of weight status within and between populations" (WHO 2000, part 1, 6). Developed by a Belgian mathematician in the nineteenth century, what makes the BMI such a useful measurement tool is that it can be calculated using only a person's height and weight. Moreover, studies have shown that it correlates well with more reliable but complex measures of body fat (US CDC 2010b). It is "calculated by dividing a person's weight in kilograms by height in meters squared" (*Diet and Fitness* 2010). It can also be calculated using pounds and inches by multiplying the weight in pounds by 704.5 then dividing the result by height in inches twice. BMI is now such a common measure that BMI calculator charts are readily available (*Diet and Fitness* 2010).

The accepted but arbitrarily established convention is that those with a BMI below 18.5 are considered underweight and between 18.5 and 24.9 are at a healthy or normal weight. Those with a BMI between 25 and 29.9 are considered overweight and those with BMIs over 30 are considered obese (US CDC 2010a).

Although BMI establishes an indicator of obesity that allows for comparison, it has many limitations. The CDC advises that, while BMI may be a "fairly reliable indicator of body fatness for most people," it "does not measure body fat directly" (US CDC 2010b). Similar to the CDC, WHO states that BMI is a "useful" but "crude" measure of obesity (WHO 2000, part 1, 7). "It can be used to estimate the prevalence of obesity within a population" but it cannot "account for the wide variation in body fat distribution and may not correspond to the same degree of fatness or associated health risks in different individuals" (7). Many also advise that the location of body fat is as significant as how much body fat an individual has. Abdominal body fat, usually measured by waist circumference, is a strong "predictor of risk for obesity related diseases" (US CDC 2010b). For this reason, some obesity experts suggest waist circumference or a waist-hip ratio calculation as an additional measure of body fat (*Diet and Fitness* 2010).

Using BMI as a measure of obesity in children raises a number of issues. Since children's body composition varies as they age and also differs for males and females, BMI ranges for children and teens must "take into account normal differences in body fat between boys and girls and differences in body fat at various ages" (US CDC 2010a). As a result, the CDC opted not to use absolute thresholds or ranges for children but instead use age and sex specific percentiles plotted on CDC growth charts. "The percentile indicates the relative position of the child's BMI number among children of the same sex and age" (US CDC 2010c). For each gender beginning at age two years, "overweight is defined as a BMI at or above the 85th percentile and lower than the 95th percentile" and "obesity is defined as a BMI at or above the 95th percentile for children of the same age and sex" (US CDC 2010d). The CDC periodically adjusts its growth charts for children and adolescents. Similar to adults, both the CDC and the American Academy of Pediatrics advise that BMI is not a diagnostic tool. They suggest that other assessment tools be used to determine if excess fat poses a health risk in children and teens (US CDC 2010c).

Obesity's Health Risks

Obesity alone is not a negative health outcome. Many who are obese suffer no negative health outcomes attributable to their obesity. Beginning in the 1990s, however, a considerable amount of research established obesity as a risk factor for a variety of diseases and conditions. These include Type 2 diabetes, metabolic syndrome, hypertension, coronary artery disease, respiratory disorders, several types of cancers, osteoarthritis, liver and gall bladder disease, and infertility in both men and women (Kopelman 2007).

One of the strongest links research has produced is between obesity and Type 2 diabetes. The CDC reported that from 1990 to 1998 the prevalence of diabetes in the population increased from 4.9 to 6.5 percent, an increase of 33 percent. What additionally troubled public health officials was that those individuals diagnosed with diabetes were younger than those in the past. Formerly, Type 2 diabetes was most common in those older than age forty-five years. The increase reported for the 1990s was greatest for those in their thirties (Grady 2000). According to some experts, "more than 80 percent of cases of Type 2 diabetes can be attributed to being overweight or obese" (Web MD 2010).

More recently, links have been found between obesity and certain types of cancer. A 2003 study reported in the *New England Journal of Medicine* "found a direct relationship between the amount of excess weight and the risk of death from most cancers" (Brody 2003). For men, the study reported that a BMI between 30 and 35 doubled the risk of dying from liver cancer, while a BMI over 35 increased the risk to four and a half times those with BMIs below 25. For women the risk of death from breast cancer increased 60 percent for those with BMIs from 30 to 35 and 70 percent for those with BMIs over 35. The study cited the "lack of physical activity" associated with being obese as an important factor in the increased risk (Brody 2003).

For children and adolescents, the negative health impacts of obesity can occur during childhood, but there is some research suggesting that some of the consequences of childhood obesity may not occur until adulthood. Obese children and teens are at risk for cardiovascular disease including "high cholesterol levels, high blood pressure and abnormal glucose tolerance" (US CDC 2010e). Obese children are also at an increased risk for asthma, sleep apnea, and Type 2 diabetes. In 2002 the *New England Journal of Medicine* reported that "one in four extremely obese children under the age of 10 and one in five obese adolescents under that age of 18" had impaired glucose tolerance, a precursor to Type 2 diabetes (Reuters Health 2002). Four years later, research published in the *Journal of the American Medical Association* reported that children who have obesity-related diabetes "face a much higher risk of kidney failure and death by middle age than people who develop diabetes as adults" (Associated Press 2006).

Obesity Prevalence

The CDC began tracking the weight of the population in the 1960s. From the 1960s through 1980, the CDC reported that about 24 percent of men and 27 percent of women were "significantly overweight" (Booth 1991). The CDC also reported, however, that during this period the overweight figures for minorities, especially African American women, were higher at 44 percent (Booth 1991). In 1994 the CDC reported a significant increase in the number of overweight Americans from 1980 through 1991, with about a third of the population being overweight. For black non-Hispanic women the rate was 49.5 percent (Burros 1994). That same year, the CDC also reported that slightly more than 20 percent of teenagers were overweight compared to 15 percent in the 1970s (Russell 1994). In 1995 it was reported that 11 percent of all children aged six to seventeen were overweight compared to 5 percent in 1965 (*New York Times* 1995).

In the late 1990s, CDC reports began making a distinction between overweight and obese, according to the previously mention BMI thresholds. With its new standard measures (BMI $\geq$ 25 is overweight; BMI $\geq$ 30 is obese), the CDC was able to examine the National Health and Nutrition Examination Survey

(NHANES) from prior years and track the increase in obesity among adults and children. For adults, 13.4 percent were obese in the early 1960s. This increased to only 15 percent by 1980 but had increased to 23.3 percent in 1994 and 30.5 percent in 2000. In 2000, 64.5 percent of the population was reported to be overweight (Flegal et al. 2002). There were significant differences in obesity prevalence across population groups. While non-Hispanic whites had an obesity prevalence of 28.7 percent, African American obesity prevalence was at 39.9 percent, and Mexican American prevalence was at 34.4 percent. Women were slightly more obese than men, but the differences in prevalence for race and ethnicity were much greater for women than for men in 2000. The CDC also reported that extreme obesity (BMI $\geq$ 40) also increased from 2.9 to 4.7 percent of the population from 1994 to 2000 (Flegal et al. 2002).

In 2006, using the NHANES, the CDC reported that between 1999 and 2004 only a slight increase in adult obesity occurred from 30.5 to 32.2 percent. Among women there was no reported increase in obesity and among men an increase from 27.5 percent in 1999 to 31.1 percent. The percentage of those reported to be overweight increased slightly to 66.3 percent (Odgen et al. 2006). For the NHANES conducted in 2007–8, the reported adult obesity prevalence was 33.8 percent, a slight increase from 2004. The CDC analysts concluded that compared to the 1990s, "the increases in the prevalence of obesity previously observed do not appear to be continuing at the same rate over the past 10 years particularly for women and possibly for men" (Flegal et al. 2010, 235).

For children the NHANES allows for obesity prevalence (BMI $\geq$ 95th percentile on the appropriate age and gender growth chart) comparisons going back to the 1970s. At that point obesity prevalence was 5 percent for those children aged 2–5 years, 4 percent for those children aged 6–11 years, and 6.1 percent for adolescents aged 12–19 years. The only difference between boys and girls was in the middle group where the obesity prevalence for boys was 4.3 percent and for girls 3.6 percent (Ogden et al. 2002). By 2000 the CDC was reporting a childhood obesity prevalence of 13.9 percent. The prevalence for children ages 2–5 years was 10.3 percent, for children ages 6–11 years the prevalence was 15.1 percent, and for adolescents ages 12–19 years, the prevalence was 14.9 percent. In the 2–5 years age group, the girls were slightly more obese than the boys and in the 6–11 year age group, the boys were slightly more obese than the girls. There was no gender difference in prevalence among adolescents (Ogden et al. 2002; Odgen et al. 2006). By 2004 overall child obesity prevalence increased to 17.1 percent. Prevalence for the 2–5 year age group increased to 13.9 percent, for the 6–11 year age group prevalence increased to 18.8 percent, and for adolescents ages 12–19 years, the prevalence was 17.4 percent. The obesity prevalence rate for non-Hispanic black youths was 20 percent and for Mexican American youths 19.2 percent (Ogden et al. 2006). Between 2004 and 2006, there were no significant changes in child obesity prevalence (Ogden et al. 2008). Similarly in 2008, no significant increases in overweight prevalence were found (Ogden et al. 2010). In 2013 the CDC reported that nineteen states had reported decreases in obesity rates for preschool aged children between 2008 and 2011. New York was one of the nineteen states with a decrease of .3 percent. No specific cause was cited for the decrease (US CDC 2013).

While the leveling off of obesity prevalence for children is certainly a positive sign, there are still some troubling aspects, as the report failed to explain why (Parker-Pope 2008). In addition, a 2004 cross-national study of adolescent obesity in industrialized countries found U.S. adolescents at the top (Nagourney 2004). Most important, the prevalence figures leveled off at their highest rates. Almost a third of U.S. children and more than a third of adults are obese. And among some racial and ethnic groups, the prevalence figures are even higher.

In 2012 Mayor Bloomberg reported that 60 percent of New Yorkers and 40 percent of public school children were overweight or obese (NYC Office of the Mayor 2012). But New York City has not collected data on obesity comparable to that collected by the CDC. It did conduct a Health and Nutrition Examination Survey (HANES) in 2004. HANES covered adults twenty years of age and older. As a result it has limited but not absolute comparability with the CDC's NHANES for 2003–4. Other than that, the only data the NYC Department of Health and Mental Hygiene (DOHMH) have collected on obesity are from a Community Health Survey (CHS) that has been conducted since 2002 and a Youth Risk Behavior Survey (YRBS) conducted in odd years beginning in 1997 (Norton 2010). The CHS relies on self-reported height and weight to calculate BMI and is of limited reliability, although it can be used to track trends over time. The NYC YRBS is conducted in conjunction with the CDC. It is based on a self-administered anonymous questionnaire completed by a sample of New York City public high school students (NYC DOHMH 2010a). New York City does not have obesity prevalence measures for the 1990s, the period during which national obesity prevalence increased significantly.

New York City's 2004 HANES reported that 25.6 percent of the population was obese and 61.7 percent was overweight (NYC DOHMH 2010b). The 2003–4 CDC NHANES reported that 32.2 percent of the population was obese and 66.3 percent was overweight (Ogden et al. 2006). If one assumes comparability of the two samples, this suggests that the city's adult obesity problem was less severe than the nation at large (NYC DOHMH 2010b). Similar to the nation, the 2004 NYC HANES reports differences in obesity prevalence among ethnic and racial minorities. While non-Hispanic white obesity was reported at 21.8 percent, non-Hispanic black obesity was reported at 32.4 percent, and Hispanic obesity was reported at 32.5 percent. The 2004 HANES reported New York Asian obesity at 6.6 percent (NYC DOHMH 2010b).

New York City's Community Health Survey has tracked BMI, based on self-reported height and weight, since 2002. For 2004, the year in which the city also conducted its first and only HANES, CHS reported obesity prevalence at 21.7 percent, approximately 4 percentage points below the HANES prevalence measure of 25.6. Overweight prevalence according to the 2004 CHS was at 55.1 percent compared to 61.7 percent reported by the 2004 HANES. Between 2002 and 2008, the CHS obesity prevalence measures indicated a stabilization of obesity, similar to earlier discussed national trends; although the 2008 obesity prevalence of 22.6 percent is the highest, 4.2 percentage points higher than that reported in 2002 (NYC DOHMH 2010c).

Similar to the 2004 HANES, the city CHS indicated significant variation in obesity prevalence among racial and ethnic groups. In 2002 white non-Hispanic obesity was at 14.2 percent, black non-Hispanic obesity at 25.7 percent, Hispanic obesity at 22.9 percent, and Asian obesity at 5.1 percent. The relative differences among racial and ethnic groups hold for the 2008 CHS although prevalence for each group increased by approximately 2 percentage points. Disaggregated CHS obesity prevalence measures also indicated differences among income groups. Dividing neighborhoods into high, medium, and low poverty, the 2002 CHS reported a 23.7 percent obesity prevalence for high-poverty neighborhoods, a 17.7 percent prevalence for medium-poverty neighborhoods, and 13.5 percent obesity prevalence for low-poverty neighborhoods. For the 2008 CHS, the relative racial and ethnic differences were similar, but all three neighborhood income groups increased by several percentage points (NYC DOHMH 2010c).

The city's Youth Risk Behavior Survey has included obesity prevalence measures since 1999 and is conducted every odd year. Surveying public high schools students in the city, with BMI based on self-reported height and weight, the obesity prevalence measures from 1999 through 2007 also indicated stability in obesity prevalence. In 1999 reported obesity prevalence was 9 percent. This increased to 13.3 percent in 2003 but decreased to 11.5 percent in 2007 (NYC DOHMH 2010d).

In 2003 DOHMH and the city Department of Education conducted a survey of a "representative" sample of public elementary school children (NYC DOHMH 2003). Taking height and weight measures from each child, the survey was able to calculate BMI. The results indicated that 24 percent of city public school children were obese and 43 percent were overweight. When disaggregated for race and ethnicity, the survey found that 16 percent of white students, 23 percent of African American students, 31 percent of Hispanic students, and 14 percent of Asian students were obese (NYC DOHMH 2003). Compared to CDC figures for elementary school children nationwide in 2000, New York City elementary school children were much more obese than the nationwide elementary school student body (Perez-Pena 2003).

In 2009 city health officials examined the fitness records of those city children enrolled in kindergarten through eighth grade who participated in the Department of Education's NYC Fitnessgram program during 2007–8. They found that 21 percent of the students were obese and 39 percent were obese or overweight. Disaggregating for race and ethnicity, white and Asian students tended to be less obese, Hispanic students tended to be more obese, and black students' obesity percentage was equal to the aggregate percentage (NYC DOHMH 2009a). A year later, the same program reported that the number of obese or overweight students in New York City schools had increased by 1 percent. Compared to CDC data for children nationwide, New York City schoolchildren have more of a weight problem than other children by approximately 5 percent (Hartocollis 2010c). In 2011, however, the Fitnessgram program reported a 5.5 percent decrease in obesity among New York City schoolchildren. Decreases occurred across all grades and races. While noting that the decrease was small, DOHMH Commissioner Farley noted, "What's impressive is the fact that it's falling at all" (Hartocollis 2011).

The Fitnessgram Program offers the possibility of actually measuring the incidence of obesity by systematically measuring BMI throughout the NYC schools. Since 2007, because the Fitnessgram program has been expanded and now covers a majority of New York City public school students, the city has the ability to gauge obesity more accurately over time (NYC Department of Education 2013).

The Causes of Obesity

For the political system to develop and employ public health policy tools to combat obesity, the causes of obesity and its recent increase must be understood. Though medical research can explain how people gain weight, evidence-based research explaining the reasons behind the increase in obesity over the past three decades is limited. Exacerbating this challenge to develop an effective public health policy is a consensus that obesity is the result of genetic, sociocultural, economic, and environmental factors and also political causes. Even more problematic are views that the roots of obesity can be found in individual lifestyle choices and the resulting at-risk behaviors.

Most obesity researchers agree that genetics plays a role in individual obesity. One study of parents and their biological children who were adopted found a relationship between the BMIs of the two groups. The same study found no BMI relationship between parents and their adopted children (Kolata 2007). Nevertheless, genetics cannot explain the recent increase in obesity since there has been no significant change in the gene pool in that short amount of time.

Much of the recent discussion on the causes of obesity has centered on the decline of physical activity on the part of population. The roots of this decline are multifaceted and are related to both long- and short-term factors. And while much of the focus has been on children and adolescents, the decline in physical activity applies to adults as well. Throughout the 1990s, the CDC documented the decline in self-reported exercise among adults (Wetzstein 1997). That the United States has over the past several decades become a much more sedentary society is suggested in the changing nature of not only labor in the United States but also leisure time activities. Fewer Americans make their living doing physical labor. Computers and new technology have replaced physical labor not only at work but, along with television, as a primary source of recreation. Obesity experts admit that while more exercise will not cure the obesity problem, it can make obese and overweight individuals healthier and may help them lose enough weight to decrease risk factors for various diseases and conditions (Krucoff 1997).

In 2010 a study conducted at Temple University found that "sixth graders who participated in a school-based health program were less obese by eighth grade than a group of similar children who did not" (Rabin 2010). The program included physical activity as well as healthier eating (Rabin 2010). But faced with budget cuts, schools at all levels have cut back on physical education. And one survey conducted by the CDC in the 1990s found that the majority of gym classes that remained emphasized traditional sports more than "lifetime fitness activities such as jogging, aerobic dance, and swimming" (Cohen 2000). A 1990 Youth Risk Behavior Survey reported that "only 37 percent of high school students reported getting at least 20 minutes of vigorous exercise three or more times a week" (Russell 1994). In 1984, 60 percent of high school students reported exercising regularly (Russell 1994). After-school activities have also been affected. With both parents working, many more children are "often confined indoors after school for safety reasons" (Brody 2004a).

Children today spend more hours watching television or at the computer than previous generations. The increased time children spend with media and technology is either the cause of less physical activity or the result, possibly both (Hillier 2008). Research has found a relationship between how much television a child watches and the likelihood of being overweight (Finholm 1997). A small sample study of California schoolchildren conducted in the late 1990s found that children who reported watching less television and ate fewer meals in front of the television experienced a decrease in their BMI (Robinson 1999). A long-term study of more than a thousand children in New Zealand concluded the amount of "time children spend watching television is a better predictor of obesity than what they eat or how much physical activity they get" (Bakalar 2005b). A more recent study involving adults found that those who "cut their viewing in half for three weeks used about 120 more calories a day" than a group of adults who continued their normal viewing habits (Rabin 2009).

The higher prevalence of obesity among minority children in urban areas has led to research focusing on the "built environment" and its impact on obesity (Lopez and Hynes 2006). Except for those who live in rural areas, the environment within which most Americans live is manmade. It is dominated by varying types of land use, buildings of various heights and densities, and transportation systems (Perdue 2008). Implicit in the concept of the built environment is the hypothesis that "neighborhood conditions represent the broader social and community contexts within which individual behaviors such as physical inactivity, sedentary activities, and poor diet might occur, thus leading to increased obesity risk" (Singh et al. 2010, 504). It includes land use issues such as proximity to supermarkets, parks, and jobs as well as negative land uses such as toxic facilities, abandoned buildings, and vacant lots. It also considers infrastructure such as sidewalks, street trees, lighting, and mass transit. Finally it considers social environmental issues such as poverty, segregation, and crime (Lopez and Hynes 2006).

Research on the built environment suggests that inner cities include additional risk factors for being obese and overweight (Lopez and Hynes 2006). Many low-income inner-city neighborhoods contain environmentally hazardous facilities, as well as abandoned buildings and vacant lots. Combined with higher-than-average crimes rates, these communities are neither safe nor attractive for walking or play. Crime and inner-city toxicities also keep adults and children inside, discouraging physical activity (Lopez and Hynes 2006).

Data from the 2007 CDC National Survey of Children's Health have, in part, confirmed the hypotheses about the impact of the built environment on obesity (Singh et al. 2010). The study found that "the odds of a child's being obese or overweight were 20–60% higher among children in neighborhoods with the most unfavorable social conditions such as unsafe surroundings, poor housing, and no access to sidewalks, parks and recreation centers than among children not facing such conditions" (Singh et al. 2010, 503). The study found that children who lived in communities with the most unfavorable social conditions were more likely to watch television and engage in recreational computer use more than two hours per day and more likely to be physically inactive than those children living in communities with more favorable social conditions. "Obesity and overweight prevalence increased consistently in relation to fewer neighborhood amenities and less health promoting built environments" (507). This relationship remained even after controlling for socioeconomic status, although the relationships were strongest for the lowest-income households (Singh et al. 2010).

A limited study of the impact of New York City's built environment on obesity was conducted in 2002 using data collected from a sample of adult volunteers recruited from all five boroughs, organized by census tracts (Rundle et al. 2007). The study found that tracts that were more pedestrian friendly had lower BMIs. Pedestrian friendly was defined as being more population dense, having greater access to mass transit, and having a more even mix of residential and commercial land uses (Rundle et al. 2007).

Another primary focus for those seeking the causes of the recent increase in obesity is America's changing eating habits. In 1999 the federal government reported that 45 percent of a household's food budget was spent on food eaten away from the home (Moore 1999). Another study reported that 30 percent of family meals are prepared outside the home, "regardless of family income" (Squires 1998). "In 1970, 26% of food dollars was spent on food prepared outside the home" (Dumanovsky et al. 2009). By 1981 this had increased to 40 percent and by 2001 it was almost half (Dumanovsky et al. 2009).

Another recent change in American eating habits is snacking, especially by children and adolescents. A study reported in 2010 that there had been a significant increase in children's snacking habits, "eating occasions outside meals," from the late 1970s to the early 2000s (Piernas and Popkin 2010, 401). The study reported that children were eating three snacks per day and that snacking was providing children with almost 30 percent of their daily calorie intake. Moreover, the study reported a change in the content of the snacks being consumed with more "energy dense" salty snacks, sweetened caloric beverages, and increased portion sizes (Piernas and Popkin 2010).

A primary culprit in the increased prevalence of obesity has been the fast-food industry with its inexpensive high-calorie meals. In the 1990s many of the fast-food chains increased their portion sizes in order to compete with other chains. A 2004 U.S. Department of Agriculture and Harvard Medical School study reported that more than 30 percent of children ate fast food regularly; and that the typical fast-food meal contained "187 more calories, 9 more grams of fat, 26 more grams of added sugars, 228 more grams of sugar-sweetened drinks and less fiber, milk, fruits, and nonstarchy vegetables than non fast-food meals" (Brody 2004a).

Although it was not a variable in the "built environment" studies, access to healthy food is a factor in the built environment's impact on obesity. Studies have documented that "proximity to stores stocking healthier food choices has measurable effects on health," and some have hypothesized that one reason for higher obesity rates among low-income residents of the inner city is that those residents face "barriers to achieving a healthy diet" (Perdue 2008).

The existence of "food deserts" in low-income neighborhoods and their impact on health has been documented (Rothstein and Dehesdin 2010). One study found that "for each additional supermarket located in a census tract, fruit and vegetable consumption increased by as much as 32 percent" (McMillan 2004). And other studies have found that the presence of supermarkets in census tracts is associated with a lower prevalence of obesity, while the presence of convenience stores was associated with a higher prevalence (Morland et al. 2006). The distribution of fast-food restaurants, convenience stores, and supermarkets that sell fresh produce "varies considerably by neighborhood" and lower-income neighborhoods have much less access to healthy foods than higher-income neighborhoods (Hillier 2008). A 2007 study by the NYC DOHMH found that "stores in Harlem were half as likely to stock low-fat dairy products and seven times less likely to sell common vegetables than stores twenty blocks south on the Upper East Side of Manhattan" (NYC DOHMH 2007). The small grocery stores and convenience stores that populate the low-income urban neighborhoods do not stock the healthiest and freshest foods. They tend to overstock energy dense, high-caloric foods (Perdue 2008). Lacking automobiles, inner-city residents must either use mass transportation to purchase more nutritious food or rely on the smaller stores in their neighborhoods that lack the fresh produce and the greater variety of foods offered by larger supermarkets located elsewhere in the city or suburbs.

In low-income inner-city neighborhoods, food insecurity, "the limited or uncertain availability of nutritionally adequate and safe foods," has been linked to an increased risk of obesity (Adams et al. 2003). While this link may seem "counterintuitive," food insecurity that occurs in neighborhoods where the amount and variety of food for purchase are limited may result in the "consumption of high energy low cost foods" (Adams et al. 2003). According to Joel Berg, executive director of the New York City Coalition Against Hunger:

> Hunger and obesity are flip sides of the same malnutrition coin. While some of the hungriest and poorest Americans eat so little that they lose weight, many others with a marginally better ability to get food, eat food of such poor nutritional quality that they gain weight. Nutritious foods are frequently more expensive than less nutritious alternatives. In October, 2007, a gallon of milk cost $3.84 on average, but two liters of cola were $1.23. Potatoes cost 52 cents per pound but lettuce cost $1.49, broccoli $1.53 and strawberries $2. (Berg 2008)

East Harlem, a neighborhood where food insecurity is present, has the highest obesity prevalence in the city. The neighboring Upper East Side, with low food insecurity, has the lowest obesity prevalence in the city. The Upper East Side has more grocery stores and green markets giving those residents "more nutritious choices" (Crawford 2005). "East Harlem has more bodegas, fast food restaurants and emergency food programs," many of which rely on surplus donations that may not be the most nutritious (Crawford 2005).

Another reason why obesity prevalence is greater among low-income Americans is the cost of eating healthy. The "inflation adjusted price of a McDonald's quarter-pounder with cheese . . . fell 5.44 percent from 1990 to 2007 . . . but the inflation adjusted price of fruit and vegetables . . . rose 17 percent from just 1997 to 2003" (Singer 2010).

The concern over childhood obesity has also focused on the role that parents play in their children's weight. Because of the increasing amount of food that children eat outside the home, parents clearly have less control over what their children eat than in the past, but parents still have considerable control over what and how much their children eat (Brody 2005). One study involving preschoolers found that "the most important factor in the amount children eat is the amount put in front of them" (Bakalar 2005a). Another study noted the significance of parental and cultural attitudes toward eating as a possible determinant of childhood weight problems (Charbonneau 2002).

In addition to fast-food restaurants, the food industry has also been implicated in the increase in obesity rates, especially among children. One aspect of the role of the food industry in increasing obesity has been changes in the food produced. In the 1970s corn surpluses resulted in the production of high-fructose corn syrup, a low-cost sweetener. Many food and drink companies, including Coca Cola and Pepsi, jumped at the chance to lower their production costs without decreasing quality. But some have suggested that the body metabolizes fructose differently from natural sugars, resulting in greater fat storage (Kakutani 2003). There is a debate about how much high-fructose corn syrup contributes to obesity compared to other sugars. Some have argued that "when it comes to calories and weight gain, it makes no difference if the sweetener was derived from corn syrup, sugar cane, beets or fruit juice concentrate" (Brody 2009). Yet other research has found that, unlike glucose that is processed by the liver and used or stored depending on whether the body needs it, fructose "bypasses the process and ends up being quickly converted to body fat" (*New York Times* 2008a). Others have suggested that "fructose can blunt feelings of satiety" and cause overeating (Brody 2004b).

A second aspect of the industry's role in increasing obesity prevalence is marketing. The food industry produces sales well in excess of a trillion dollars. It spends a great deal of money "to promote consumption of high calorie processed foods" (Ebbeling et al. 2002, 478). In 2002 the food industry spent $10 billion in direct media advertising and another $20 billion on indirect marketing; the latter includes toys and games given away at fast-food restaurants and advertising on school logos and scoreboards (Duenwald 2002). As far back as the 1960s, the food industry began targeting children in its advertising campaigns, dominating children's television advertising. While there are documented links between watching television and childhood weight gain, there has been no direct link established between the food advertising aimed at children and obesity (Ives 2004). Some companies have voluntarily decided to cease any advertising to children younger than twelve years (Neuman 2010).

A third element of the food industry's involvement in increased obesity prevalence is portion size. A 2002 study by Young and Nestle reported that "marketplace portion sizes" have not only increased over time but were now exceeding "standard serving sizes by at least a factor of 2" and in some cases as much as a factor of eight (Young and Nestle 2003, 231). Both the U.S. Department of Agriculture (USDA) through its food guide pyramid and the Food and Drug Administration (FDA), through its food labeling, have established standard serving sizes. The study by Young and Nestle (2003) examined not only popular restaurant foods but also a sample of packaged foods found in grocery stores. They also researched changing serving size directions in popular cookbooks. They found that for all categories of food examined, the marketplace portion size exceeded the standard serving size defined by the USDA and the FDA. But even more significant, they found that the marketplace portion sizes offered over time had increased. Since the 1970s, the eight-ounce soda became the twelve-ounce soda and, in some fast-food and convenience stores, the twenty-ounce soda or, in some cases, sixty-four-ounce. The two-ounce muffin of the 1970s became the six- or seven-ounce muffin today (Duenwald 2002). Although the Young and Nestle (2003) study could not draw a direct link between people consuming these larger marketplace portions and obesity, "the trend toward larger marketplace portions has occurred in parallel with rising rates of obesity," possibly due to increased energy content of portion sizes (Young and Nestle 2003, 233; Nestle 2003).

Recently, some food companies have admitted partial responsibility for the increasing obesity prevalence, and a few have changed their behavior in limited ways. In 2005 Proctor and Gamble and Kraft Foods introduced one-hundred-calorie packs of many of their snack foods, all of which contained fewer calories than their previously individually packaged snack foods (Warner 2005a). In 2011 McDonald's announced that it was reducing the size of the portion of french fries in its Happy Meal and adding fruit in order to reduce the calories by 20 percent (Strom 2011). Coca-Cola enlisted several sports figures and funded a nationwide middle school program emphasizing "exercise and healthy living" (Warner 2005b). Some snack food producers have made changes in their packaging, and some soft drink companies voluntarily decided to stop selling sodas in school cafeterias and vending machines (Strom 2007). In 2006, the Better Business Bureau created the Children's Food and Beverage Advertising Initiative, a self-regulating program designed to address the type of food advertising targeted to children under twelve. Despite the obvious limitations of a corporate self-regulating program, many of the largest food producers have joined (Better Business Bureau 2014).

New York City's Programs to Combat Obesity

Because of the multifactorial nature of obesity causation, any attempt to combat obesity must involve a variety of public health tools with multiple targets. Similar to asthma, obesity provides another example of the necessity of seeking "health in all policies" (World Health Organization 2010). Moreover, the probability that any one tool will be successful in decreasing the prevalence of obesity is relatively small. Beginning in 2008, obesity rates in the city leveled off for some population groups and declined for preschool age children. Whether any program was related to these shifts is not clear.

Table 5.1 displays the tools currently being used by the city to combat obesity. In 2012 Mayor Bloomberg convened a multiagency Obesity Task Force, which later that year issued a report, Reversing the Epidemic, with twenty-six proposals to further the city's antiobesity programming (NYC Obesity Task Force 2012). Not all of its proposals have been adopted. For example, because of intransigence at other levels of government or the city's own political system, tools such as taxes on sugared food and drinks and zoning to limit fast-food outlet location have not been employed by the city. The city has, though, employed a two-pronged approach in other respects, implementing some programs citywide while other programs are targeted to areas of high obesity prevalence (Van Wye 2010).

TABLE 5.1
Public Policy Tools Addressing Obesity

MONITORING AND SCREENING
New York City
Department of Education, Fitnessgram: Assesses student health-related fitness (including BMI), which schools then share with parents
Federal government
CDC: Has played the primary role in defining and measuring obesity

EDUCATION (PREVENTION/PUBLIC)
New York City
Department of Health and Mental Hygiene
Campaigns against sugared beverages
DOHMH staff (together with local nonprofit groups): Host cooking demonstrations to provide nutritional information to customers as part of bodega program
DOHMH staff: Hold nutrition education workshops and cooking demonstrations at select farmers markets
DOHMH: Works with community organizations to raise nutritional awareness and promote the purchase healthier foods (at area bodegas)
Department of Education
Encourages schools to communicate with parents about constitutes healthy lunches and snacks
Sends letter to parents seeking to enlist them in the fight against obesity
New York State
Targets Just Say Yes to Fruits and Vegetables Program to food stamp recipients
Federal government
FDA's 1990 Nutrition Labeling and Education Act: Requires nutrition labels, including calories on packaged foods
Surgeon General's report (2010): "Call to Action to Prevent Overweight and Obesity"

Michelle Obama, Let's Move Campaign: Fosters more childhood physical activity, less TV/video time

National Heart, Lung and Blood Institute: We Can Program

Nonprofit groups

Community organizations: Participate in Healthy Bodega program by helping to raise nutritional awareness

EDUCATION (DAY CARE TRAINING STAFF, SCHOOLTEACHERS, STUDENTS)

New York City

Department of Health and Mental Hygiene: Staff offer day care staff training on nutrition via workshops, newsletters, and a curricula tool kit and encourage increasing physical activity in children

DOHMH and the Department of Education's Move to Improve Program: Trains teachers to integrate physical activity into all areas of classroom activities

New York State

Eat Well Play Hard Program: Supports DOHMH staff in offering nutrition lessons for children in childcare settings; extended to third grade

Healthy Kids, Healthy New York: Sponsors after-school initiative tool kit

Active8Kids program, State Department of Health, and Department of Education: Instills in children (before age 8) a daily regimen that includes nutritious eating, physical activity, and less TV and video game time

Tool kit for school administrators, teachers, and parents

Nonprofit groups (example)

New York Academy of Medicine Healthy Eating Active Living Program: Geared toward schools in low-income communities

EDUCATION (BODEGA OWNERS AND GREEN CART VENDORS)

New York City

Department of Health and Mental Hygiene

Healthy Bodega Initiative, DOHMH: Educates bodega owners to carry more nutritious and fresh foods and provides bodega owners with training on dealing with fresh produce and improving store layouts and food displays to accommodate new products

DOHMH staff: Assist bodegas in applying for licenses to sell fresh produce in front of stores

Green Cart Program, DOHMH staff: Hold workshops in several languages to teach prospective green cart owners how to complete the permit application, how to purchase produce and attract customers, and how to run a small business

Compiles Green Cart regulations on location and products sold

REGULATIONS (BUSINESS, RESTAURANTS)

New York City

Department of Health and Mental Hygiene: Imposes calorie-posting requirements on restaurants with 15 or more locations nationally (fines for noncompliance)

Federal government

Federal Trade Commission: Children's Advertising Review Unit

TABLE 5.1 (continued)

REGULATIONS (BODEGAS)

New York City

Department of Health and Mental Hygiene

Healthy Bodegas Initiative, DOHMH: Works with participating bodega owners who agree to stock and sell a variety of wholesome foods and display nutritious foods prominently in their stores

Star Bodega Program, DOHMH: Convinces a few bodegas to carry low-calorie drinks, whole-grain bread, and low-sodium canned vegetables and soup

Shop Healthy NYC: Encourages and educates food retailers in selected communities to stock and sell more healthy foods and encourages community groups to support participating retailers

REGULATIONS (FARMERS' MARKETS)

New York City

Department of Health and Mental Hygiene and Human Resources Administration: Encourage farmers' markets to accept food stamps and electronic benefit cards

REGULATIONS/INCENTIVES (GROCERY STORES)

New York City

Department of City Planning, Food Retail Expansion to Support Health (FRESH): Hopes to create new grocery stores in underserved areas; provides zoning and financial incentives to property owners, developers, and grocery store operators in those parts of the city underserved by grocery stores

Nonprofit groups

Food Trust: Works to persuade supermarkets to move to poor neighborhoods (funded in part by a grant from the Robert Wood Johnson Foundation)

REGULATIONS (CHILDCARE CENTERS)

New York City

Department of Health and Mental Hygiene: Mandates day care centers, as part of the permitting process, to adhere to a variety of regulations with the goal of early childhood education regarding healthy habits to combat obesity:

Minimum amount of physical activity per day

Limitations on television viewing

Regulations on fruit juice and low-fat milk

New York State

Child and Adult Care Food Program: Establishes minimum standards for meals and snacks at adult and child care centers

Monitors food service programs

REGULATIONS (PUBLIC SCHOOLS)

New York City

Department of Education

Issues regulations governing the fat content of breakfasts, lunches, and snacks served at schools to limit total fat, saturated fat, use of hydrogenated oils, and high fructose corn syrup (partly in response to federal regulations)

Issues regulations on the sale of food on school premises, including vending machines, school stores, or fundraising activities:
Nutritional standards for approved snacks and beverages
Chewing gum, candy prohibited
Develops program that promotes nutritional education and physical activity (partly in response to federal regulations related to school meal programs)
New York State
Active8Kids Program
Regulations governing food served in schools
Federal government
Instructs school districts that participate in federal subsidized school meal programs to develop and implement a wellness policy (2004)
USDA standards for food served in schools, amended by Healthy, Hunger Free Kids Act (2010) and subsequent regulations

REGULATIONS (CITY AGENCIES)
New York City
All city agencies: Issue regulations for food purchased and served by all city agencies, including those contracting with city agencies and child care centers (includes vending machines)
Department of Design and Construction with DOHMH and Department of City Planning: Issues active design building regulations

SERVICE PROVISION
New York City
Department of Parks and Recreation
Shape Up New York Program: Offers an array of free noncompetitive family fitness classes at recreation centers and community centers throughout the city
Department of Education
Fitnessgram reports: Sent to parents to suggest ways in which child can improve healthy eating and exercise
Department of Health and Mental Hygiene
Healthy Bodegas Initiative
Gives bodegas free packages of apples and carrots to sell to customers
Supplies bodega owners with posters for their windows—Shop Healthy Here
DOHMH staff together with local nonprofit groups, as part of bodega programs: Host cooking demonstrations
Green Cart Program: Establishes new mobile food vending permits for carts that sell fresh fruits and vegetables in communities where little or no fresh produce is sold
Health Bucks Program: Distributes, through community organizations, coupons redeemable at farmers markets
MarketRide: Provides transportation from senior centers to grocery stores and farmers markets
New York State
Child and Adult Care Food Program
Reimburses cost of meals and snacks for qualifying individuals
Improves the nutritional quality of meals and snacks served in participating child and adult day care programs

TABLE 5.1 (continued)

Nonprofit groups
    Distribution of Health Bucks
Federal government
    Food stamp program
    Healthy Food Financing Initiative
        Funds efforts by communities to help bring grocery stores to underserved areas
        Assists those communities in developing ways to enhance access to nutritious foods
    Farmers Market Nutrition Program
        Allows the use of WIC coupons at farmers markets

FINANCIAL ASSISTANCE
New York City
    Grants financial incentives to developers building qualifying grocery stores in under-
        served areas
    Offers Green Cart microloans
    Provides Health Bucks subsidy
New York State
    Provides loan fund for developers/businesses building qualifying grocery stores in un-
        derserved areas (supported by Goldman Sachs)
Federal government
    CDC: Supports state and local prevention programs through the Putting Prevention to
        Work Program (supplemented by American Recovery Act)
    U.S. Department of Agriculture: Supports the school breakfast and lunch program
        with additional subsidies for fresh fruit and vegetables; NYS Child and Adult Care
        Food Program and the Just Say Yes to Fruits and Vegetables Program (food stamp
        recipients)
    Healthy Food Financing Initiative (2010)
Nonprofit groups
    Charitable organizations: Underwrite the cost of the Green Cart Program
    Just Food: Supports Community Supported Agriculture in low-income communities

Educating Citizens to Eat Better through
Private-Sector Regulation

The key to decreasing the prevalence of obesity is getting people to eat both less food and better food. For the political system to be successful, obese people must be informed that they are eating in a self-destructive way and then be given the information to make better choices. Because of the political system's limited legal and political ability to regulate individual and family behavior, the city is attempting to educate families and individuals about healthy choices. But in or-der to educate individuals in public eating establishments, those venues must be mandated to cooperate with city education programs. Restaurants make a profit by selling more food, so city regulations with the goal of getting individuals to eat better or less are not in the interest of businesses whose goal it is to sell as much food as possible, regardless of its health impacts. Since some of the most energy- or caloric-intense eating is associated with fast-food restaurants, public health officials saw the possibility of concentrating their mandate on a small number of restaurants, limiting the political opposition and overall cost of the program.

The mandating of calorie posting in fast-food restaurants is based on the assumption that "if consumers were provided with caloric information at fast food restaurants, many might select lower calorie items" (Farley et al. 2009, w1098). Mandating calorie posting was also based on the fact that few restaurants were providing customers with prominent "point of sale information about the ingredients or calories" in the foods being purchased and on the assumption that few restaurants would do this voluntarily (Rutkow et al. 2008). In 2007, prior to the implementation of the city calorie posting regulation, the DOHMH surveyed more than seven thousand customers at 167 randomly selected restaurants. With the exception of Subway restaurants, which were already prominently posting calorie information, fewer than 5 percent of respondents "reported seeing calorie information in restaurants where they had made a purchase" (Farley et al. 2009, w1099).

In late 2006 the Board of Health amended the city's health code requiring that certain fast-food restaurants "prominently post information on the caloric content of foods on their menus and menu boards" (Farley et al. 2009, w1099). The regulation applied only to those restaurants that on a voluntary basis had already made caloric "information available to the public in places other than their menus (e.g., the internet, tray liners, pamphlets)" (Rutkow et al. 2008). The board considered requiring several pieces of information about food items, including total fat, saturated fat, and sodium, but ultimately decided that caloric content was the "single most important piece of information for consumers" (Farley et al. 2009, w1101). The regulation did allow restaurants to supply additional nutritional information if they wanted to do so.

The regulation was opposed by the restaurant industry, which used both the city council and the courts in an attempt to block the implementation of the regulation. In addition to the belief that any information that would result in people purchasing less food was not in the interest of the industry, the New York State Restaurant Association (NYSRA) argued that "the laboratory testing to measure the calorie content of food items would be costly" (Farley et al. 2009, w1104). It also argued that providing calorie content information for all the food items available in some restaurants would be "impractical" (Farley et al 2009, w1104). The Board of Health's regulation did ease the burden somewhat by allowing restaurants to provide a calorie range on items where patrons can combine or customize their purchases (Farley et al. 2009).

The NYSRA sued the city in federal court, claiming that city's regulation was preempted by the federal Nutrition Labeling and Education Act (NLEA) and also violated the First Amendment of the U.S. Constitution. The federal court threw out the First Amendment claim but ruled in favor of the NYSRA on the preemption claim. While the NLEA regulations promulgated by the FDA have been interpreted as not applying to nutritional labeling by restaurants, they have been interpreted as applying to voluntary nutritional claims made by restaurants. Since the NLEA gives the FDA the right to regulate nutritional claims, the NLEA preempted "New York City from regulating 'nutrient content claims, including claims made by restaurants'" (Rutkow et al. 2008). The court reasoned that since those restaurants in New York City, subject to the Board of Health's calorie-posting mandate, were the same restaurants that were voluntarily providing their customers with nutritional information, this information could be categorized as a nutritional claim rather than a required disclosure. Therefore they could not be regulated by the city since those restaurants' claims were already regulated by the FDA (Rutkow et al. 2008).

In its ruling, the court made clear that if the city were to require nutritional disclosures by a larger, different group of restaurants, that regulation would not be preempted by NLEA. Rather than appeal the federal court's decision, the city decided to take the court's advice by rewriting the calorie-posting regulation. In late 2007 the revised regulation was reissued. The substance of the regulation was identical to one issued in 2006, requiring the posting of calorie content on all menus and menu boards. But this time it was applied to all restaurants in the city with fifteen or more locations nationally, not just those which were voluntarily supplying the information to consumers in some format (Rutkow et al. 2008).

Following the issuance of the revised regulation, the NYSRA sued the city again in federal court, this time claiming that even though the city was requiring all restaurants within a certain class to comply with the regulation, the calorie content information being required still qualified as a "claim" and therefore the city's attempted regulation should again be preempted by the federal NLEA. The federal court this time ruled in the favor of the city finding that what the city was requiring did not constitute voluntary claims (Rutkow et al. 2008). The NYSRA appealed the ruling, but the courts gave the city permission to implement the ruling pending appeal. The U.S. Court of Appeals ruled in favor of the city in February 2009, once again finding that the revised calorie-posting rule did not violate the First Amendment of the Constitution and was not preempted by the NLEA (Chan 2009).

Implementation began in July 2008. The restaurants in the city subject to the regulation composed approximately 10 percent of the city's restaurants (Amar 2009). "Restaurants that fail to comply with the rule can be fined $200 for first-time violations and as much as $2000 for repeat violations," but this type of violation has no bearing on routine restaurant health inspections (Amar 2009). Most restaurants complied with the regulation. The NYSRA reported that complaints from its members on the new regulation were few (Amar 2009). There was nothing in the Board of Health rule that guaranteed the accuracy of the calorie postings. While the federal NLEA requires that calorie postings on packaged foods "be within 20 percent of the food's actual content," there was no equivalent precision requirement in the city's restaurant calorie-positing rule (Jerome 2008). Some laboratory analysis of fast-food chain calorie counts found discrepancies by as much as 55 percent (Jerome 2008).

Given how recently the calorie-posting rule went into effect, there are no comprehensive evaluations of how effective they have been in reducing the caloric intake of those who frequent restaurant chains subject to the posting rule. In 2007 the DOHMH collected data on eating habits from a random sample of fast-food restaurants in the city. These data create a baseline against which data can be compared once it has been collected (Dumanovsky et al. 2009). A follow-up study in spring 2009 found that the number of customers who reported seeing calorie information increased from 27 percent two months prior to the calories posting rule to 64 percent two months after the rule went into effect (Huang and Dumanovsky 2009).

Two limited studies have been completed examining the impact of the rule. One study examined customer receipts and survey responses at a few fast-food restaurants in low-income neighborhoods in the city and in Newark, New Jersey, both before and after the calorie-posting rule went into effect (Elbel et al. 2009). The study confirmed that once the calorie content of food was posted on the menu and menu board, many more respondents reported seeing the information as opposed to when it was supplied on tray liners or in less visible parts of the restaurant. But the study also concluded that while 27.7 percent of the respondents who noticed the calorie postings "said the information influenced their choices," no decrease in the number of calories purchased was seen after the implementation of the rule (Elbel et al. 2009, w1110). A second study conducted exclusively at 222 Starbucks throughout the city, as well as Starbucks in Boston and Philadelphia, found that "after the law took effect, New York customers ordered 14 percent fewer calories from food than before" (Hartocollis 2010a). Most of the calorie decline came from customers buying less food or buying lower-calorie food items. When drinks were factored into the results, the total decline in calories from before the calorie posting to after was only 6 percent, but New Yorkers were still purchasing fewer calories than Starbucks patrons in Boston or Philadelphia (Hartocollis 2010a).

Promoting Access to Nutritious Food in Low-Income Neighborhoods

Although aggregate obesity prevalence for New York City is not as high as the nation, low-income minority residents of the city bear a disproportionate share of obesity prevalence, with rates much higher than the city and nation overall. City public health officials have responded with a campaign to attack obesity in low-income neighborhoods on several fronts. One of the more recent campaigns has been to change the food environment of low-income neighborhoods by providing them and their residents with greater access to more nutritious foods (Van Wye 2010).

The assumption behind this policy is that these neighborhoods, populated primarily by small food stores and fast-food restaurants, do not have the same access to fresh produce and nutritious food choices that exist in middle- and upper-income communities of the city. In 2004 researchers examined food stores in East Harlem and the Upper East Side looking for five recommended healthy foods for diabetics. "Only 18 percent of the East Harlem stores had all five of the recommended foods, compared with 58 percent of the Upper East Side stores" (Robinson 2005). In 2006 the New York Coalition Against Hunger examined the availability of food resources across the city. It "found that residents of low-income neighborhoods are forced to choose between bodegas and unhealthy restaurants because they lack access to larger grocery stores and farmers markets common in affluent areas" (Brustein and Robinson 2006).

One of the programs the city has implemented to increase access to nutritious foods in low-income neighborhoods is the Healthy Bodegas Initiative. This program, begun in 2006, has been targeted at communities in three boroughs: East and Central Harlem, the South Bronx, and North and Central Brooklyn. DOHMH commissioner Frieden stated "bodegas are essential food providers in our communities, but healthy options are often unavailable" (Santora 2006). The bodegas, small food stores, in these communities offer "fewer healthy options than supermarkets" but are the primary supplier of groceries in the communities (NYC DOHMH 2010e, 1). NYC DOHMH defined bodega as a store having two cash registers and that sells mostly food, including milk, but does not specialize in one item. As part of the program, officials in DOHMH work with bodega owners to carry more healthy foods. To participate in the program, bodegas had to agree to "stock and sell a variety of wholesome foods," "display nutritious foods prominently in their store," and "label and promote healthful items" (2). DOHMH has acted to increase demand for healthy food by working with community organizations and area residents to "raise nutritional awareness and promote the purchase of healthier foods" (1).

In the first stage of the program, participating bodegas agreed to carry low-fat milk as well as "display posters promoting low fat milk and distribute health information to customers" (2). DOHMH staff also promoted low-fat milk through "community organizations, health centers, schools and health fairs" (2). At the peak of the program, more than one thousand bodegas were participating in the milk program. In 2010 DOHMH reported that "21% of participating bodegas started carrying low-fat milk for the first time . . . 45% reported an increase in low-fat milk sales," and "70% of stores reported an increase in demand for low-fat milk" (2).

In the second phase of the program, DOHMH worked with more than five hundred bodegas in Harlem, the South Bronx, and North and Central Brooklyn to carry more fresh fruit and vegetables. One survey of bodegas in Harlem found that fewer than 5 percent carried fresh vegetables and many did not sell fruit (Campanile 2006). At the outset of the program bodegas in some communities were given free packages of apples and carrots so that they could sell them to customers for fifty cents and "buy one, get one free." When their free supply ran out, bodega owners were able to buy an additional limited supply of the snacks at half price as long as they continued to offer customers two for the price of one (Campanile 2006). DOHMH staff provided bodega owners with training on dealing with fresh produce and improving store layouts and food displays to accommodate the new products. To promote the program and inform the community, participating bodegas were given posters for their windows that stated "Shop Healthy Here" (NYC DOHMH 2010e). They also connected bodega owners with local fresh produce distributors. As a result of the program "53% of participating bodegas started stocking a wider variety of fruits and vegetables . . . 46% started carrying more fruits and vegetables . . . 32% reported that more customers bought fruit." In addition, "26% reported more customers bought vegetables" (3).

In 2008 DOHMH's Star Bodega program convinced a select number of bodegas to carry "low-calorie drinks, whole grain bread, low-sodium canned vegetables and soup, and unsweetened canned fruit" in addition to healthier snack foods, fresh produce, and low-fat milk (3). To promote the bodegas, DOHMH staff together with local nonprofit groups hosted cooking demonstrations to "provide nutrition information to customers and people passing by. Staff also helped owners apply for stoop-line licenses to sell fresh produce in front of stores" (3). Fifty-five bodegas participated in the program. Most were offering more nutritious food and reported that customers were buying it (NYC DOHMH 2010e). DOHMH staff also worked with community organizations to develop relationships with bodegas as a means to increase and maintain the supply of healthy foods sold and increase the demand for nutritious foods in the neighborhood (NYC DOHMH 2010e).

Despite the number of bodegas that participated in the program, the Healthy Bodegas Initiative did have problems. Some bodegas did not have sufficient shelf space for fresh produce, and other bodega owners were simply unwilling devote any space to a product whose shelf life was short (Gross 2008). Some bodega owners noted that even with DOHMH assistance, fresh fruits and vegetables are more expensive than the foods that the bodegas normally carry (Gross 2008).

In 2012 the bodega programs were renamed Shop Healthy NYC. More-targeted programs were initiated in two neighborhoods in the Bronx. The goals of the program were to get food stores in these neighborhoods to reduce un-healthy food advertising as well as to stock and more prominently display healthy foods, including fresh fruit and vegetables, healthy snacks, low-sodium canned goods, and water and low-calorie drinks. Staff members from the DOHMH ed-ucate storeowners about healthy foods and help the owners "stock and promote these foods" (NYC DOHMH 20013). Community groups are "encouraged to Adopt-a-Shop and support retailers who are increasing access to healthy foods as well as assist in recruiting small stores to participate in the program" (NYC DOHMH 2013). Because of the success of the program, it was expanded to three additional Bronx neighborhoods in 2013. Shop Healthy is also attempting to ex-pand access to more nutritious foods through its MarketRide program that pro-vides seniors from participating senior centers with transportation to and from nearby supermarkets or farmers' markets (NYC Food 2013).

A second program the city implemented in 2008 to increase access to food in low-income neighborhoods is the Green Cart Program. The goal of the pro-gram is to establish "1000 new mobile food vending permits for carts that will sell fresh fruits and vegetables" in communities where little or no fresh produce is sold (NYC Office of the Mayor 2008). Many affluent areas of the city were already served by street vendors selling fresh produce as well as the usual array of green grocers. Although the goal of the program was to place the carts in neighborhoods isolated from supermarkets, the major opposition from the pro-gram came from representatives of the food industry, which believed that green cart vendors outside their stores would "undercut their prices" (Danis 2008). Green grocers, many of whom are Korean, rallied on the steps of City Hall as a vote on the legislation neared. A spokesperson for the Small Business Congress, which represents the green grocers, stated that the green carts would threaten the livelihood of his members, many of whom already had profit margins as low as 3 percent (Zimmer 2008). The city council also expressed concern that the new green cart regulations on location, products sold, and food safety would be poorly enforced by the DOHMH or the police (NYC Council 2008).

The Green Cart Program was assisted by a $1.5 million grant from a chari-table organization used to "help green cart operators get up and running" (NYC Office of the Mayor 2008). The funding was used to "develop a branded and functional cart designed to help customers recognize green carts . . . to estab-lish a relationship with non-profit wholesalers that will result in a dedicated sup-ply of high quality and low cost produce . . . to create a loan fund . . . to help cart operators cover start up costs," and "to launch a coordinated marketing campaign to promote Green Carts" (NYC Office of the Mayor 2008). Green cart vendors who applied for and received permits were given access to microloans for startup purchases such as $2,000 for the cart (Collins 2009).

DOHMH staff held workshops, in English, Spanish, and Bengali, to teach prospective green cart owners how to complete the permit application, how to purchase produce and attract customers, and how to run a small business (NYC DOHMH 2010f). Most of the green cart vendors were immigrants (Collins 2009). In the first year of the program, 248 permits were allotted for green carts. The carts were placed in those parts of the city where surveys reported the lowest percentage of individuals responding that they had eaten fruit or vegetables on the previous day (NYC DOHMH 2009b).

A third program that the city uses to change the food environment in low-income neighborhoods is promotional activities surrounding farmers' markets. In the past decade, the number of farmers' markets in the city has increased, some of which are located near low-income communities. The city's farmers' market program has several facets. First, the city is encouraging farmers' markets to accept food stamps and electronic benefit cards in hopes that those who are eligible for food assistance will shop at farmers' markets (NYC DOHMH 2010g). Second, the city promotes food shopping at farmers' markets through its Health Bucks Program. Health Bucks are coupons redeemable at participating farmers' markets. They are distributed through community organizations in designated high-need areas of the city. Organizations must apply for and then distribute them to their constituents. Participating organizations must promote the use of the Health Bucks as well as track their use reporting back to DOHMH. At participating farmers' markets, individuals who spend five dollars in food stamps or with electronic benefit cards receive two dollars in Health Bucks, increasing their purchasing power (NYC DOHMH 2010h). In 2009 the city Health Bucks program produced $220,000 in sales of fresh produce. The DOHMH reported that the food stamp–Health Buck incentive has increased food stamps sales significantly at a number of farmers' markets (NYC DOHMH 2010i). Finally, through the city's Stellar Farmers' Market program, DOHMH staff members hold "nutrition education workshops and cooking demonstrations at select farmers markets" throughout the city with the goal of targeting food stamp recipients (NYC DOHMH 2010i).

Another way the city is attempting to increase access to nutritious food in low-income neighborhoods is by creating an economic environment conducive to larger grocery stores locating in these communities. In the past, restrictive zoning and parking limitations, in addition to low-income populations, resulted in fewer large grocery stores locating in the inner city. At times, bodegas themselves have organized to oppose city attempts to assist large grocery chains in locating in low-income neighborhoods. This was the case in the 1990s when a local development corporation, along with the city, sought to locate a Pathmark grocery store in East Harlem (McMillan 2004).

In 2009 the city and state announced the initiation of the Food Retail Expansion to Support Health (FRESH) Program. "The program provides zoning and financial incentives to property owners, developers and grocery store operators" in areas of the city "underserved by grocery stores" (NYC Economic Development Corporation 2009). The goal of the program is to create fifteen new grocery stores and upgrade ten existing ones. To be eligible, new grocery stores or those being renovated must "provide a minimum of six thousand square feet of retail space for a general line of food and nonfood grocery products intended for home preparation . . . provide at least 30 percent of retail space for perishable goods that may include dairy, fresh produce, fresh meats, fish and frozen foods," and provide at least five hundred square feet of retail space for fresh produce" (NYC Five Borough Economic Opportunity Plan 2009).

The FRESH zoning regulations allow "residential buildings to be slightly larger than otherwise permitted if they have a neighborhood grocery store on the ground floor" (NYC Economic Development Corporation 2009). Parking requirements will also be relaxed for some grocery stores that locate on pedestrian-oriented streets. Finally, grocery stores up to a certain size will be able to locate in FRESH-designated communities zoned for light manufacturing without having to obtain a special permit (NYC Economic Development Corporation 2009).

The FRESH Program includes financial incentives such as "real estate tax abatements, mortgage recording tax waivers and sales tax exemptions on purchases of materials used to acquire property or to construct, renovate or equip grocery stores" (NYC Economic Development Corporation 2009). This is designed to aid not only in grocery store construction but also in possible store expansion or improvement, such as upgrading refrigeration (NYC Economic Development Corporation 2009). New York State is also assisting this effort through the establishment of a loan fund, Healthy Food and Healthy Communities, supported by Goldman Sachs. And the federal government recently began subsidizing these efforts through the Healthy Food Financing Initiative.

Early in 2010, the city announced the first two grocery stores to receive benefits under the FRESH Program. Both are located in the Bronx (Lennard and McGeeghan 2010). A third grocery store in the Bronx was approved for support under the FRESH Program later in 2010 (NYC Economic Development Corporation 2010). Nonprofit groups such as the Food Trust and foundations have also been involved in the effort to "persuade supermarket operators to return to poor neighborhoods" (Strom 2007). By 2011 ten projects had been approved and several more were under consideration (NYC Office of the Mayor 2011).

Despite the implementation of the FRESH Program, the city has not fully employed zoning or tax incentives in the cause of increasing access to nutritious

food or decreasing obesity. The zoning code could be used to discourage or prohibit fast-food restaurants by "capping" the number of those restaurants allowed
to locate in some communities. This was proposed by a member of the city council but did not receive sufficient support. In 2008 the Los Angeles city council
"passed a bill to place a one year moratorium on the development of new fast
food restaurants in South Los Angeles," a low-income community with high obesity levels (Emerson 2009). New York City and State currently issue tax incentives for businesses locating in low-income areas of the city, but this includes
fast-food restaurants. Some have proposed the modification of the city's Industrial and Commercial Abatement Program, eliminating incentives for fast-food
restaurants to locate in low-income communities (Emerson 2009).

Education

Education is a primary tool utilized by the city to combat obesity. More than
most public health issues, combating obesity relies on individuals changing their
behavior. Education may be the only way to facilitate this change. Short of removing nonnutritious foods from the shelves of grocery stores and limiting access to restaurants and other outlets for unhealthy foods, the city is relying on
its residents to make healthy choices about how much and what to eat and engaging in physical activity. But in order to make healthy choices, individuals must
be supplied with the information that leads them to make the appropriate decision. Education includes mass education efforts targeted to all New Yorkers
but also includes efforts to target messages about obesity and eating healthy to
those New York City citizens and communities that are most at-risk.

The city's calorie-positing laws are one of the major pieces of the city's antiobesity education campaign. Of course, they impose a regulatory burden on the restaurant industry to supply the information even though the intent is public education. In addition to mandating that the private sector provide the public with
education, the city has embarked on its own public antiobesity education efforts. Much of the city's education efforts have been targeted against sugared
beverages. The primary media for the campaigns have been subway posters, brochures, websites, and videos posted on the internet. In 2009 the city's anti–
sugared beverage campaign adopted the theme "Are you pouring on the pounds?"
(NYC DOHMH 2009c). The campaign urged New Yorkers to "cut back on soda
and other sugary beverages" and "go with water, seltzer or low-fat milk instead"
(NYC DOHMH 2009c). In 2010 DOHMH continued the campaign with a
new poster displaying a cup of a sugared soda, claiming "Your kid just ate 26
packs of sugar" (NYC DOHMH 2010j). The point of the campaign was to educate New Yorkers that the sugar content of a thirty-two-ounce soda was equivalent to twenty-six packets of sugar. A twenty-ounce bottle of soda contained
the equivalent of sixteen packs of sugar (NYC DOHMH 2010j).

Much of the city's antiobesity education efforts are aimed at low-income minority communities, where obesity prevalence is highest. Much of the educational activity in at-risk communities is channeled through community organizations participating in these programs in cooperation with DOHMH staff.

Day Care and the Schools:
Combining Education and Regulation

A segment of the city's education efforts is focused on the city's youngest residents, those who attend group childcare centers licensed by DOHMH. As part of the licensing process, day care centers have been mandated to adhere to regulations with the goal of educating children regarding healthy habits to combat obesity. These mandates include a minimum amount of physical activity per day, limitations on television viewing, and regulations on how much fruit juice children can be served, low-fat milk requirements for those over two years of age, and the availability of water (NYC DOHMH 2010k). To further facilitate these mandates, DOHMH offers day care staff training on nutrition through a one-day training workshop, a curricula tool kit, and newsletters. As part of the city's Eat Well Play Hard Program, funded and supported by New York State, DOHMH staff members also make themselves available for nutrition lessons for children in childcare settings. The lessons are directed at children three to four years old and include the "importance of family meals, appropriate portion sizes, fun ways to be physically active as a family, and how to include fruits, vegetables and low-fat dairy into meals and snacks without increasing costs" (NYC DOHMH 2010l).

Part of the city's early childhood antiobesity campaign is also focused on increasing physical activity. Workshops and training for childcare center staff are focused on demonstrating "developmentally appropriate games and activities that staff can use in small spaces to get children moving" (NYC DOHMH 2010l). As part of the Eat Well Play Hard Program, this training has been extended to teachers working with children through the third grade (NYC DOHMH 2010l). Through DOHMH cooperation with other city agencies, the campaign to increase physical activity has been expanded to older children and adults as well. In conjunction with the Department of Parks and Recreation, the city sponsors the Shape Up New York Program, which offers an array of free noncompetitive family fitness classes at recreation and community centers throughout the city. These include step aerobics, walking, working with weights, and stretching (NYC DOHMH 2010m).

One of the principal agencies involved in the city's campaign to reduce childhood overweight and obesity rates is the Department of Education (DOE). Unlike attempts by DOHMH to educate the general public to eat healthier foods as a means of decreasing obesity, the DOE has much greater control over the food sold and provided to children on school property. With this control, DOE has attempted to regulate school food consumption to reduce obesity through a variety of mechanisms. First, DOE has issued regulations governing the fat content of breakfasts, lunches, and snacks served at schools by school personnel. Regulations limit total fat, saturated fat, hydrogenated oils, and high-fructose corn syrup. In addition, fresh fruit and vegetables are now part of the school meal diet. Some of the DOE changes have been in response to federal regulations since the federal government subsidizes the school breakfast and lunch programs. With a few exceptions for those with special diet needs, only low-fat or fat-free milk is served. All new food items are tested in a central test kitchen before they are approved for use in schools (NYC DOE 2010c). Second, DOE has implemented new menus in an attempt to change the food culture in the schools. In 2010, there were almost six hundred salad bars in school cafeterias; by 2013, there were more than a thousand (Cohen 2013).

A second set of regulations issued by DOE controls the sale of food on school premises through vending machines, school stores, or school fundraising activities that take place during school hours. The regulations include nutritional standards for approved snacks and beverages that limit total calories, fat as a percentage of total calories, saturated fats and transfats, and sodium. Fruit products with no added sugar as well as dried fruits and nuts are exempt. Items such as chewing gum, candy, water ices with no fruit or fruit juice, and foods with artificial sweeteners are prohibited (NYC DOE 2010c). The city schools have a number of programs, some in cooperation with community-based organizations, which educate children about nutrition and healthy eating through growing fruits and vegetables on school grounds.

DOE also encourages schools to communicate with parents about healthy eating. This might include communication on what constitutes healthy lunches and snacks as well as those foods that do not meet the DOE's nutrition standards (NYC DOE 2010c). In 2009 DOHMH and DOE sent a joint letter to the parents of city schoolchildren urging them to help combat obesity by using 1 percent or fat-free milk instead of whole milk for all children two years of age and older (NYC DOHMH/DOE 2009).

DOE also promotes physical activity and physical education, but unlike the food and nutrition regulations mandated by DOE, the physical education guidelines are recommendations (NYC DOE 2010c). Daily physical activity in the schools is encouraged but not required. In some schools, promoting physical education is difficult since gymnasiums have been converted to classrooms to address overcrowding. To compensate for the lack of daily physical education, DOE attempts to integrate physical activity into the everyday classroom setting. In conjunction with DOHMH, DOE participates in the Move To Improve Program, which trains teachers to "integrate physical activity into all areas of classroom academics" (NYC DOHMH 2010l).

To get parents involved in their child's physical activity, in the early 2000s DOE initiated the Fitnessgram program. This "consists of a series of exercises that measure" each child's "health related fitness, including body composition, muscular strength, flexibility, muscular endurance and aerobic capacity" (NYC DOE 2010a). The Fitnessgram report, sent to parents, as well as supplied to children in the third grade and above, summarizes each student's performance based on individual improvement as opposed to a standardized norm. But the report does suggest ways in which the child can achieve the "Health Fitness Zone," which is a measure relative to optimal performance for their age and gender (NYC DOE 2010b).

As in the case of asthma, DOHMH District Public Health Offices (DPHO) have a major role in mobilizing and educating areas of the city where obesity rates are high. Unlike asthma, however, DPHOs have had to first mobilize and build constituencies among community groups in order to more effectively attack the obesity problem (Hayes 2014). Nonprofit organizations have teamed up with the DPHOs and the schools in high-obesity neighborhoods in an attempt to develop new programs to attack the problem. One example is the New York Academy of Medicine's (NYAM) Healthy Eating Active Living (HEAL) Program implemented in several schools in East Harlem and the South Bronx. The overall goal of the program has been to "build school capacity" to change the school culture toward one that promotes health (Eichel 2011). The program includes establishing school wellness councils, curriculum development, professional development for teachers and staff, parent education, and schoolwide health promotion events (Eichel 2011). There has been some discussion to use the Fitnessgram Program to evaluate the impact of HEAL on the target schools. At the same time, however, cutbacks in school budgets and staff as well as the loss of school parent coordinators threaten the success of this and other such programs (Eichel 2011). NYAM was also one of the principal founders of Designing a Strong and Healthy New York (DASH), a coalition of nonprofits seeking to provide technical assistance and training to local governments across the state on issues related to healthy food system reform and designing the built environment to promote physical activity (New York Academy of Medicine 2013). In another example, the Community Health Care Association of New York State joined with DOHMH to form the New York City Obesity Prevention and Management Consortium. The goal of this effort was to attack childhood obesity through federally qualified health centers in the city's underserved neighborhoods (Community Health Care Association of New York State 2014).

At the initiation of Mayor Bloomberg in 2007, and with the assistance of the nonprofit Trust for Public Land, the Departments of Education and Parks and Recreation collaborated to implement the Schoolyards to Playgrounds program. The goal of the program is to convert hundreds of schoolyards, unused and sometimes locked on weekends and after school, into playgrounds for the surrounding community, when school is not in session. The impetus for the program came from Mayor Bloomberg's PlaNYC, which included the goal of increasing the opportunities for healthy activities by providing every New Yorker a park or park-like space within ten minutes of home (NYC Office of the Mayor 2007).

The city has also issued standards for food purchased and served by all city agencies, including those contracting with city agencies and childcare centers. The standards include regulations on transfats and caloric and sodium content limitations. The standards also promote the availability of fresh fruit and vegetables as well as water as a beverage (NYC Office of the Mayor NYC 2010). The city has also issued standards for vending machines in all city agencies, although these standards are not as stringent as vending machine standards issued for city schools (NYC Office of the Mayor 2009a).

Finally, as a result of the 2012 Task Force on Obesity, in 2013 the Mayor Bloomberg issued an executive order and the city council introduced legislation promoting "active design." The goal of these initiatives is to promote physical activity through the design of buildings and public spaces. For instance, in new or newly renovated buildings, stairways would be more prominent and user friendly to encourage greater use of the stairs as opposed to elevators. The executive order applied only to city-owned buildings but the legislation is designed to apply the principles of active design to all buildings being constructed or renovated in the city (NYC Office of the Mayor 2013).

The City Proposal to Bar the Use of Food Stamps to Buy Sodas and Ban the Sale of Large Sugary Beverages

In late 2010, the Bloomberg administration sought federal permission "to bar New York City's 1.7 million recipients of food stamps from using them to buy soda or other sugared drinks . . . The ban would affect beverages with more than 10 calories per 8 ounces, and would exclude fruit juices without added sugar, milk products and milk substitutes" (Hartocollis 2010d). The proposal stated that the ban would last for two years so that officials could examine its impact and then take further action (Frazier 2010). In 2004 the USDA, which administers the food stamp program, denied a request by Minnesota to ban junk food purchases by food stamp recipients. Congress also debated restricting food stamp purchases but never took any action.

In response to the city's proposal, a spokesperson for the New York City Coalition Against Hunger stated that the city was punishing poor people. "It's sending a message to low-income people that they are uniquely the only people in America who don't know how to take care of the family . . . The problem isn't that they're making poor choices, the problem is that they can't afford nutritious food" (quoted in Frazier 2010). Thomas Farley, the DOHMH commissioner, noted that food stamp recipients "could still purchase soda if they choose" but with their own money (Hartocollis 2010d). The proposal was supported by various groups including the Citizens' Committee for Children, the United Way of New York City, and the Center for Science in the Public Interest (Hartocollis 2010e).

In August 2011, the federal government rejected the city's proposal to bar food stamp users from purchasing soft drinks and beverages with too much sugar. One of the reasons stated for the rejection was that the proposal would have been too complicated to implement since the federal government would have had to communicate to grocers which drinks were allowed to be purchased with food stamps and which were not. At the same time, many viewed the decision by the USDA as a victory for the soft drink industry that lobbied against the city's proposal, as well as grocery stores, which complained that it would have been difficult for stores in the city to program their registers differently from those outside the city (McGeehan 2011).

At the mayor's initiation, in 2012, the New York City Board of Health issued a regulation that barred the sale of most sugary drinks larger than sixteen ounces. Mayor Bloomberg called the regulation the biggest step any city had taken to date to curb obesity. The regulation was scheduled to take effect in early 2013. The ban covered only those retail establishments in the city that received inspection grades from DOHMH (Grynbaum 2012a). In response to the Board of Health ruling, the beverage industry, together with several New York restaurant and business groups, sued the city. The suit contended that the Board of Health did not have the authority to "ratify the new rules unilaterally" (Grynbaum 2012b). The beverage industry and its allies prevailed in their suit at the two lower levels of the New York State courts. And in 2014, the New York State Court of Appeals ruled in their favor.

Economic Development and Obesity in New York City

Similar to many other public health issues, and as previously discussed, economic development is linked to the obesity problem. Economic development has freed much of the population from physical labor as the primary occupational activity. More recently, economic development has produced and made accessible a range of leisure activities that require little, if any, physical activity. While all of these developments have been welcomed, they have resulted in a decline in physical activity on the part of the population, in terms of both daily work and leisure time. In addition, economic development and particularly urbanization and suburbanization have separated much of the population from its food supply and made it dependent upon a profit-motivated food industry. Finally, as noted earlier, in parts of the city, economic development has produced a "built environment" that discourages physical activity through the absence of parks, environmental degradation, and crime, particularly in low-income communities. Economic development alone is not responsible for obesity. There were obese individuals before the industrial revolution, and there are many normal and below weight individuals today. Yet economic development and its negative externalities have both created the food deserts that exist in parts of the city and exacerbated the problems of limited food choices, in addition to the impact they have on decreasing physical activity.

Race in the City and Obesity

As previously noted, the prevalence of obesity is higher in low-income minority populated communities of the city. Obesity has become one of a number of health indicators demonstrating disparate health outcomes across socioeconomic classes and ethnic and racial groups in the city. As such, it is possible that obesity, similar to asthma, could have become a contentious political issue. But this did not happen. Why? Unlike asthma, with the obesity problem city officials did not need to be prodded by minority leaders and community groups to take action. With little attention being paid to obesity by the minority and low-income communities, the city embarked upon a range of programmatic activities to combat obesity.

Minority communities have not yet placed obesity high on their public health agenda. There are several possible explanations. First, as diffuse as the causes for asthma are, the causal factors related to obesity are even more diffuse and less visible. Minority groups and leaders were able to single out bus depots, idling school buses, and waste transfer stations as sources of asthma, even if these sources were not the entire story behind high asthma rates in minority communities. Aside from fast-food restaurants or bodegas, there are no visible sources that can serve as rallying points for the fight against obesity in these low-income communities. And in low-income communities, many bodegas and fast-food restaurants are minority owned and a source of employment in the community.

Second, the negative health impacts of asthma were tangible. The costs of asthma on the community and the individual could be easily observed and calculated. The negative impacts of obesity are less visible and more long term. Because of the multifactorial nature of diabetes or heart problems, the link between individual obesity and the onset of negative health cannot always be demonstrated, even though medical evidence has confirmed the link, and epidemiological correlation has confirmed the relationship at the community level.

Third, much more than asthma, obesity is viewed as a self-inflicted health problem. Like smoking and unlike asthma, obesity is viewed by many as an individual failing, either by adults themselves or by adults as parents. And despite the myriad of systemic causes of obesity, including television, the food industry, and the built environment, much of the public health response to obesity is based on the concept of individual responsibility. Given the multifactorial nature of obesity, the current state of evidence-based research, and the way the issue has been defined, minority leaders have a host of other health issues that they can use to highlight continued health disparities and discrimination in society. At present the causes of obesity are simply too widespread to mount a campaign of blame or responsibility.

New York State's Support of the City's Antiobesity Programs

New York State assists the city with both funding and programmatic support for the city's campaign against obesity, but the state does not play a leading role. The city has taken the lead in addressing obesity, and state programming is secondary to the array of programs being implemented by the city. With financial support from the CDC, the state constructed a strategic plan for overweight and obesity prevention. The report discussed the possible causes of obesity as well as strategies for intervention (NYS Department of Health [DOH] 2006). The city does receive state funding for some of its programs (Van Wye 2010). As previously noted, the city participates in the state's Eat Well Play Hard program targeted at childcare centers and designed both to increase physical activity and to promote the consumption of fresh fruit and vegetables among children older than two years of age (NYS DOH 2005).

Many childcare and senior care centers in the city also participate in the state's Child and Adult Care Food Program. Funded in part by the USDA, this program seeks to improve the "nutritional quality of meals and snacks served in participating child and adult day care programs. It establishes minimum standards for meals and snacks served, provides reimbursement for qualifying meals and snacks, and mandates ongoing monitoring of food service programs and training program staff" (NYS DOH 2005). The USDA also subsidizes New York State's Just Say Yes to Fruits and Vegetables Program. Just Say Yes is a nutrition education program targeted to food stamp recipients. The program funds nutritionists to "conduct nutrition educational sessions focusing on increasing fruits and vegetables" in the diet, food safety, and thrifty shopping (NYS DOH2010a). In the city, Just Say Yes has vans that appear at farmers' markets. Its staff conducts nutrition education sessions at food pantries, health fairs, and commodity food surplus centers (NYS DOH 2010b).

In 2005 the state DOH in conjunction with the state DOE embarked on the Activ8Kids Program implemented through local school systems. The goal of the program is to instill in children, before the age of eight years, a daily regimen that would include "consuming at least five fruits and vegetables; engaging in at least one hour of physical activity; and reducing screen time (TV and video games) to fewer than two hours" (NYS DOH 2007). To promote the program, the Department of Health produced a tool kit for use by local education agencies in the state. The tool kit gives school administrators, teachers, and parents information to assess the "school nutrition and physical activity environment; develop school wellness policies"; develop "nutrition guidelines for snacks, vending and fundraising"; and develop "best practices for promoting lifelong physical activity through school activities" (NYS DOH 2007). In 2008 the state published an additional tool kit geared toward after-school programs, Healthy Kids, Healthy New York (NYS DOH 2008).

In 2009 Governor Paterson proposed a tax on sugared sodas. The tax would levy one penny for every ounce of sugared soda and other sugared drinks (Hartocollis 2010b). Tax revenues would be used to offset the state's increasing health and medical care costs; but it was certainly hoped that many, induced by the increasing cost of sugared drinks, would purchase less. This proposal, similar to taxes on cigarettes, represented a new tool in the campaign against obesity but certainly not a new weapon in the public health arsenal. While advocates ran advertisements on television supporting the tax in which pediatricians spoke about the risks of diabetes in children, the beverage industry together with antitax advocates ran a much more compelling ad with a mother urging the public to keep Albany from meddling in family grocery shopping (Hartocollis 2010b). The proposal failed.

Federal Government Involvement in Antiobesity Activity

The federal government has a significant role in the nation's and city's antiobesity activities. The federal government's policies to promote nutrition predate the recognition of obesity as a public health problem. The 1990 Nutrition Labeling and Education Act required nutrition labels, including calories, on packaged foods. As a public health tool, the regulation was based on the simple premise that consumers were entitled to accurate information about what they were purchasing (Brownell et al. 2010). The FDA, the Federal Trade Commission (FTC), and the USDA all play a role in food marketing, although only recently has their regulatory authority been mobilized in a concerted effort to combat obesity. In 2006 the FTC urged "food companies to develop products that are more nutritious and to review and revise its marketing practices" (Warner 2006). At the same time, the FTC's Children's Advertising Review Unit began to consider "minimum nutrition standards for foods advertised to children" (Warner 2006).

The CDC continues to play the primary role in measuring the prevalence of obesity and has also funded antiobesity promotional activities as well as supporting city activities. Federal funding has been significant for the city in its fight against obesity. As far back as the mid-1980s, the CDC was funding its own advertising campaigns promoting physical activity and good nutrition (Burros 1996). And a CDC grant supported the production of the state's strategic plan for obesity and overweight prevention. The CDC also funds a great deal of the city's community-based antiobesity activities through the Communities

Putting Prevention to Work grant program (Van Wye 2010). The city has received millions of dollars from this program and received an additional $15 million as part of the 2009 American Recovery and Reinvestment Act (U.S. American Recovery and Reinvestment Act 2010). At the state level grants from the USDA support the state Just Say Yes and Child and Adult Care Food programs.

Efforts by the surgeon general and by First Lady Michelle Obama to publicize the issue have been extremely important in increased public attention and action. As the leading public health official in the country, the surgeon general has limited media attention and limited ability to publicize health issues nationally.

Surgeon General David Satcher's 2010 report, "The Surgeon General's Call to Action to Prevent Overweight and Obesity," gave legitimacy to obesity as a public health issue (U.S. Department of Health and Human Services 2010). The report documented the increase in obesity prevalence to date and current research on health risks. It then laid out focal points and strategies to combat obesity. As other research and reports have acknowledged, the surgeon general's 2001 report recognized that much of the fight against obesity would have to be fought by families, schools, and communities. As a result it was critical to provide these institutions with information and access to appropriate resources (U.S. Department of Health and Human Services 2010). Although the surgeon general's report increased the legitimacy of the issue as well as the media attention the issue was receiving, it is difficult to assess what impact the report had on state and local government action.

In 2004 Congress used the reauthorization of Women, Infants and Children (WIC) program to establish a requirement that "school districts that participate in federally funded school meal programs" develop and implement wellness policy (NYC DOE 2010c). New York City's Department of Education responded by developing a program that addressed nutritional quality of school meals, nutrition education and promotion, and physical activity and education. The policy engaged parents, teachers, students, and food service providers (NYC DOE 2010c). USDA also approved the use of WIC coupons at farmers' markets, as part of the federal Farmers Market Nutrition Program (McMillan 2004).

Probably the most influential role the federal government has played in the fight against obesity has been in the area of education and child nutrition. For decades, the USDA in conjunction with the Department of Health and Human Services (formerly Health, Education and Welfare) has issued dietary guidelines and has set minimum standards for food served in school cafeterias. For many years, health advocates have accused these federal agencies of issuing guidelines that cater more to the needs of the farm lobby than the health of Americans (Brody 2011).

In 2004, amendments to the federal Women, Infants and Children (WIC) nutrition program "established a requirement for school districts that participate in federally funded school meal programs to develop and implement a wellness policy," including "guidelines to promote student health and reduce childhood obesity" (NYC DOE 2010c, 2). In 2010 Congress passed and the president signed the Healthy, Hunger Free Kids Act. As a result of this law, in 2012 the Obama administration announced new rules and funding "that added more fruits and green vegetables" to federally subsidized school breakfasts and lunches (Nixon 2014; United States Department of Agriculture 2014). The new regulations also reduced the amount of salt and fat in school meals (Nixon 2014). Early in 2011 the USDA and Department of Health and Human Services issued "science based" Dietary Guidelines for Americans. The new guidelines, replacing the old food pyramid, "offer a wide variety of dietary options to help" Americans "eat better for fewer calories" (Brody 2011). As an educational device, the new guidelines will only be effective to the extent that families and those who have influence over food and meal choices employ the guidelines daily.

But there are inconsistencies in federal food and nutrition policy. While one branch of USDA is pushing new science-based food guidelines another branch of the department is promoting consumption of many of the products being discouraged by the guidelines (Moss 2010). Dairy Management, a nonprofit "marketing creation" of the USDA is supported by a "government mandated fee on the dairy industry" as well as a directly subsidy from USDA. Dairy Management is one of many USDA programs that promote consumption of U.S.-produced commodities regardless of their contribution to nutrition and antiobesity (Moss 2010). In the past Dairy Management has spent millions of dollars on advertising that promotes "the notion that people could lose weight by consuming more dairy products," a message that contradicts the new USDA dietary guidelines (Moss 2010). Probably the most visible promotion was the "Got Milk" campaign of the 1990s that was credited with "slowing the decline in milk consumption." In one instance, a USDA brochure urged pizza lovers to request half the cheese normally provided "even as Dairy Management worked with pizza chains . . . to increase cheese" (Moss 2010). Recently, some of Dairy Management's promotions have been curtailed by the FTC response to complaints by health and nutrition groups that many of the nutrition claims being made by Dairy Management promotions are false (Moss 2010).

The most recent assistance the federal government has given the city in its fight against obesity is the public attention by First Lady Michelle Obama. Early in the Obama presidency, Michelle Obama began the discussion on obesity and health when she created a vegetable garden on the White House grounds with the help of a local Washington, D.C., elementary school. Then, in early February, 2010, she announced the initiation of a national campaign, Let's Move, with "the goal of solving the challenge of childhood obesity within a generation" (White House 2010). At the announcement, the First Lady was joined by the secretaries of Agriculture, Education, Labor, and Interior, as well as the surgeon general. Members of Congress, mayors, and leaders from the medical, media, sports, entertainment, and business communities were also present. Supporting the Let's Move campaign, President Obama simultaneously created a Task Force on Childhood Obesity and gave it the responsibility to "conduct a review of every single program and policy relating to child nutrition and physical activity and develop a national action plan that maximized federal resources and set concrete benchmarks toward the First Lady's national goal" (White House 2010).

The Let's Move campaign seeks to involve parents, schools, state and local officials, communities, and children in the fight against childhood obesity. The focus of the program is on fostering more childhood physical activity, including less time in front of computers and televisions, and getting children to eat more nutritious foods, including smaller portion sizes. The Let's Move website lists strategies and programming for each of the five identified stakeholders in the First Lady's campaign (Let's Move 2010). In conjunction with the campaign, several major media companies, including Walt Disney, NBC, and Universal, committed to join the First Lady in increasing public awareness of obesity through the creation of public service announcements. Other nongovernmental groups including the American Beverage Association, the American Academy of Pediatrics, and the School Nutrition Association also joined the campaign (White House 2010).

Several executive branch agencies were also involved in the campaign. The FDA agreed to begin working with food retailers and manufacturers "to adopt new nutritionally sound and consumer friendly front of package labeling" (White House 2010). The USDA committed to revamping its food pyramid to encourage healthier food choices. Even before the Obama administration launched the Let's Move campaign, in 2005 the federal National Health, Lung and Blood Institute (NHLBI) of the National Institutes of Health initiated the We Can program, offering parents and communities resources to promote healthy eating and increased physical activity among children (US NHLBI 2013). In 2009 the New York City Children's Museum, with the assistance of the We Can program, began work on an evidence-based curriculum guide to combat childhood obesity (NYC Office of the Mayor 2009b).

In 2011 Obama administration began funding the Healthy Food Financing Initiative. Administered jointly by the Departments of Treasury, Agriculture, and Health and Human Services, the program is designed to invest funds "to help bring grocery stores to underserved areas and help places such as convenience stores and bodegas carry healthy food options," similar to New York City's program (White House 2010). Although New York City did not receive funding for the 2011 fiscal year, it did receive more than $3 million in funding for both fiscal years 2012 and 2013 (Healthy Food Access Portal 2014). Earlier, the Clinton administration launched the New Markets Tax Credit program in 2000 offering grocery store developers tax incentives. Critics have suggested that by itself the incentive is not large enough to induce grocery store location in low-income areas; but along with city efforts, the tax incentive could be helpful (McMillan 2004). Finally, the U.S. Department of Education worked with Congress in revamping part of the Elementary and Secondary School Act to provide funding to schools to develop plans to get children more active in and outside of school (White House 2010).

Conclusion

Obesity is the most recent major public health issues to be addressed by the city, state, and national governments. According to some recent measures, obesity rates appear to leveling off, and there have been some small declines in some populations, but it is probably too soon to tell whether any of the public health interventions have had an impact on obesity prevalence. Just as important, because of the variety of tools that have been employed by the city in the fight against obesity, it will be difficult to determine whether or to what extent any single tool has worked. There are simply too many tools employed simultaneously to isolate the effects of any single program.

Even more than the number of public health tools employed to address obesity, the number of possible sources of increased obesity prevalence confounds the formulation and implementation of policy, let alone the assessment of which tools are working. Surgeon General David Satcher stated that "the best approach to combating obesity is through physical activity" (Krucoff 1997). Throughout the course of the antiobesity campaign, there have been a group of health professionals who have argued that the focus of government policy should be on maintaining a level of fitness, regardless of one's weight. They argue that although exercise may not make someone thin, it will make him or her healthier (Krucoff 1997).

The built environment of low-income minority neighborhoods creates a range of potential independent variables influencing obesity. Some of these variables, including crime, the proliferation of fast-food restaurants, the popularity of computers and video games, and the lack of accessible parks and public spaces are more easily manipulated than others.

"Until recently, American approaches to diet, physical activity, and obesity have largely focused on the individual" (Brownell et al. 2010, 382). While public health policy tools can mediate many of the diffuse sources of obesity prevalence, ultimately it is individual behavior and the behavior of parents that may have the greatest impact on obesity. The tools available to public health policy makers are frequently perceived as "forcing people to behave in certain ways" (Brownell et al. 2010, 382). Yet much of public health policy making involves a blend of tools that focus on the individual, while recognizing collective responsibility (Brownell et al. 2010). In combating obesity, the challenge for public health policy is to educate individuals and families to make more intelligent choices, while structuring an environment that inhibits the least healthy choices and encourages the healthiest.

CHAPTER SIX

THE FIRST APPEARANCE OF WEST NILE VIRUS

West Nile virus arrived in the New York City metropolitan area in 1999. Approximately sixty individuals with the disease required hospitalization, seven of whom died (Mostashari et al. 2001). In the city, there were forty-four hospitalized and four fatalities (NYC Department of Health and Mental Hygiene 2003). For a short time, West Nile virus concerned public health officials and the public at large. It was the first known appearance of this disease in North America. "In 2003, West Nile Virus caused the largest outbreak of neuroinvasive disease ever recorded in the Western Hemisphere, with 9862 cases reported overall, including 264 deaths" (New York City Department of Health and Mental Hygiene [DOHMH] 2010a, 7). Mortality and morbidity rates, however, have remained low. But the disease's rapid spread throughout the country is evidence that West Nile virus will be a public health concern for many years (NYC DOHMH 2003).

Because it never affected many people, West Nile virus was never given the crisis status that AIDS, obesity, and asthma received among urban public health officials. Nevertheless, because the disease had never been seen in the North America before and could kill, it concerned the public. Just as important, West Nile virus and the city's response to its arrival illustrate the workings of the public health infrastructure in ways unlike the responses to other public health concerns. The appearance of West Nile virus in New York City can almost be treated as two distinct events. Its appearance in the city in the late summer of 1999 elicited an emergency response on the part of the city's public health system. With little knowledge of what it was dealing with and no time to plan, the city adopted emergency tools dominated heavily by the citywide spraying of pesticides to eliminate adult mosquitoes carrying the virus. Although the city's pesticide spraying was supported by state and federal authorities, there was a significant negative public reaction. Because the city learned from the 1999 experience with the virus and had the time to plan, its response to the anticipated appearance of West Nile virus during the summer of 2000 was far more comprehensive and premised on the city's hope to avoid citywide pesticide spraying if at all possible.

Among the public health issues facing the city recently, West Nile virus is unique. For the most part, neither the incidence of the disease nor the city's public health policy response had any racial, ethnic, or class aspects. In addition, the disease was neither caused by or had an impact on the city's economic development activities. Given the origin of West Nile virus in Africa and the Middle East, however, its appearance underscores the impact of international travel and global commerce on public health (Nash et al. 2001). As an important global city, New York City is susceptible to the introduction of new organisms, including human pathogens (Fish 2007).

Since 1999 West Nile virus has spread over much of the continental United States, generally following a westward progression. In 2005 mosquitoes carrying the disease were found in every state except Hawaii, Alaska, and Washington (Duenwald 2005). Nationally, West Nile virus deaths peaked at 177 in 2006. In 2009 there were 729 reported cases nationally with 32 deaths (U.S. Centers for Disease Control and Prevention 2010). In 2003 an official from the Centers for Disease Control (CDC) stated, "West Nile is probably never going to be one of our leading public health threats. But even if it continues like it is now, and West Nile kills about three hundred people a year, that's three hundred people, and you can't say that West Nile doesn't matter" (Perez-Pena 2003).

West Nile Virus

"West Nile Virus is a member of the Japanese encephalitis virus serocomplex," which contains a number of medically significant viruses linked to human encephalitis (Petersen and Marfin 2002). There is a close genetic relationship between West Nile virus and a virus isolated earlier in Israel, but how it got from the Middle East to North America remains unknown (Petersen and Roehrig 2001).

Most humans get West Nile virus through Culex mosquito bites, with the incubation period normally ranging from two days to two weeks. West Nile virus is kept alive through a mosquito-bird-mosquito cycle. The outbreak of West Nile virus in the city was preceded by "anecdotal reports of an extensive die-off among American crows and several other bird species in the most affected boroughs" of the city (Marfin et al. 2001, 730). This was the first time that "significant bird mortality" was attributed to the outbreak of the disease. Reasons for this are also not known (Hayes 2001). Because the disease was first misdiagnosed as St. Louis encephalitis, no connection was initially made between the bird deaths and the outbreak in humans (Nash et al. 2001). West Nile virus cannot be contracted by casual contact or caring for someone who is infected (NYC DOHMH 2010c).

The disease cycle lasts roughly from the spring through the early fall corresponding to the reproductive cycle of female mosquitoes (Petersen et al. 2003). To date, no one knows what percentage of those who are bitten by a mosquito carrying West Nile virus actually contract the disease; but a survey of one community in New York believed to be heavily infested with mosquitoes carrying the disease found that 20 percent of those infected developed the virus (Peterson and Roehrig 2001). The virus survives in the city over the winter through either surviving mosquitoes or infected birds that remain in the area during the winter months. There is also the possibility that the virus is reintroduced into an area each spring through migratory birds that are infected (NYC DOHMH 2010a). There is no vaccine for West Nile virus.

For the most part, West Nile virus produces mild flulike symptoms that last from three to six days. "The risk that a person will develop severe West Nile" virus from a mosquito bite is low, and most infections in humans are not clinically apparent (Altman 2002). "About twenty percent of infected people experience mild non-specific symptoms that resemble influenza, making diagnosis difficult without a blood test" (Altman 2002). For those with more overt manifestations, symptoms include muscle weakness, "malaise, anorexia, nausea, vomiting, eye pain, headache, myalgia and rash" (Petersen et al. 2003, 526). Diagnosis of West Nile virus relies on "clinical suspicion and on results of specific laboratory tests" (Petersen and Marfin 2002, E176). The most effective diagnostic method is detection of the West Nile virus antibody in the blood or spinal fluid (Petersen and Marfin 2002).

Older individuals have tended to experience more severe symptoms, including neurological diseases, such as encephalitis and inflammation of the brain; and meningitis, an inflammation of the spinal cord and brain. In addition, "advanced age is the most important risk factor for death" from the disease (Petersen et al. 2003, 526). For those who require hospitalization but survive, "substantial morbidity may follow" (526). "At discharge, fewer than half of patients hospitalized in New York and New Jersey in 2000 had returned to their previous functional level, and only one third were fully ambulatory" (Peterson et al. 2003). Among those who were hospitalized, one-year follow-up examinations found persistent fatigue and memory loss among a slight majority of patients, and difficulty walking, muscle weakness, and depression among a substantial minority (Petersen and Marfin 2002).

West Nile Virus Prevalence

In July and August 1999, New York City's health community became aware of a mosquito-borne illness affecting older New Yorkers. In late August, a disease specialist at Flushing Hospital Medical Center reported to the city's Department of Health (DOH) that two elderly patients had been identified with symptoms that looked like a neurological illness. Further investigation by the DOH found six additional cases of encephalitis in Queens, all within a sixteen-square-mile area. The eight individuals, between the ages of fifty-eight and eighty-seven years all had fever followed by "changes in mental status. All but one had severe muscle weakness," and four required ventilator support (Nash et al. 2001, 1807). Interviews with the eight individuals revealed no common exposure, but all reported engaging in outdoor activities around their homes (Nash et al. 2001). The initial diagnosis by public health experts was that these

individuals had St. Louis encephalitis, a virus that belongs to a larger group identified as Japanese encephalitis (Nash et al. 2001).

The city Department of Health's Bureau of Communicable Disease told
Flushing Hospital to send samples to the state Department of Health. The
city's Department of Health took blood samples as well and forwarded them
to the Centers for Disease Control, the federal agency responsible for identifying and monitoring diseases (Cohen 1999). The illness was first identified as
St. Louis encephalitis, a disease that occurs primarily in the southeastern
United States. The identity of the disease was later changed to West Nile virus,
a disease that is indigenous to Asia and Africa. The virus had appeared in Europe on a few occasions but had never been identified in the Western Hemisphere (Cohen 1999).

Shortly before the discovery of encephalitis in Queens, there were reports
of a substantial number of deaths among birds in the New York City area.
Since St. Louis encephalitis does not normally kill birds, no immediate link was
made between the bird deaths and the eight Queens patients hospitalized with
encephalitis (Nash et al. 2001).

By mid-September, there were fourteen confirmed cases of West Nile virus
with three cases resulting in deaths of elderly individuals in the city. Suburban
jurisdictions also began reporting cases of the virus (Lombardi 1999a). By the
end of the summer, there were sixty-one reported cases of the virus, with seven
fatalities, in the metropolitan area (Mahoney 2000). In 2000 the city's epicen-
ter for the disease was Staten Island where ten of the twenty-one persons hospitalized in the Northeast United States lived (Marfin et al. 2001).

Although the number of West Nile virus cases the city has experienced since
1999 remains small (table 6.1), the death rate of approximately 15 percent is still
noteworthy and has remained a cause of alarm among city health officials. In
addition, the median age of those reported with the disease has been over sixty
years of age in all but two of the years for which data are available, suggesting
that the elderly continue to be the most vulnerable group.

Overall, the total number of West Nile virus cases reported annually by
DOHMH has declined since its initial outbreak in 1999. This corresponds with
the declining number of birds found with the disease reported in table 6.1; but
it does not correspond to the number of pools found with infected mosquitoes.
Fewer humans are being reported with West Nile virus, and fewer birds are being detected with West Nile virus, but mosquitoes are still being detected with
the disease. Several reasons have been suggested by researchers at departments
of health in the metropolitan area for the decline in cases. First, "aggressive mosquito and larval control activities, particularly on Staten Island, may have reduced the infected mosquito population enough to diminish the virus' transmission to humans," despite the continued discovery of pools with infected

TABLE 6.1
West Nile Virus in New York City, 1999–2010

Year	Total Cases	Neuro-invasive Cases	Fever Only	Median Age	Deaths	Death Rate (%)	Birds Detected	Mosquito Pools Found
1999	47	45	2	71.0	4	9		
2000	14	14	0	62.0	1	7		
2001	9	7	2	51.0	1	14	242	234
2002	29	28	1	72.0	3	11	185	197
2003	32	31	1	67.0	7	23	170	275
2004	5	2	3	34.0	0		43	185
2005	14	11	3	61.0	2	18	41	122
2006	12	8	4	64.5	2	25	74	197
2007	18	13	5	75.0	5	38	30	174
2008	15	8	7	64.0	1	13	0	197
2009	3	3	0	63.0	0		0	40
2010	17	15	2				0	367

Sources: New York City Department of Health. 2010. West Nile Virus: Reported, Suspected, Confirmed Cases and Rates; New York City Department of Health. 2001–10. West Nile Virus: Positive Results Summaries.

mosquitoes (Weiss et al. 2001, 657). Second, the indigenous bird population may have established immunity to the virus over time preventing the mosquito-bird-mosquito transmission of the virus (Weiss et al. 2001).

New York City Takes Action against West Nile Virus

Table 6.2 lists the public health policy tools employed by the city to combat West Nile virus. Within two or three years of the initial outbreak, the city developed a comprehensive and traditional response to the virus. The most visible and the most controversial tool used by the city in its campaign against West Nile virus was pesticide spraying to eradicate adult mosquitoes. In fact, this was the city's first response to the virus. Pesticide spraying was initiated on September 9, 1999, before the West Nile virus was identified. Officials at the federal CDC explained that since St. Louis encephalitis and West Nile virus were both mosquito-borne viruses, mosquito spraying was appropriate regardless of the disease's identity (Nasci 1999).

Even though the citywide spraying of pesticide malathion was defended by both the U.S. Environmental Protection Agency (EPA) and the New York State Department of Environmental Protection, city officials were criticized by some citizens and groups, including the Sierra Club and New York Public Interest Research Group, for its use of a toxic pesticide. A few critics of pesticide spraying argued that, because of the limited incidence of West Nile virus and the few deaths, the health risks created by citywide pesticide spraying far outweighed the risks from the virus. City officials, including borough presidents, also criticized

TABLE 6.2
Public Policy Tools Addressing West Nile Virus

MONITORING AND SCREENING
New York City
    Hospital reporting to NYC Department of Health
    Department of Health
        Active surveillance
            Contacts sentinel hospitals every2 weeks (DOH staff)
            Directs hospitals to submit spinal fluid samples of suspected cases
            Directs hospitals to send blood samples to NYS DOH
        Passive surveillance
            Encourages physicians to report suspicious cases
            Arranges for transportation of specimens to DOH lab (stopped in 2005)
            Offers Seroprevalence survey in Queens and Staten Island
            Monitors individuals with virus
            Monitors dead birds
            Monitors mosquito collection from traps set across city
            Hunts for mosquito breeding areas (DOH staff)
New York State
    NYS DOH lab: Tests specimens
Federal government
    CDC: Adds West Nile virus to national notification list for encephalitis
    CDC: Develops ArbNet surveillance system

EDUCATION
New York City
    Mayor's office (Giuliani) with DOH commissioner
        Addresses public concerns about disease in a press conferences
    Department of Health
        Posts question-and-answer list about West Nile virus on website
        Publishes daily pesticide spraying schedule
        Distributes mosquito control brochures (eight languages)
        Posts pesticide spraying hotline
        Initiates public education campaign to increase awareness about disease

EDUCATION (PUBLIC/PREVENTION)
New York City
    Department of Health
        Asks public to report dead bird sightings to DOH
        Mosquito Proof NYC Campaign:
            Subway and bus posters
            Radio and TV spots
            311 phone line or online connection for public to report standing water
            Requests for residents to address standing water on their own property
            Public education to avoid mosquito bites
        Community notification of pesticide spraying

EDUCATION (HEALTH/MEDICAL PERSONNEL)
New York City
    Department of Health
        Presents information to health/medical personnel
        Contacts physicians via faxes, brochures, and email alerts
        Emails advisories to all hospitals each spring
        Provides hotline for medical personnel regarding pesticide spraying

REGULATIONS (PREVENTION)
New York City
    Department of Health, Board of Health (BOH): Issues regulations that standing water
        is a public nuisance. DOH allowed to address standing water on all property and fine
        landowners who fail to address standing water

REGULATIONS (PESTICIDE SPRAYING)
New York State
    NYS Department of Conservation (NYSDEC): Issues pesticide spraying permits
    NYSDEC: Monitors pesticide spraying
Federal government
    CDC: Monitors pesticide spraying and issues recommendations for implementation

SERVICE DELIVERY
New York City
    Department of Parks and Recreation
        Sends out personnel to search for dead birds
    Department of Sanitation
        Remediates pools of water on vacant lots (discarded tires)
        Uses mosquito fish in sewage treatment plants
    Department of Health
        Conducts pesticide spraying

FINANCIAL ASSISTANCE
Federal government
    CDC: Provides financial support for DOH surveillance and control activities

the Department of Health for not clarifying or keeping to the announced pesticide spraying schedules (NYC Council 1999).

Initially, Mayor Giuliani and his administration took a fairly cavalier attitude toward pesticide spraying. In early September 1999, the Mayor proclaimed "there is no point in not spraying because there is no harm in spraying" (New York City Office of the Mayor 1999). Several months later Commissioner of Health Neil Cohen noted that, although the city was unable to discover any adverse impacts of malathion by examining emergency room visits or calls, the Department of Health was certainly aware that some people were being adversely affected by exposure to the pesticide (Cohen 2000a).

In April 2000 the city commissioner of health announced that, if the city did resort to spraying for mosquitoes, it would use a less toxic pesticide than malathion (Steinhauer 2000a). Ultimately, the city chose to use the pesticide Anvil, containing the active agent sumithrin. DOHMH has continued to use this pesticide through 2010. According to the department, sumithrin is effective against adult mosquitoes but "exhibits very low mammalian toxicity" and "does not bioaccumulate in the environment" (NYC DOHMH 2010a, 24). The pesticide is applied in small quantities and degrades in sunlight so spraying must be done at night. Additionally, the commissioner of health stated that the city would conduct only targeted spraying in those parts of the city where the virus was found (Cohen 2000b).

Since both the state and federal governments have regulations on the application of pesticides, city spraying was monitored by both the U.S. Environmental Protection Agency and the New York State Department of Environmental Conservation (NYC DOHMH 2010a). There were both state and federal regulations prohibiting the city from spraying pesticides in wetlands or marshlands. But the U.S. National Parks Service had jurisdiction of Gateway National Recreation Area on Staten Island. After Mayor Giuliani criticized the regulations as valuing fish more than humans, both federal and state environmental officials offered to waive the regulations and allow the city to spray (Lueck 2000).

In July 2000, after several dead crows infected with West Nile virus were found on Staten Island, the city announced that it would spray part of the borough in an attempt to kill the mosquitoes before they could infect humans. The CDC recommended that spraying should take place across a two-mile radius of every infected bird found (Toy 2000). Urging the public not to panic, the mayor noted that no humans had been reported with the virus (Lipton 2000a). Spraying would be done by trucks, rather than by helicopter or plane. There was consensus within the environmental community that Anvil, the pesticide used by the city in 2000, was considerably less harmful than malathion. But there was still disagreement whether Anvil was harmless. At one press conference, Mayor Giuliani suggested that one would have to drink the pesticide in order for it to cause harm. Most agreed that there had been little research into the pesticide's long-term effects on humans (Colangelo 2000).

The spraying was spread to Queens when infected birds were found there later in July 2000. Although the city was not using malathion, a coalition of environmental groups sued the city claiming that city officials violated federal law. The suit alleged that the city violated the federal Clean Water Act procedures (Steinhauer 2000b). The suit was not settled until late in 2002 when a Federal District Court judge ruled in favor of the city, noting that the plaintiffs "had failed to identify incidents that would amount to anything more than technical violations of labeling requirements" (Kelley 2002).

As more infected birds and mosquitoes were found, the city's spraying efforts were expanded and spraying from the air was resumed. In late July, the city closed Central Park for the night, canceling a concert by the New York Philharmonic, in order to spray after infected mosquitoes were found in the park (Lipton 2000b). Environmental groups went to court to seek a temporary restraining order to stop the expanded spraying but failed (Kershaw 2000). For several weeks, Commissioner of Health Neil Cohen became a fixture at mayoral news conferences, standing next to or behind the Mayor, answering questions and attempting to calm the public. Some environmentalists accused the mayor and the city of overreacting to the West Nile virus presence, but one federal official complimented the mayor stating: "He has been able to convey in very practical terms what the issues are for the public . . . And that is something scientists sometimes have difficulty doing" (quoted in Lipton 2000c). And even though the mayor was openly critical of those who expressed concern about the city's massive pesticide spraying strategy, he advised New Yorkers to "seal their windows, take in their pets and turn off air conditioners on spraying nights" (Lipton 2000c). In addition, the New York City Police Department advised its patrolman to avoid any trucks spraying the pesticide (Colangelo et al. 2001).

Because of the continued controversy surrounding the application of pesticides, DOH began to notify communities of adulticide spraying in advance of spraying in order to give the public "sufficient time to take any necessary precautions to reduce pesticide exposure" (NYC DOHMH 2010a, 26). By mid-August, the city was publishing a daily spraying schedule (Chen 2000). In 2001 the DOH did conduct an environmental impact study on the pesticides being used. "The study concluded that at the relatively low levels at which adulticides are applied, the occurrence of adverse public health effect to the population . . . would not be considered significant when compared to the potential risk to the public from West Nile Virus" (NYC DOHMH 2010a, 5). In 2003 environmental advocates reporting on New York City's routine use of pesticides noted that pesticide use for West Nile virus constituted approximately 1 percent of the city's use of pesticides (Quinn 2003).

The city's pesticide spraying policy during the summers of 2001 and 2002 was quite similar to the response in 2000. In May 2001, city officials suggested that they would adopt a more "conservative" approach to the virus, implying that they would not resort to spraying as fast as they had in previous years (Cardwell 2001). While not ruling out spraying entirely, Health Commissioner Neil Cohen noted that a dead bird would not "trigger a spraying response" (Cardwell 2001). Cohen also stated that the city would attempt to enforce nuisance laws to deal with standing water, including the levying of fines (Cardwell 2001). But when a Staten Island man contracted the virus in early August, the city resumed spraying. In 2001 there were seven reported cases of the virus in the city, with no deaths (Chen

2002). In 2002 the city resorted to spraying in July after it found mosquito samples and one bird that tested positive for the virus (Lueck 2002). In 2002 the city used approximately twice as much pesticide as it had in 2001, although it was still less than it used in 1999 or 2000 (Colangelo 2003). In 2005 the city council voted to "direct city agencies to reduce the use of harmful pesticides on municipal property, and substitute, whenever possible, nontoxic pest control methods" (DePalma 2005). There is little evidence that this resolution had any significant impact on the behavior of DOHMH.

After the 1999 outbreak of West Nile virus and the city's emergency response, the city's public health officials were able to use the winter months to plan a more comprehensive multitiered response to the virus. The response included three elements: surveillance of humans, birds, and mosquitoes; vector (mosquito control activities), including pesticide spraying; and public education (Cohen 2000a).

Following the emergence and identification of West Nile virus, New York City, New York State, and neighboring jurisdictions established both active and passive surveillance systems to track the disease. Hospital-based active surveillance involved two types of activities. First, DOHMH contacted relevant hospital personnel at "sentinel" hospitals every two weeks to "ascertain potential cases meeting clinical criteria" (Weiss et al. 2001, 654). These personnel included "neurologists, infectious disease consultants, intensive care physicians and chief medical residents" (654). Second, DOHMH directed twelve hospitals to submit spinal fluid specimens of those individuals who were suspected of having West Nile virus. DOHMH also instituted "enhanced passive surveillance" encouraging physicians to report to DOHMH any suspected cases. Hospital surveillance identified fifty-nine individuals, seven of whom died and a few reporting mild symptoms; but the actual numbers of those with the virus who had either mild or no symptoms was never known (Mostashari et al. 2001). DOHMH also established a hospital nurses hotline to allow nurses to report suspicious cases as well. In addition, DOHMH staff conducted surveys of pharmacies to ascertain whether pharmaceutical use might indicate outbreaks of the virus (Cohen 2000a).

To support the surveillance effort, DOHMH disseminated testing procedures via presentations by Health Department medical staff and contacted more than sixty-five thousand city physicians through brochures, faxes, and email alerts where possible (Weiss et al. 2001). Every year since the onset of the disease, the department has sent out email advisories to all hospitals beginning in June reminding relevant medical personnel of the need to report suspected cases of West Nile virus (NYC DOHMH 2010a). DOHMH's Bureau of Communicable Disease staff conducted more than one hundred presentations to health professionals (NYC DOHMH 2003).

To address these new efforts, DOHMH established a special West Nile virus office within the Communicable Disease Program (Weiss et al. 2001). Up until 2005, DOHMH actively participated in the transportation of suspected West Nile virus specimens to the DOHMH laboratory for rapid testing. Since 2006, DOHMH has simply encouraged providers with suspect specimens to arrange for transportation of these specimens to commercial laboratories (NYC DOHMH 2010a). By 2010, with the prevalence of the disease declining in the city, DOHMH informed physicians that DOH laboratories would no longer conduct testing for West Nile virus; nor would they be shipping spinal fluid samples to the state laboratories. Medical personnel, however, were still being urged to test for West Nile virus when cases with suspicious symptoms were discovered. Moreover, DOHMH informed physicians that the department was still available for consultation (NYC DOHMH 2010c).

As a result of the virus outbreak and in conjunction with action taken by the city's DOHMH and other state and local health departments in the metropolitan areas, the CDC added West Nile virus to the list of "nationally notifiable" encephalitis strains (Peterson and Marfin 2002). The CDC developed and implemented ArboNet, a West Nile virus "surveillance system designed to provide data to monitor the geographic and temporal spread" of the virus as well as to "identify areas at increased risk for human infections" (Marfin et al. 2001, 730). This system involved not only enhanced passive and active human surveillance but also bird surveillance and monitoring, mosquito surveillance, and "equine and non-human mammal surveillance" (730). Veterinary surveillance had identified the virus in horses in the northeast United States (Marfin et al. 2001).

In the early fall of 1999, shortly after the outbreak had peaked in the metropolitan area, DOHMH conducted a seroprevalence survey in northern Queens, where the prevalence of the virus was greatest. Seroprevalence "refers to the testing of blood for antibodies to an infectious organism" (NYC DOH 2001). Because of the variety of the virus symptoms and the number of virus victims with mild or no symptoms, it was important for public health officials to understand West Nile virus prevalence in affected communities. Selecting a sample of affected blocks in the community "residents were invited to participate . . . by responding to a questionnaire and providing a blood sample" (Mostashari et al. 2001, 261). Participants remained anonymous. In the 1,861 households visited, 1,069 adults were present, and 470 agreed to participate. The survey found 19 people with signs of the virus, 6 of whom recalled a fever in the recent past. The greatest prevalence was found among those who spent more than two hours outdoors in the evening. From the sample, the DOH study estimated that between 2 and 6 percent of the community's population was infected with West Nile virus (Mostashari et al. 2001).

A similar DOH survey was conducted on Staten Island in 2000, with the assistance of the CDC. That survey concluded that 0.5 percent of the population aged twelve years and older had probably been infected with West Nile virus (NYC DOH 2001).

Once an individual contracted the disease, the DOHMH, in conjunction with a hospital or the individual's physician, continued to monitor the individual's illness. In the case of West Nile virus, the DOH was not involved in the treatment of the illness when contracted by individuals. The disease was treated through the private health care system for those who could afford it or who had public health insurance. Those needing hospitalization, without health insurance or the ability to pay, received care via one of the city's public hospitals.

In addition to human surveillance, the city adopted a program of bird or animal and mosquito surveillance that supported the city's vector control program. The goal of vector control was to control the adult mosquito population in order reduce the need for pesticide spraying. Early on in the outbreak, DOH concluded that the virus could be detected in birds and mosquitoes weeks before there was a risk to human health. As a result, DOH began to track reports of dead birds, especially crows, in order to target those communities where the virus would appear (NYC DOHMH 2003). The Parks Department sent out teams searching for dead birds (Jacobs 1999). And the public was enlisted in the effort to report dead birds so they could be tested. In addition, every year since the onset of the virus, DOH staff collected mosquitoes from traps set at locations across the city and each year tested thousands of mosquitoes for the virus.

The city also sent out Health Department employees and others to hunt for mosquito breeding areas (Revkin 2000). In 2009, 4,480 sites were visited by city inspectors and checked for breeding (NYC DOHMH 2010a). In addition, the city's Board of Health, an appointed body, issued a resolution that standing water, a likely point of mosquito breeding, was considered to be a public nuisance. This allowed the DOH employees to deal with standing water, regardless of location. It also allowed the Health Department to levy fines on property owners who did not rid their property of standing water (Cohen 2001). "In 2009, 1079 Notice of Violations were" sent to property owners who failed to respond to department requests to address standing water on their property (NYC DOHMH 2010a, 21).

DOH discovered that pools of water in tires, particularly on vacant lots, were also a popular mosquito breeding ground. To get rid of them, the department enlisted the help of the Department of Sanitation, which had the responsibility to remediate these lots (NYC DOHMH 2010a).

Beginning in 2000, in those areas where standing water could not be emptied or drained, DOH used a larvacide. In conjunction with the NYC Departments of Environmental Protection, Parks and Recreation, the NYC Housing Authority, and with a permit issued by the New York State Department of Environmental Conservation, the city applied larvacide in street corner storm drains, parks, sewage treatment plants, and other large bodies of standing water (NYC

DOHMH 2003). The chemical used was not toxic to humans or the "natural enemies of mosquito larvae" (NYC DOHMH 2003, 19). The chemical caused a disease in mosquito larvae by "interfering with normal digestion and triggering the larvae to stop feeding" (NYC DOHMH 2003, 19). In the city's wastewater treatment facilities, where there were large pools of water, mosquito-larvae-eating fish were introduced (Cohen 2000b).

A final major tool used in the city's fight against West Nile virus was public education. As with other public health threats, education was critical in assuaging public fears about West Nile virus. While the low prevalence of the virus did not produce mass panic, there was concern about a disease with which the public was unfamiliar. Education was also significant in enlisting the public's help in combating the disease. Once DOH gained sufficient knowledge about the virus, it posted a series of questions and answers on its website to inform the public of who was most susceptible to West Nile virus and what individuals could do to prevent mosquito bites, the most practical way of avoiding the virus (NYC DOHMH 2010f).

Because of the press attention that the illness received and the initial uncertainty as to the illness's identity and how many people would be affected, the Health Department used Mayor Giuliani to calm the public but also to enlist the help of the public in attacking the virus. Mayor Giuliani's involvement gave the Health Department's activities additional legitimacy as well as extra importance and urgency, possibly at the risk of panicking the public. Public participation was critical not only in assisting individuals in protecting themselves from the disease but also in contributing to the overall public effort in eradicating the virus.

As previously noted, physicians and relevant hospital personnel were the first individuals whose cooperation was sought by DOH. They were a critical component in the surveillance and reporting of the disease. Beyond medical personnel however, DOH education efforts enlisted the public in several ways. Every year since the onset of the disease, DOHMH has launched a "public education campaign to increase awareness" of West Nile virus (NYC DOHMH 2010a, 9). The two primary goals of the department's education efforts were to get the public to take measures against mosquito bites and to enlist the public's help in eliminating mosquito breeding grounds (NYC DOHMH 2010a).

To assist DOH in locating where the virus might appear, it asked the public to report dead birds, with the exception of pigeons, so that they could be tested. The department established a hotline to report dead birds. In the days following the opening of the phone lines, hundreds of calls came in from the public identifying dead birds (Cohen 2000a). Over time, as the prevalence of the disease declined, the public was asked not to report findings of single dead birds but to continue to report findings of ten or more dead birds of any species and three or more dead water birds (NYC DOHMH 2010b). Finally, in 2008, concluding that dead birds no longer served as a viable indicator of West Nile virus activity, DOH discontinued this type of surveillance (NYC DOHMH 2010b).

Public help was also enlisted in the eradication of mosquitoes and the prevention of mosquito breeding. In 2000 DOH initiated a public campaign, Mosquito-Proof NYC. Posters in English and Spanish appeared on subways and buses, public service messages were aired on radio and television, and fact sheets in seventeen different languages were disseminated (NYC DOHMH 2003). The public was also asked to report to DOH any sightings of standing water, places where mosquitoes were known to breed. This could be done through either dialing the city's 311 Citizen Service Center or, beginning in 2009, filing a confidential report online (NYC DOHMH 2010e). Citizens who noticed puddles of standing water were urged to call the Health Department. In 2002 more than 7,500 mosquito pools and more than 2,000 complaints of standing water were reported to DOH (NYC DOHMH 2003). In 2009 the city received 5,163 complaints of standing water from the city's 311 Citizen Service Center, through the DOH website, from community leaders and groups, or from surveys conducted by inspectors (NYC DOHMH 2010a). Citizens were also asked to address standing water on their own property including birdbaths, swimming pools, and gutters (NYC DOHMH 2003). Calling on citizens to help the city, Commissioner of Health Neil Cohen stated, "We can only truly succeed in significantly reducing mosquitoes if everyone pitches in to mosquito proof New York City by eliminating areas of standing water where mosquitoes lay their eggs" (quoted in Steinhauer 2000a).

DOH also advised citizens what they could do on their own to reduce mosquitoes around their homes and communities as well as protecting themselves from possible mosquito bites. The advice included the removal of standing water around the home, the wearing of protective clothing, limiting outdoor activity in the evening, and the proper use of insect repellent (NYC DOHMH 2010d). In some cases the messages were targeted to the most vulnerable populations. In early September 2002 Commissioner of Health Frieden urged those New Yorkers over the age of fifty years to wear long pants and long sleeves when going outside (Newman 2002). Those city residents who conserve rainwater were advised to cover water barrels with tight fitting lids (NYC DOHMH 2003).

West Nile Virus and Economic Development

While economic development is directly responsible for some public health threats, West Nile virus is linked to economic development in only the most limited global perspective. West Nile virus arrived in North America because it was able to survive intercontinental travel. Researchers do not know, however, whether it came by boat or plane. Not knowing how long the virus might survive in an insect or avian host, it is possible that the virus could have survived nineteenth- or maybe even eighteenth-century international travel, making the link to contemporary economic development effects even more remote.

West Nile Virus, Race, and Ethnicity

The appearance of West Nile virus in New York City had limited implications for the city's racial and ethnic diversity. The disease did not impact any specific racial or ethnic group. The city's public education response, however, included brochures and posters in eight different languages (Cohen 2000a). Because of the need to get as many residents of the city as possible involved in the elimination of mosquitoes, a multilingual campaign was necessary. There is no evidence that the city's ethnic and racial diversity was an inhibiting or complicating factor in the response to the virus.

West Nile Virus and Intergovernmental Relations

The relationship between the DOH, the New York State Department of Health, and the CDC during the West Nile virus outbreak illustrates intergovernmental public health policy at its most routine and cooperative. As previously discussed, the CDC, the State Department of Health, and DOH worked cooperatively to identify and report the virus as well as engage in surveillance. Both state and federal laboratories participated in testing specimens; although it was ultimately veterinarians at the Bronx Zoo who correctly identified the virus (NYC Council 1999).

As previously noted, both the federal and state environmental authorities publicly approved of the city's use of pesticides, and the city cited this support when critics attacked the city's decision to engage in citywide spraying. The State Department of Environmental Conservation monitored the city's application of pesticide (Cohen 1999).

In 2000 CDC designated West Nile virus as a nationally reportable disease, establishing its permanent interest in the presence of the disease (Petersen and Marfin 2002). The joint federal-city activities were part of a series of standard operating procedures established years before and utilized on numerous occasions in response to a variety of diseases and public health threats. In addition to the CDC, the U.S. Environmental Protection Agency provided the regulatory infrastructure for the city's use of pesticides in dealing with adult mosquitoes (Petersen and Marfin 2002).

The city requested aid from the federal government to help defray the costs of responding to the West Nile virus. Over the years, the city received a modest amount of funding from the CDC for surveillance and control of the virus. In both 2007 and 2008, however, the CDC budget for West Nile virus was cut almost in half. The city lost federal funding as a result. But by that time the virus was not affecting the city as much as it had in 1990–2000 and had spread across the country affecting many other jurisdictions, which were also receiving CDC funding. What might have been most significant about the CDC funding cuts was that some of the funding had gone to training and recruiting students in medical entomology at universities across the country. The budget cuts resulted in these programs being curtailed (Fish 2007).

In 1999 the city's director of emergency management asked Governor Pataki to request a presidential disaster declaration from President Clinton in order to qualify the city, and surrounding suburbs, for additional federal aid (Lombardi 1999b). The disaster declaration was never issued.

Despite the overall focus on cooperation between the various levels of government, some aspects of the case were reflective of tension between the levels of government. Initially, both the state and the city pursued separate attempts to identify the illness, without consulting each other. The city turned to the federal CDC for help identifying the illness. Unlike many local health departments that work through their state departments of health, the city keeps its own records and reports statistics directly to the CDC. The CDC laboratories act as a resource for information about diseases on which states and cities have no information. New York State health officials, apparently not convinced of the CDC's St. Louis encephalitis identification, pursued their own route through a private laboratory in California. Tension between the state and city health establishments dated back to the 1980s when the state and city commissioners of health differed over the response to the AIDS crisis (Steinhauer 1999).

Conclusion

West Nile virus was identified shortly after its arrival in the New York metropolitan area. Much of the mystery in the initial identification of the virus was that the disease had never been seen in the Western Hemisphere. But this lack of knowledge that resulted in the misidentification of West Nile virus as St. Louis encephalitis had no impact on the number of cases, the treatment of those already reported cases, or the public health policy tools adopted.

Except for those cases that required hospitalization, continuous surveillance of the virus was problematic because many of those stricken with the virus never developed symptoms that required a physician's or hospital's care. In the early years of the virus's appearance, the NYC DOH, in cooperation with the CDC did conduct local studies to better understand the prevalence of the disease among the entire public, but this did not appear to affect overall policy in combating the disease.

There is no vaccine for West Nile virus, so it cannot be prevented via immunization. There is also no standard treatment for West Nile virus except for standard protocols in dealing with encephalitis, the most severe manifestation of the virus's symptoms. As a result, public health authorities focused on dealing with how the disease was transmitted to humans, through mosquitoes. This too was not without its risks, both political and medical. To combat mosquitoes, DOH used locally applied larvacides, and the EPA approved adult mosquito pesticides of low toxicity; but some community leaders and environmental groups were critical of pesticide use and unsuccessfully sued to prohibit its use. City council oversight hearings on the city's response to West Nile virus were at times conflictual and combative as environmental advocates and some members of the council used these hearings to criticize the administration's use of pesticides and failure to adequately inform communities about when spraying would occur.

As the number of West Nile cases in the metropolitan area declined and as the public became convinced that the number of serious cases would never reach levels that would create panic, public concern over West Nile virus subsided. Nevertheless, it remains on the DOHMH watch list, and the application of larvacides and pesticides still takes place as infected mosquitoes are identified. The virus cannot be eliminated, but it appears as if it can be managed.

Compared to many current public health issues, West Nile virus is not a complex public health problem. Once it was identified and its source discovered, the solution to preventing West Nile virus was simple, although not easily implemented. Public health authorities know that preventing individuals from being bitten by a mosquito carrying the virus can eliminate the virus in the population, although there is no public health tool that can guarantee that individuals will not be bitten. The elimination of standing water, public education, and the application of larvacides and pesticides have certainly decreased the likelihood that those living in the city will contract the virus. But it is not precisely clear to what extent the risk has been reduced, or whether the benefits of risk reduction are worth the cost. Given current knowledge about the virus, West Nile virus is a single-factor public health problem. This makes the virus a far simpler problem to understand, but not necessarily a far simpler problem to resolve, if the single factor—in this case, mosquitoes carrying the virus—cannot be comprehensively addressed by available knowledge on which public health tools are based.

CHAPTER SEVEN

CONCLUSION

A primary purpose of this book is to explore the meaning of public policy by examining the tools employed by public health policy makers in formulating and implementing solutions to public health threats. By focusing on the use of public policy tools across five public health issues, this within-case case study seeks to examine how the same tools were employed under different but similar conditions. In addition, this work examines how those forces that influence urban public policy in general affect the use of public health policy-making tools specifically. In doing so, this examination finds that, while knowledge is critical for the formulation and implementation of public health policy, other forces influence how this knowledge is employed. But in all five cases, knowledge about the threat, however incomplete, is at the center of policy formulation and implementation.

This concluding chapter attempts to address two issues. First, how does the use of public policy tools differ across the five cases examined? Are different tools being utilized by public health policy makers across the five examples? Or, are the same public health policy tools being employed but in very different ways?

Second, this chapter revisits the analytical frameworks discussed in the introduction. What factors influence the choice of tools being used by public health policy makers? Public health policy represents a clash of forces in explaining the choice of public policy tools. On the one hand, there are forces that affect the overall urban political milieu. These include the need of urban political systems to promote economic development, those systems' dependency on the state and federal levels (i.e., intergovernmental relations), and the growing racial and ethnic diversity that cities are experiencing. On the other hand, more than other areas of urban public policy, public health policy is steeped in medical or health policy making that is driven by knowledge of causes and solutions. How do these two sets of forces interact in explaining public health policy tools?

The Tools and Their Usage
Monitoring and Surveillance

In order for the city to know how serious a public health threat is, there must be a means by which it can be measured. The ability to measure the existence of a threat relies on several components. First, there must be consensus within the medical and public health community on a clinically diagnosable medical definition of a condition that can be categorized as a public health threat. The federal Centers for Disease Control and Prevention (CDC) is recognized as the agency with the authority to establish definitions of public health threats. Second, unless the condition can be measured unobtrusively, individuals must agree to be screened. At times this has raised privacy issues. For the CDC, of the five public health conditions discussed in this volume, the least controversial condition to clinically diagnose and obtain community consensus was West Nile virus. Once the virus was identified and labeled, there was no controversy over its existence. The disease carried no stigma, and much of the monitoring involved birds and mosquitoes, not humans.

In the case of childhood lead paint poisoning, the CDC altered the definition over time, lowering the threshold of dangerous lead in the bloodstream as research was better able to recognize the negative health impact. With HIV/AIDS as well, the CDC was able to produce a diagnosable medical definition of the condition but altered the definition in the mid 1980s as more symptoms were recognized as being caused by the disease. With obesity there is a general consensus on a clinical definition of obesity based on the concept of body-mass index (BMI). But this definition has its critics, who have argued that some of those whose BMIs are above the obesity threshold should not be labeled obese. In the case of asthma, because of the variety of symptoms and the fact that many of the symptoms were similar to other conditions, there is no agreed-upon clinical definition that can be diagnosed. As a result, the CDC and local public health authorities measure asthma when its symptoms become severe enough to require an emergency room visit or hospitalization.

Normally, consensus on a medical definition is accompanied by a test allowing public health authorities and other medical personnel to assess whether any person has the condition. In most cases, an agreed-upon definition of the condition is due to a laboratory-established method for measuring the existence of the condition and its severity. This was the case with West Nile virus and lead poisoning. With obesity, BMI is easily measured outside of a laboratory, given that height and weight measurements are all that is needed. With HIV/AIDS, while the virus was first identified in the early 1980s, a test was not available to detect the disease in individuals until 1985. Finally, with asthma, there is no test.

Of course, the mere existence of a test or measure to detect the presence of a public health threat does not, by itself, allow public health authorities to monitor the prevalence of a public health threat in the community. Three additional steps must be fulfilled: venues must be established where the test can be administered; individuals at risk must show up at the venues to be tested; and the results of the tests must be reported to public health authorities. Because of the structure of health care delivery in this country, public health authorities are dependent upon a private health care delivery system for much of the surveillance of public health threats.

Of the five public health threats discussed in this volume, the only one with mandated screening is lead poisoning. Since the mid-1990s, New York State has required that all one- and two-years-olds, the most at-risk population, be screened through a blood test in both public and private settings. The samples are tested in state-certified labs. The fact that the mandated population is children makes the mandate enforceable because it is in the interest of parents to have their infant seen by a physician and physicians are well aware of the screening mandate. In addition, the tests as part of normal infant health care are covered by both public and private insurance. Because there is little or no stigma attached to the condition and treatment is available, physicians are encouraged to test and report the findings as is mandated by law.

With HIV/AIDS, there is no mandate that the most at-risk in the population be screened. Given that they are adults, and some of them very difficult to reach, how would such a mandate be enforced? New York State does mandate screening of newborns. For all others, the state and city encourage screening. The new consent protocol introduced in 2010 employs an opt-out and does much less to discourage testing than the earlier protocol. Of course, the availability of life-saving pharmaceuticals and significantly decreased discrimination against homosexuals has created an environment more conducive for getting tested.

For West Nile virus, only those reporting suspicious symptoms are screened, and all those who test positive are reported. Because of the nature of the disease and how it is contracted, these procedures are not controversial. But the Department of Health and Mental Hygiene (DOHMH) did seek a random sample of blood from residents in areas where the incidence of the virus was high in order to examine how many were carrying the virus. For asthma, there is no mandatory screening or reporting because there is no test. Although there is no mandatory reporting, DOHMH does collect hospital data on asthma admissions and emergency department visits. In addition, the New York City schools request asthma information on school health forms. Similar to asthma, there is no mandatory screening or testing with obesity. Most obesity data come from surveys in which BMI is calculated from self-reported weight and height. The expansion of the NYC public schools Fitnessgram Program should give the city a much more reliable assessment of childhood obesity over time.

Education

Education may be the tool most often used by the public health establishment. It is not as controversial as regulation because it lacks the coercive element of forcing people to change their behavior. And it does not involve the direct delivery of services, generally viewed as the purview of the health or medical profession or social services bureaucracies. Despite its appearance of simplicity and a lack of political controversy, the provision of information as a public health tool can be both complicated and controversial.

It is complicated because such a pervasive tool in the public health field can serve a variety of purposes. First, not all public health education is aimed at each and every citizen. Very different publics can be the targets of public health education. These include the general public, those at-risk persons, and those who can help prevent the threat from occurring or spreading. Second, education can have various purposes in public health policy. On the most general level, the provision of information to the public can serve to ease public fear and to assist in prevention. But on a much more targeted level, education can be geared toward getting certain individuals to take specific action toward preventing their own victimization or the victimization of others. In this capacity the provision of public health education is based on the assumption that if provided with understandable information, people will use that information to change their behavior and decrease behaviors that place them, or their children, at greater risk.

In the cases of both HIV/AIDS and West Nile virus, public health education was used to assuage public fear. In dealing with the public for this purpose, action by public health officials is not sufficient. More-visible elected officials are needed. At mayoral press conferences where public health issues are being addressed, the commissioner of DOHMH is usually beside the mayor, specifically to respond to technical questions beyond the mayor's expertise.

In the case of West Nile virus, because the disease was fatal for some, the mayor needed to address the city and at the very least clarify the at-risk groups. In the face of scientific ignorance and uncertainty in the case of HIV/AIDS, the fact that the disease's contagiousness was unexplained produced something close to a public panic. The mayor was called upon to address these public fears, with limited knowledge. Then, as knowledge about the disease's contagion was made available by the research community, the mayor was called upon integrate this knowledge into the public realm, further quelling public fears.

West Nile virus also created some unique public health education challenges because of the DOHMH's engaging in pesticide spraying in selected areas of the city. For some of the public, the pesticide spraying was as much a cause of concern as the virus itself. As a result, DOHMH and the mayor spent a great deal of time educating the public on safety issues with regard to the pesticide being used. The department also established a hotline to answer the public's questions on pesticide spraying and safety.

In the case of obesity, Mayor Bloomberg, through his press conferences, attempted to raise the degree of public awareness about this citywide public health threat, believing that the public was too complacent in responding to the condition. DOHMH also produced a citywide campaign to increase awareness of asthma. This was done to inform those suffering from asthma, or their parents, that resources were available to manage the condition.

The other major function served by citywide public health education is prevention. DOHMH educational campaigns attempt to make the public aware of public health threats and then provide information and encouragement that will enable the public to take steps to prevent the condition from occurring. Here a distinction is being made between public education campaigns that are citywide and those that are targeted to smaller at-risk groups. For instance, in the wake of the discovery that HIV was passed primarily through bodily fluid during sexual relations, DOHMH and even the U.S. surgeon general launched public campaigns promoting the use of condoms and safe sex. With regard to HIV/AIDS there were some who needed the message more, but local and national public health authorities deemed that everyone could profit from the information. For some, this education campaign was controversial. At the national level, and to a much lesser extent in the city, there were those who believed any educational campaign conveying a sexual message was unwelcome.

Similar to HIV/AIDS, DOHMH (assisted by the mayor), the CDC, and Michelle Obama have embarked upon a major educational campaign in response to obesity. However, unlike HIV/AIDS, where the deaths of AIDS victims provided immediate awareness of a problem to the public, with obesity the public first had to be educated that obesity was a problem. Both local and national campaigns linked obesity with diabetes and other negative health outcomes. At the same time, educational campaigns provided the prevention information: eat less, eat better, and exercise more. Beyond that, DOHMH has run campaigns against sugared beverages, and since the 1990s the federal government has attempted to educate all consumers through the promulgation of better food labeling.

Providing the public with calorie information at some of the city's restaurants is one of the more controversial attempts at citywide public health education. The controversy was created by the need for regulations requiring selected restaurants to provide this information, most of which would not have provided it if not required by law. The Patient Protection and Affordable Care Act mandates that more restaurants provide calorie information, but the regulations have not yet been issued.

With West Nile virus, initially citizens were also asked by DOHMH to notify the department about dead bird sightings. In addition, the city embarked on an educational campaign to get citizens to help eradicate mosquitoes by addressing standing water not only on their own property but also anywhere in the city by calling the DOHMH when standing water was found. Finally, city public service announcements attempted to educate the public on the best ways to avoid mosquito bites. In the case of asthma, despite the inconclusive science surrounding the condition, DOHMH did conduct a citywide campaign to promote awareness. In addition, the campaign attempted to educate parents that the disease could be managed and that asthma attacks could be decreased by limiting exposure to some substances.

With lead-based paint poisoning, there was no citywide awareness campaign. Although many children could be at risk, their parents lacked the knowledge and technology to both detect and prevent the existence of lead paint poisoning in the home. The lead paint poisoning message was much more effectively targeted to a smaller group, landlords and those doing housing rehabilitation, who owned the property and therefore were ultimately responsible for abating lead poisoning.

In promulgating citywide public health education, the city has a variety of mechanisms by which to disseminate information. As previously noted, for the most serious public health threats, mayoral press conferences were utilized. These press conferences are held almost daily and are well attended by the print, cable, and internet media. In instances when public health threats are extant, attendance increases. Any statement by the mayor will receive maximum public exposure and therefore provides an effective means to reach the public. Just as important, there is an expectation on the part of the public that the mayor, as chief executive and chief of state for the city, will address public threats and provide citizens with both assurance and a sense that the city is moving to quell the threat.

Beyond mayoral press conferences, the city has other less dramatic means to disseminate information to the public. Television and radio public-service announcements have been a typical means by which public health authorities have gotten their message out. These were used with HIV/AIDS, West Nile virus, and obesity. Sensitive messages, such as safe sex, have to be carefully crafted to go out over the airwaves. With HIV/AIDS, the airwaves were not used for the most controversial messages. In a city where many ride mass transit, subways, bus shelters, and billboards have become standard venues for public health education campaigns. Finally, the internet and the city's own website has become a means by which mass public health education has been attempted. Of course, in order for this to be successful, the public must be attracted to, and have access to, the website.

Public health education is at times targeted to smaller groups. These groups may be at-risk groups or groups that have a specific role to play in prevention. In attempting to reach these groups, the same mechanisms that public health authorities use in educating the mass public may not be effective. Targeted communication of public health information is also dependent on the nature of the group being contacted. To the extent that the group is centralized or organized, the information may be more easily conveyed.

HIV/AIDS provides three examples. The three most at-risk groups were male homosexuals, IV drug users and their partners, and youths. To a limited extent these groups were centrally located. Many homosexuals had settled in a specific part of the city; and IV drug users, although more decentralized throughout the city than homosexuals, inhabited those parts of the city where drug use would be least conspicuous and where the rest of the community would be least resistant to their presence or less able than other more affluent communities to effectively protest.

Of the at-risk groups, youths were the easiest community to target through the schools. The DOHMH, partnering with the public schools and community groups, conducted HIV/AIDS education in the high schools. But the abstinence curriculum forced many of the community health groups to sever their relations with the schools. Ultimately the state and city developed an HIV/AIDS curriculum guide, which together with the distribution of condoms provided a politically feasible program of prevention education.

Before the AIDS outbreak, the homosexual community in New York City was organized to a limited degree. Much of the organization was focused on antidiscrimination efforts. In addition, the gay community was organized, but less formally, around its social life centered on gay bars, bathhouses, and an emerging print media. The formation of Gay Men's Health Crisis (GMHC) shortly after the initial cases of AIDS were publicized was a significant event in the battle against AIDS. GMHC awareness and prevention education preceded that of DOHMH. Early on, in its own HIV/AIDS prevention education efforts, DOHMH realized that groups in the gay community, such as GMHC, were far more effective in delivering HIV/AIDS prevention education to its community than DOHMH. Groups such as GMHC had far more credibility in the gay community than city officials. Initially GMHC had more knowledge of the disease and could craft a message that was far more focused, if not blunt.

Because of their lack of affluence and the multiple disabilities created by their drug use, IV drug users never had the capability or desire to organize. The drug abuse rehabilitation community, however, provided a setting in which HIV prevention education did take place. But drug rehabilitation in New York City was underfunded. As a result, the drug rehabilitation centers never offered the scope to engage in comprehensive prevention education citywide.

Much of the drug use took place in minority communities or on the periphery of these communities; and most IV drug users and ultimately AIDS victims in the city were minorities. Minority churches were the most consistent and stable organizational force in minority communities and certainly offered the best possible institutional mechanism for delivering HIV/AIDS prevention education in the minority community, to both IV drug users and homosexuals. But the leadership of minority churches was resistant to play a major role in HIV/AIDS prevention education for the first decade of the disease.

A few community groups conducted outreach to the minority communities using peer street participants, but this was never a comprehensive enough effort to reach the entire at-risk minority community. Minority churches and their social program affiliates finally began to seriously address HIV/AIDS and began to promote prevention in the mid-1990s, when the disease had already taken a serious toll in their communities.

Other groups targeted by public health education are those which have a major role to play in prevention. In the case of lead paint poisoning, regulations required landlords and those developers engaging in housing rehabilitation to inspect housing and abate where unsafe lead paint was found. In addition, these landlords and developers were required to inform tenants not only of their rights but also of the landlord's responsibilities. In conveying these regulatory responsibilities, DOHMH and the Department of Housing Preservation and Development (HPD) had a relatively easy time reaching landlords and developers. They were a well-organized and highly attentive public with regard to lead paint regulations. Because of their significant financial interest in the regulations, landlords and developers participated in the legislative process and so were well aware of the legislative outcome. The existence of landlord and developer professional associations facilitated their education on the content of the regulations.

The other group that public health authorities attempted to reach in the battle of lead paint poisoning was the small contractors or subcontractors who would be performing the lead paint abatement work. The goal was not only to eradicate lead in the environment leading to a lead-safe home but also to conduct this type of rehabilitative work in a safe way. New York State provided most of the education and training programs in its role as occupational licensing authority.

As with HIV/AIDS, in dealing with childhood obesity, DOHMH has partnered with the public schools to inform not only children but also parents about the health impacts of obesity and what can be done to prevent it. The State Department of Education has also been involved in school antiobesity programming. The schools, decentralized at the community level, are well organized to reach children and their parents. Teacher training, workshops, and curriculum guides have all been employed in the antiobesity efforts. Seeking to get an earlier start, DOHMH has included day care staff in some of the antiobesity training and workshops.

Schools also assisted public health officials and the medical community in educating parents and children about the management of asthma. Schools themselves became a focal point in the asthma educational process, especially since asthma attacks were so disruptive to the educational process. DOHMH ran programs to train teachers to recognize asthma symptoms and help students manage the disease.

In addressing both asthma and obesity, DOHMH has also been assisted by other groups in the community. With asthma, groups such as the Harlem Children's Zone and the Reducing Indoor Allergens Study Team in northern Manhattan have engaged in parent education and have gone into homes of child asthma sufferers and educated parents as to how to create an environment that can reduce asthma attack aggravating symptoms. With obesity, because of the increased salience of obesity and food nutrition issues, various groups have become active in antiobesity and nutrition education at the community level. For instance, some community groups are working with DOHMH's bodega and farmers' market initiatives to provide demonstrations and education programs at these venues. And the New York Academy of Medicine has been the source of obesity education in schools in some communities.

Finally, the medical profession and other health professionals are frequently a target of public health education. Since the medical community is frequently involved in screening for diseases, it is already in communication with public health authorities. In addition, most of the members of the medical community are organized and easily identified because of state licensing procedures and the overall organization of the medical profession. Although physicians routinely receive communications from the New York State Department of Health and DOHMH, public health threats often give rise to nonroutine forms of education. In the case of asthma, DOHMH undertook the task of educating physicians on the most current methods for treating the condition. Because of GMHC's knowledge of the HIV/AIDS and its sensitivity in dealing with it, early on in the AIDS outbreak the city contracted with the group to educate medical professionals and other allied professions in dealing with AIDS patients. Ultimately, however, New York State, through the AIDS Institute, the HIV Clinical Education Initiative, and the HIV Care Networks, provided a great deal of health professional education. The CDC's AIDS clearinghouse also played a role in educating physicians and other health professionals.

Regulation

The underlying assumption of much of public health policy's education tool is that provided with the proper information, citizens and relevant groups will voluntarily behave in ways that will maximize the public's health. The use of the regulation tool as part of public health policy is based on the assumption that education alone will not work or has not worked. What education hopes to achieve voluntarily regulation aims to achieve through the coercive power of the state. In the United States, the power to regulate on behalf of public health rests in the police power, which resides primarily at the state level. States can cede some of the police power to their local governments through home rule, and this is certainly the case in the public health arena.

Since regulations attempt to force people to behave in ways they otherwise might not, they are the most controversial tool in the public health arsenal. And since public health issues are, in some cases, related to lifestyle choices, many individuals view attempts to regulate this type of behavior as a violation of their right to privacy or to live their life the way they choose. Similar to education, however, the degree of controversy surrounding regulations is a function of who is being regulated and precisely what the targets of regulation are being forced to do.

The regulation of business has deep roots in the history of public health, dating back to ancient Rome's regulation of the public markets. Business practice for decades, if not centuries, has underscored the need for the regulation of business to achieve public health ends. At the same time, business interests have successfully used their political power to push back against public-sector regulation attempts.

Of the five examples discussed in this study, lead paint provides the clearest example of business regulation. Regulations composed the bulk of the public health policy response to the problem. The real estate industry was the primary target of regulations. Under New York City's law, landlords in multiple unit (more than three apartments) buildings were required to annually inspect apartments for lead paint hazards. They were required to take prompt action to abate lead paint hazards when they were found. And they were required to relocate the residents of the apartment, at the landlord's cost, when the abatement work could not take place safely with the residents remaining in the home.

On a secondary level, the small lead abatement subcontracting industry that emerged to address the problem was also subject to licensing, mandatory training, and the regulation of specific abatement procedures, primarily by the state.

Public policy toward both obesity and HIV/AIDS involves the use of business regulations as well, but in these cases the regulations occupy a smaller segment of public health policy. In the case of obesity, the restaurant calorie-posting requirements constituted one of the more visible and controversial pieces of recent public health policy. Note, however, that this regulation was a vehicle to further educate consumers about the caloric content of foods being purchased. Unlike lead paint abatement regulations, the calorie-posting regulations have no impact on public health unless the relevant restaurant patrons make different food choices as a result of the information with which they are being provided. In 2012–13 the Bloomberg administration's attempts to regulate the size of sugary drinks sold at many food establishments in the city was met with opposition by the beverage industry and their allies. These groups have been successful, to date, in defeating this regulatory proposal.

Public health policy toward obesity also included regulations on bodegas that are participating in one of the city's programs to offer and more prominently display nutritious foods in low-income neighborhoods. But these regulations governed participating bodegas only, and those bodegas received incentives to participate. In addition, nonprofit organizations running day care centers in the city had to agree to a set of minimum standards on physical activity, television viewing, and serving fruit juice and low-fat milk, all as part of the permitting process.

In the case of HIV/AIDS, public health policy sought to regulate sexual activity in business establishments. Using its police power, the state and city banned at-risk behaviors at bars, bathhouses, clubs, and movie theaters frequented by gay males, threatening the owners of those establishments with closure if the at-risk behaviors went unmonitored. Several bathhouses and movie theaters were closed. Public health policy dealing with West Nile virus has not used business regulations. As a mosquito- or bird-borne virus, West Nile virus is not the result of private-sector activity. The only regulation promulgated as a result of West Nile virus was the elimination of standing water on private property to decrease mosquito breeding.

The one area where private-sector activities have been regulated as a mechanism to reduce asthma or asthma attacks is air quality. Federal, state, and local air quality regulations dealing with both vehicle and stationary emissions have increased air quality. Note, however, that many of these regulations were promulgated long before asthma became a public health issue. Moreover, vehicle and other emission regulations address a host of public health and other problems, not just asthma. Beginning in the 1990s, the city took steps to regulate diesel fuel emissions of its own vehicle fleet as well as the vehicle fleets of those entities doing business with the city, such as school bus companies and private trash carters. New York City's attempts to "green" its yellow taxi fleet contributes to air quality and asthma reduction; but most yellow cabs, "green" or not, do not travel into those parts of the city where asthma rates are highest. The move by the state to regulate the use of ultralow sulfur diesel fuel and compressed natural gas in the Metropolitan Transit Authority's bus fleet has also been significant.

Physicians and, to a lesser extent, hospitals constitute a special group of businesses that have been the subject of public health regulations. Two of the regulations imposed on physicians throughout much of the recent history of public health policy are testing and reporting. Physicians and hospitals have been cooperating with public health authorities for more than a century, so testing and reporting mandates are not seen as controversial or overly burdensome. They are part of medical practice. In the case of lead poisoning, physicians and hospitals were mandated by the state to test infants. With HIV/AIDS, physicians were given a protocol to strongly recommend testing to their patients. They were also given a protocol to strongly recommend partner notification. And with West Nile virus, physicians were instructed to test when symptoms suggested the possibility of the disease.

For the most part, mandates or recommendations to test have been accompanied by mandates to report conditions when discovered. In the case of asthma, hospitals have been mandated to report admissions and emergency room visits as a result of asthma attacks. And in the early days of HIV/AIDS, hospital reporting of AIDS admissions was one of the only ways in which the city DOHMH and the CDC could establish data on the prevalence of the disease. As HIV/AIDS testing became more decentralized, physicians were initially mandated to report cases anonymously and later report patient names with the promise of confidentiality.

With HIV/AIDS, however, in the early years of the disease there was reluctance on the part of some physicians to report cases when discovered. Even when mandated to report cases anonymously, some physicians went out their way to protect their patients' privacy by not reporting, especially since there was no cure and little could be done for the patient. Once medicine was developed that could allow an individual to live a long life with HIV, one of the major reasons for not being tested disappeared. Yet the gay community and civil libertarians still argued that individuals could not be coerced into being tested. Nor could they be coerced into divulging the names of all their sexual partners.

The most controversial target of public health regulations is individual at-risk behaviors. Regulating individual behavior in the interest of public health raises a number of issues. First, in some cases individual behavior, even that which may not be healthy, is constitutionally protected. The right to privacy and substantive rights affirmed as part of the Fourteenth Amendment's "liberty" interest include individual behaviors. Second, even if regulating individual behavior were not constitutionally protected, it would be politically difficult to regulate. While the "nanny state" can legislate where some unhealthful behaviors can and cannot take place, it has been unsuccessful it eradicating these behaviors entirely.

Third, the state has in the past criminalized unhealthful behaviors. But almost a century of regulation of individual behavior suggests that enforcement of laws banning individual behavior is problematic at best and quite possibly ineffective. Laws banning drug possession did not eliminate IV drug use. Laws may be able to ban certain behaviors in specific places that can be monitored. But eliminating individual behavior everywhere presents the state with an enforcement dilemma. As a result, most state restrictions on individual behavior are attached to places where that behavior can be observed and controlled.

In the case of HIV/AIDS, obesity, and some of the indoor triggers that aggravate asthma (e.g., smoking), individual behavior is at the root of the public health threat. In the cases of asthma and obesity, it may be the parents' behavior or inaction that is placing children at risk. But there are significant limits, legal and political, on the state's and city's ability to regulate at-risk behaviors, especially when they take place in the home.

As a result, the state has sought to regulate at-risk behavior when and where it is legally, politically, and administratively possible to do so. In addition, using antismoking policy as a model, the Bloomberg administration proposed to tax some foods directly connected with obesity, but it has failed to get any of these proposals enacted.

In the case of HIV/AIDS, the state and city used their abilities to regulate business frequented by gay males to curb at-risk behavior. With obesity, the city is using the public school system to control overeating and nonnutritious eating as best it can.

Mandatory testing and reporting regulations are much more feasible when dealing with children. Parents have an interest in having their children seen by health professionals, and health professionals have a history of cooperating with public health authorities. As a result, mandatory testing of infants for lead poisoning and the reporting of results to state and local health authorities were never seen as controversial.

Direct Provision of Services

The public health profession has a long history of providing health services to at-risk populations. For the most part the direct provision of services by the public health establishment has not been controversial. There was little or no conflict between the public health community and the medical profession over the delivery of services. First, the public health infrastructure never sought to deliver a comprehensive range of health care services to middle- and upper-class citizens. Rather, on those few occasions when the public health profession sought to deliver a comprehensive array of services, it was to low-income populations, groups not sought after as clients by the medical profession. The advent of Medicare and Medicaid decreased public health involvement in the delivery of health care to indigent populations.

Second, most of the public health forays into the delivery of health services were disease or condition specific. And when the medical profession moved into these areas, the public health community decreased its involvement. For instance, the public health establishment initially took on the responsibility of mass vaccinations for polio and some communicable diseases. But in most cases it slowly retreated as the delivery of private health care assumed this responsibility for middle-class and affluent populations. More recently it has played a critical role in educating the public about the benefits of vaccination; for example, the human papillomavirus vaccine for young girls and boys. Third, and most important, the direct delivery of health services by the public health policy makers is associated with those diseases and conditions that can best be attacked at the community level.

Of the five public health conditions addressed in this study, HIV/AIDS provides the best examples of the public health community's delivery of services. Not only did HIV/AIDS take the entire health care community by surprise, but also its prevalence grew at such an alarming rate that the health care establishment was quickly overwhelmed by the number of victims needing assistance. In the early and mid-1980s, the health care establishment in New York City was in the midst of negotiating a number of hospital closings, reducing the number of available beds.

In the absence of initial action by all three levels of government, the nonprofit sector became the vanguard of service deliverers for those with HIV/AIDS. In some cases, such as housing, the nonprofit sector remains the primary service provider. In other instances, it was eventually replaced by either New York State or New York City, assisted on occasion by federal funds. Gay Men's Health Crisis was the leader in almost all areas of service delivery. These included family and partner therapy, nutrition, basic housekeeping services, advocating for those in need of social services, and transportation.

Housing was the other major service provided to HIV/AIDS victims. The need for housing evolved because of the ability of persons with AIDS to live longer lives, housing discrimination against those with the disease, a shortage of intermediate and skilled health facility beds for persons with AIDS, the impoverishment of those with HIV/AIDS, and the need for supportive housing that could both provide shelter and deliver needed services in one setting. Housing was delivered by a range of nonprofit groups, including the AIDS Resource Center, Housing Works, preexisting nursing homes, and community-based religious institutions.

The most significant contribution of all three levels of government toward the provision of services to HIV/AIDS patients was Medicaid. If an individual with AIDS was able to qualify for Medicaid, primarily through establishing disability, he was able to access a range of medical services, including housing through licensed nursing homes. Federal Ryan White funding, once it became available, also strengthened the state and city's ability to coordinate and deliver services to HIV/AIDS victims. Federal funding directly subsidized the provision of emergency services as well as state drug treatment and mental health services provision to those with AIDS.

Once the Koch administration created the Division of AIDS Services (later known as the HIV/AIDS Services Administration) within the larger Human Resources Administration, the city slowly began to develop the capacity to assist persons with HIV/AIDS. One of the primary services provided by the division was assisting those with AIDS in receiving and coordinating all the available city services for which they qualified. These included hospitalization, case management, housing, the receipt of Medicaid and food stamps, employment and vocational assistance, and counseling for victims and their family members. As the need for housing increased, the city began contracting with nonprofit community-based groups. In 2005 the city and state established the Supportive Housing Agreement to further the commitment to house persons with AIDS who needed it. The city also provided rent subsidies to those who were eligible and established homeless shelters, or sections of shelters, for those with AIDS. Budgetary issues during both the Giuliani and Bloomberg administrations, however, frequently got in the way of the city being able to supply housing to all who needed it.

Over time, the state also assumed a significant service provision role. Funded in part by federal Ryan White funds, the state established HIV Care Networks, local associations of health care providers and community-based organizations to assist those with HIV/AIDS. Through the state's AIDS Institute, community-based services were coordinated through community organizations, including family services and home-based care. For Medicaid recipients, the state also provided persons with AIDS with special needs plans through the establishment of AIDS Designated Care Centers in some of the city's hospitals. And for AIDS victims without insurance, the state created a pool of funds to pay for medical care.

The state had practically complete control over drug rehabilitation services, which were in short supply. The state's Harm Reduction Initiative attempted to expand these services to more substance abusers and their families.

Similar to HIV/AIDS, nonprofit organizations have taken the lead in providing services to victims of other public health conditions. With lead paint poisoning, several nonprofit organizations and hospitals in the city have created lead-safe houses where families can go while their homes are being made lead safe. This type of service is in short supply. Both HPD and DOHMH provide lead paint home inspection services, but this is as much a part of the city's regulatory regime as it is a provision of a service.

Nonprofit organizations have similarly taken the lead in the provision of services related to asthma. In Harlem, northern Manhattan, and the South Bronx, nonprofit groups have gone into homes assisting families in identifying and alleviating indoor asthma triggers. Some of these same groups have also assisted families in developing asthma management plans. The city's Asthma Resource Centers have also been involved in the coordination of asthma care and management in selected communities. These centers have been involved in the distribution of spacers and peak flow meters for those asthma sufferers not eligible for Medicaid.

With obesity, the city and nonprofit, community-based organizations have both been active in providing services. The primary venue for the provision and antiobesity services is the schools. A few nonprofit groups have entered the schools with programs to combat obesity. In order to promote physical activity, the Department of Education in conjunction with the Department of Parks and Recreation is converting school playgrounds to city parks that can be used by the community on weekends and when school is not in session. The other major city service provision to combat obesity is directed toward the provision of nutritious foods to neighborhoods where these foods have been in short supply. The Shop Healthy NYC, the Green Cart Program, and the Health Bucks Program are also services designed to create greater food choices for communities where fresh produce has been in short supply. The state is also attempting to supply more nutritious foods to adult and child day care centers.

Liability

The assignment of liability as a public health policy tool is possible only when the source of the condition is singular and known. Of the five conditions or diseases discussed here, liability was employed only with lead paint poisoning. Even in this case, there was the possibility, however remote, that the source of the poisoning among some populations might be food or cookery. For this reason, landlords and even the mayor objected to that aspect of the local law. The presumption of liability created by the legislation gave victims and their families easier access to civil litigation against landlords in cases of poisoning, but it also served to motivate landlords to do all they could to remediate lead paint deterioration in their buildings. There are isolated cases of individuals infected with AIDS being criminally prosecuted for knowingly having unprotected sex with others, but this was never a component of public health policy.

The Tools Not Used

Drawing on the long history of public health policy making, there are tools that were not used in the five cases examined in this study. In some cases, use of these tools could have furthered the identification and control of the disease or condition. Public health policy, however, is not made in isolation of other public policy concerns. Those tools that would be most effective in responding to public health threats must frequently compete with other public policy goals, including individual freedom and liberty, privacy, confidentiality, and cost. Former city commissioner of health Stephen Joseph noted that "AIDS is the first major public health issue in this century for which political values rather than health requirements set the agenda" (Joseph 1992, 89). It may be that as those at risk for public health threats begin to advocate for themselves, this phenomenon may spread to future public health conditions.

Most notable on the list of unused tools is the use of quarantine, the most coercive regulatory tool. In various outbreaks, from leprosy to tuberculosis, public health has employed isolation through quarantine well into the twentieth century. It is rarely used today, though. Public health policy makers know much more about contagion today than they did previously. In the past, isolation through quarantine was a response based as much on ignorance about disease as on a disease's contagion. But as recently as the HIV/AIDS outbreak of the 1980s, before the existence of knowledge about how HIV/AIDS was spread, some policy makers called for the quarantine of persons with AIDS. In addition, throughout the later half of the twentieth century persons with disease began to advocate for themselves in the political arena, demanding more research, compassionate treatment, and rights. In the face of ignorance or inconclusive findings on disease contagion, these victims have asserted their rights to be free of restraint and to be treated in the least intrusive manner possible. Finally, in the face of potential pushback from those with disease and their advocates, an attempt on the part of public health policy makers to adopt the most appropriate, least intrusive, and most humane tools, and the general policy-making environment seeking a less regulated society, the political system is less likely to use quarantine under any circumstance.

A second tool that has been underutilized is contact tracing. As employed in cases of venereal disease, contact tracing involves the health worker asking the patient to reveal those persons with whom the patient has had sexual contact. The patient's name remains confidential, but the health worker then contacts those named individuals and urges them to be tested. All contact tracing is ultimately voluntary since patients cannot be forced to name their sexual partners. At the same time, however, the protocol and language used by the health worker in discussing the need to contact sexual partners can certainly convey a tone of authority or not. And the precise protocol to be used is usually established at the state or city level.

With HIV/AIDS, New York State's initial contact tracing protocol was weak. Because of concerns with privacy, patients were advised to engage in partner notification on their own. As a result health care workers did no contract tracing. In 2000 the protocol was strengthened. Physicians were mandated to discuss with patients those sexual or needle-sharing partners who might have been exposed to HIV. If the patient identified partners, either the physician or DOHMH would contact them. But the law made clear that individuals were not obligated to reveal the names of partners, and the confidentiality of the patient was retained. The weaknesses in the law resulted in few partners being notified.

Another underutilized tool, particularly in the case of HIV/AIDS, was mandatory testing. Early on in the outbreak of HIV/AIDS, mandatory testing was resisted both for privacy reasons and because there was no cure. Today in New York, only newborns are mandated to be tested for HIV. All others are counseled to be tested but can opt out. Unlike HIV/AIDS, mandatory testing for lead poisoning was adopted in many states. Some public health officials in New York want to employ a tuberculosis-like testing regime for HIV/AIDS where a test would be mandated for some at-risk groups. Recently, New York State rescinded mandatory tuberculosis testing for school age children.

Finally, in the fight against smoking, New York State and New York City are using taxes on tobacco to dissuade New Yorkers from smoking. Governor Patterson in the early 2000s attempted to place a tax on sugary beverages. The beverage industry was successful in defeating the measure.

Factors That Influence the Use of Specific Public Health Policy Tools

Within the confines of this discussion, there are two analytic frameworks that offer explanations as to why specific tools or a specific set of tools are adopted to address public health policy issues. One hypothesis, originating in the study of urban politics, argues that forces within the urban political milieu can explain urban public policy, including public health policy. These forces include the need of cities to adopt policies that promote economic development, the increasing ethnic and racial diversity of cities, and, within the context of urban politics in the United States, the impact on urban politics of actions taken by the state and federal governments.

The second hypothesis is based more on a rational model or an idealized perspective of medical decision making. This second hypothesis suggests that information, or the state of knowledge, on specific diseases or conditions in the public health policy arena drives the selection of the appropriate tool by policy makers. When knowledge is available to address a public health problem, it is that knowledge that determines the appropriate choice of policy tool chosen, independent of forces or influences coming from the urban political system. The availability of information on a cure for or elimination of the condition will result in public policy tools being adopted to bring about this end. In the absence of a cure or elimination of the condition, available information on how to treat debilitating symptoms or how to prevent the condition will dictate the public policy tools adopted. And in the absence of all information, public policy tools either addressing or incorporating systemic ignorance about the condition will be adopted.

It should come as no surprise that both hypotheses offer credible explanations as to why specific tools are selected. At the same time, however, the way in which the two sets of forces affect the choice of public health policy tools is quite distinct. The availability of information provides a constraint on the choice of policy tool. No knowledge or limited knowledge seriously affects a political system's ability to respond and therefore influences the type of response. What makes health policy a fascinating area of study is the fact that the existence or absence of knowledge about how to solve the problem is so significant. In most areas of urban public policy—housing, transportation, poverty, and even education—the knowledge to solve the problem is present. The primary stumbling blocks are the forces that prevent those in positions of authority from summoning the political will to employ the knowledge. In public health policy making, the forces that affect the operation of urban political systems do not have the direct or consistent impact on policy tool choice. Declining deference to expertise and the politicization of knowledge in the public policy making arena has been less of a factor in public health than in other urban public policy arenas. Nevertheless, the forces that affect urban public policy making in general do create a context within which public policy tool selection takes place; and they also at times dictate how the tools are implemented.

The five public health threats examined in this study illustrate how the state of knowledge affects the public policy rationale and the subsequent policy tools adopted. Childhood lead paint poisoning provides a case where knowledge on the cause was clear. There was a period of time in the early twentieth century when children suffered from lead poisoning, and there was limited knowledge of the cause. After the elimination of lead from gasoline in the 1970s, however, only one major source of lead in a child's environment remained, lead-based paint.

In addition, because of the source of the problem, prevention was viewed as a less intrusive and possibly less expensive solution to the problem than treating children once they were poisoned. The fact that the effects of childhood lead poisoning were potentially long term, even once blood lead levels were reduced, made the case for prevention all the more convincing. As a result regulation was employed to prevent childhood lead poisoning, despite the opposition from the lead paint industry at first and the real estate industry later.

Unlike lead paint poisoning, HIV/AIDS and West Nile virus were both diseases where knowledge of the cause was unknown at the initial outbreak. The source of West Nile virus was discovered quickly, resulting in education and regulatory tools being adopted to facilitate prevention.

The discovery of the cause of HIV/AIDS took longer. In the interim, the public health policy response could do little more than deliver appropriate services to those with the disease and formulate prevention policy based on educated guesses. In addition, even after the discovery of the causes, the fact that the disease could be contracted through distinct and lifestyle-related activities complicated the policy response. Unlike childhood lead paint poisoning and West Nile virus, HIV/AIDS prevention could not be easily achieved through regulation, so the public health policy system had to rely much more on education.

For the most part, the overall causes of obesity are known. Similar to HIV/AIDS, however, much of obesity is related to lifestyle behaviors that are difficult to regulate. As a result, obesity prevention relies heavily on education. In the case of restaurant calorie labeling, some public education requires the regulation of some businesses. And to the extent that obesity is related to the existence of food deserts or the built environment, regulation or other less coercive inducements to food suppliers have been used to a limited extent.

The lack of knowledge on the causes of asthma continues to confound the public health and medical communities. Knowledge does exist on what triggers asthma attacks and how to manage attacks well enough to prevent the need for emergency room visits or hospitalization. Asthma triggers remain so ubiquitous in the urban environment that it has been difficult to regulate them. Federal and local regulations have reduced air pollution, but the most significant improvements have been in education and provision of services that have allowed children with asthma, their parents, and schools to better manage the disease and prevent hospital visits.

Of the forces that affect urban political systems, economic development receives the most attention. Much of the recent literature on urban politics, and New York City politics as well, views economic development as the first among equals of the forces affecting how urban political systems behave. From a public health perspective, economic development is a perplexing phenomenon. On the one hand, the contemporary study of urban politics suggests that economic development may be the primary way by which urban political systems will raise sufficient revenue enabling them to respond to public health problems. On the other hand, however, economic development activities produce negative externalities in the form of pollution and other waste products, as well as lifestyle choices that not only are harmful to the urban environment but may also be the direct cause of some public health conditions, such as asthma and obesity. Thus, in some instances urban economic development can be viewed as both the cause of the problem and the source for cure of urban public health problems.

What places economic development activities in a unique position in urban political systems is the fact that they are pursued and defended by a powerful coalition of actors including developers, real estate interests, and construction and trade unions. Over the past several decades, as economic development has become one of the most viable ways of cities to maintain a positive fiscal flow, many government and elected officials have joined this coalition.

While the existence of knowledge is critical in the adoption of public health policy tools, when that knowledge points to economic development interests as the cause of the public health problem, the forces defending economic development become a significant intervening obstacle in the adoption of policy. Even with the existence of definitive knowledge about the link between economic development activities and public health problems, economic development interests will oppose the more coercive public health policy tools in favor of the least coercive. Regulations that inhibit or are perceived to inhibit economic development will be opposed in favor of less coercive measures. Even public health activities as benign as education may at times be opposed if economic development or private-sector profitability is threatened.

In the early years of the campaign against AIDS, New York City and state officials were reluctant to close bathhouses or gay bars even though they were aware of unsafe sexual practices taking place inside these establishments. San Francisco moved to close these types of establishments more than a year before the city or state took any action. When the state did act, it was only to issue regulations banning certain sexual practices from commercial venues where gay males would gather. Only after the city and state realized that these regulations were insufficient did closings take place. Reluctance by the state and city to close these places of business was as much about privacy and civil liberties as it was about not wanting to inhibit business practice.

Policy toward lead poisoning provides a clearer example. Regulations on inspection and remediation of lead paint hazards were targeted at the real estate industry and those developers involved in the rehabilitation of older housing in the city. These industries lobbied against the legislation creating the regulations. The city had comprehensive lead paint legislation as early as the 1980s, but several mayors viewed that law as unworkable, in part because of the burden it placed on developers and the real estate industry. The persistence of childhood lead paint poisoning as an issue due to the number of victimized children and the periodic lowering of the harmful blood lead level threshold kept the issue alive for two decades. As recently as 2003, the political clout of economic development interests, in part, convinced the mayor to veto comprehensive lead paint legislation, although the veto was overridden by the city council. There were two key differences between lead paint as an issue and AIDS. First, at the time of the city's most recent, and most comprehensive, lead paint poisoning law, knowledge of the impact of lead poisoning was well established and accepted. Even those in the housing industry did not dispute it. Knowledge about AIDS and its causes in the mid-1980s at the time the city started adopting policy, however, was at best very recent and at worst still being debated. Second, the primary victims of lead poisoning were innocent children, whereas persons with AIDS were viewed as victims who had engaged in risky behavior.

Asthma and obesity have also been associated with economic development, but to date both conditions are so multifactorial that the knowledge is insufficient to provide evidence for regulatory response. There are certainly air quality regulations, promulgated by all three levels of government, but most of these were legislated and implemented long before asthma became a national or local problem. At best, the link between air pollution and asthma was only a small reason for the four-decade legacy of air quality regulations.

The links between economic development and obesity (home technology such as video games, the built environment, fast food) are only a small piece of the obesity-causal puzzle. But the beverage industry has successfully rebuffed several attempts by the state and the city to implement regulations to reduce sugary beverage consumption. This has forced the city to rely more on providing the public with the knowledge that would hopefully result in engaging in healthier behavior. There are regulations requiring some food manufacturers and restaurants to provide the information in a format that the public can better understand.

Unlike economic development, there is no direct link between increasing racial and ethnic diversity and the creation of public health problems. The only possible direct connection is the danger that lax enforcement of immigration laws might have on the mobility of diseases, such as SARS earlier this century. Racial and ethnic groups with low-income constituencies, those who are most susceptible to public health problems, have been at the forefront of campaigns to get public health policy adopted. When public health threats are most visible in minority communities, and when the causes of these threats can be linked to forces external to these communities, minority leadership has advocated for the most comprehensive use of public health policy tools.

There are exceptions. As was previously noted, the prevalence of AIDS among African Americans and Latinos surpassed that of white gay males very early in the epidemic. While the gay community organized to address the disease, the minority community leaders ignored their own victims and the extent to which it was affecting their communities for almost a decade. It was not until the 1990s, as minority HIV/AIDS numbers continued to climb, that the African American and Latino communities began to play a greater role in organizing and lobbying for a greater response.

One other possible exception is that some minority groups, including the NAACP and groups representing bodega owners, joined the opposition to the Bloomberg administration's proposed cap on sugary drinks. For bodega owners, opposition was a self-interested business move. For other minority groups, opposition was due to minority-owned businesses in the community as well as recognition of past support by the beverage industry.

Their representation of the victims of public health problems, with the exception of AIDS in the 1980s, places racial and ethnic groups in the position of pursuing the most comprehensive policy solutions. And because of their legacy of successful governmental action with a variety of social and economic concerns, these groups have supported the adoption of those policy tools, such as regulation and the provision of public services, that rely on the full weight of the government or nonprofit groups to resolve a problem. In response to asthma, the minority community pushed hard for both regulations and increased services; and in some cases, minority-led community-based organizations made decisions to provide their own services to asthma sufferers when the public response as inadequate.

To curtail air pollution in communities with high rates of asthma, minority leadership attempted, unsuccessfully, to pressure the Metropolitan Transit Authority to relocate its bus depots from northern Manhattan. This problem was resolved in part as the bus fleet was converted to natural gas, ultralow sulfur diesel fuel, and hybrid technologies. To the extent, however, that facilities producing any type of noxious or hazardous waste have been located in low-income minority neighborhoods, those communities have used claims of environmental racism to identify a broader problem in the city. To abate indoor pollutants, non-profit minority-led groups in northern Manhattan and the Bronx not only assisted families with developing asthma management plans for their children but in some cases went so far as to inspect homes for the presence of indoor asthma triggers, something the city lacked the authority to do.

In those cases where less intrusive policy tools, such as education, are employed, racial and ethnic groups have pursued, not always successfully, requirements that public health educational output be provided in multilingual formats. Because of the increasing diversity of the city, public health officials have also come to accept the necessity of multilingual public health policies; although logistics and budgetary constraints do not always make this possible.

The influence of the federal and state governments on public health policy is significant, but the two levels of government have had different impacts on New York City's public health policy tool choices. As discussed earlier, out of necessity public health was a function of local government long before the formation of the modern nation-state. Unlike economic development and racial and ethnic diversity, intergovernmental relations have rarely, if ever, influenced the development of a specific public health policy tool at the local level in response to a public health threat. For the most part the federal and state levels have sought to supplement and support the local public health establishment and the tools it is employing in response to public health threats. Given their legal responsibility for their units of local government, states are far more active in this area and, on occasion, intervene directly into the public health affairs of their local governments. The federal government plays a much more limited role, and only in the face of public health threats that are national in scope does it intervene at the local level.

In the United States, public health fell under state control both because of local government's traditional role in this area and because the founders desired to keep the functions of the new national government as limited as possible. Over time, revolutions in communication, transportation, the development of a national economy, and changing political attitudes encouraged the national government to expand its role in a wide variety of policy arenas including public health. The national government did develop a role in public health policy making, but for the most part the role has remained limited. With Medicare and

Medicaid in the 1960s, however, the national government developed a large role in the financing of health insurance and, indirectly, the delivery of health care throughout the entire country. As a result, its impact on public health policy has grown considerably.

One of the areas of public health policy that is under the control of the federal government, in cooperation with the states, is disease tracking and reporting. As far back as the 1870s, the U.S. Marine Hospital Service, predecessor of the U.S. Public Health Service, was tracking specific diseases in cooperation with those states that had the capacity to accurately report. By the 1920s most states were cooperating with the Public Health Service and later the CDC in the tracking and reporting of diseases, as well as decision making on which diseases should be reported. For the states, this meant establishing a reliable network that included physicians and hospitals in order to accurately track and report designated diseases.

The CDC, the State Department of Health, and the city also cooperate in screening and monitoring for childhood lead paint poisoning and West Nile virus. State regulations require that all infants be tested for lead poisoning and that the blood lead levels above a specified threshold be reported to the state, which then reports them to the CDC. Similarly, physicians and hospitals are mandated to report cases of West Nile virus to the state as well.

The federal government plays two other roles in responding to public health threats. One, not addressed in this discussion, is research. Federal public health research is decentralized throughout the federal executive branch, including but not limited to the Centers for Disease Control and Prevention, the National Institutes of Health, United States Department of Agriculture, and the Environmental Protection Agency. These federal agencies and others support basic research into the causes of public health problems as well as more policy-oriented research examining possible solutions to public health problems. At times, however, the federal health research enterprise has been criticized for focusing too much on cure and not enough on prevention (Stevenson 2003).

The other federal role in public health policy is funding. In terms of specific policy tools federal funding covers a wide range of activities. Within this range, two funding streams are significant. First, because of the CDC's role in monitoring and screening public health conditions at the national level, much CDC intergovernmental funding supports state and local government participation in these activities. Second, Medicaid and Medicare address the basic health care needs of large numbers of low-income Americans. As such, they serve two purposes for the public health establishment. First, because of the public health sector's historical role of addressing the primary health needs of low-income citizens who cannot afford to purchase health care in the private market, Medicaid and Medicare have, in a limited way, given selected populations the ability to purchase health services on the private market. This has alleviated a major burden of the public health sector. Second, in the case of asthma, Medicaid paid for spacers and peak flow meters for low-income children. Similarly, for those children with severe cases of lead paint poisoning, Medicaid paid for hospitalization and chelation. In the case of HIV/AIDS, most persons with AIDS were not eligible for Medicaid when they were diagnosed with the disease. In many cases they had to demonstrate a state of disability for three months as a result of the disease before they could apply for Medicaid.

In terms of funding for specific policy tools, federal funding rarely if ever funds state or local regulatory regimes. But the federal government does regulate some of elements of the public health milieu directly under its jurisdiction. In the area of lead paint poisoning, the federal Department of Housing and Urban Development regulates lead paint abatement in those residential properties receiving federal assistance. The federal Food and Drug Administration regulates blood banks in an attempt to decrease the transmission of HIV-contaminated blood. And the 1990 Nutrition Labeling and Education Act requires nutrition labels, including calories on packaged foods.

Federal funding does support education and public awareness activities. Much of this is connected to the CDC's traditional role of tracking and screening. One example of this is the CDC's National AIDS Clearinghouse and the CDC program educating physicians and health professionals through the AIDS Information Line. Possibly the most unique element of the federal public health education effort is when the White House promotes a public health issue. Michelle Obama's Let's Move campaign has become a highly visible component of obesity awareness and education.

In a few cases, federal funding addresses the delivery of services. Much of this is done through Medicaid. But in a few instances, the federal government has moved beyond Medicaid in providing services in response to a public health threat or problem. In the case of Ryan White, federal funds subsidized emergency services, the purchase of insurance or drugs for persons with AIDS, and case management.

The passage of the Affordable Care Act (ACA) in 2010 presents several opportunities, as well as challenges, for continued federal involvement in public health policy. First, by giving many more access to medical care, the ACA promises to address some of the individual health issues that frequently fall under the jurisdiction of public health policy makers. Second, parts of the ACA have the potential to bring the public health and medical care communities closer together. The ACA established the National Prevention Council at the federal level involving twenty federal agencies. Chaired by the surgeon general, the council has already produced a National Prevention Strategy and Action Plan (Rein 2013). In addition the ACA funds a few Community Transformation Grants, which fund those at the local level implementing community-level programs to prevent chronic diseases (US CDC 2013). Third, however, the cost of the Affordable Care Act, at least in the short term, threatens to draw away needed federal dollars from those grant programs dedicated to public health issues such as AIDS, lead paint, and obesity.

The division of responsibilities and the use of public health policy tools by New York State and New York City are complex. In responding to childhood lead paint poisoning and obesity, the state has played a limited role. With asthma, West Nile virus, and obesity, the state had more of a role but the city still dominated. With HIV/AIDS, the state played a major role, acting as the city's partner in many facets of policy.

There are at least two reasons why New York State's involvement in policies toward HIV/AIDS was far more comprehensive than its involvement in other public health policy areas. First and foremost, AIDS was far more devastating than the four other conditions discussed here and most other health conditions addressed by local public health authorities in the later half of the twentieth century. Second, AIDS struck New York in the early 1980s as it was slowly recovering from the fiscal crisis of the mid-1970s. By itself, the city lacked the fiscal wherewithal to address the level of need it was facing. The fiscal crisis underscored the city's dependence on the state and control by the state. With AIDS, as with the fiscal crisis, the state had little choice but to get involved.

There was at least one critical area of policy, regulation of sexual activity at commercial establishments that catered to gay males, where the state took the lead in the absence of city action. For drug rehabilitation, since the state had close to a monopoly on this type of program, it remained the dominant service provider in this area. In a related area, because of state drug laws, the city and nonprofit groups needed state waivers to conduct clean needle exchanges. Because of its programmatic links with drug users through community-based service providers, the state implemented the Harm Reduction Initiative, providing services to drug users and their families.

Because of its historical function of tracking and reporting diseases, the state also took the lead role, sometimes controversial, in HIV/AIDS monitoring and testing regulations. Although it took many years for the state and city to develop screening guidelines, the state ultimately had control over decisions to make testing anonymous or confidential. It also controlled regulations on pretest counseling, the mandatory screening of all newborns, opt-in screening for pregnant women, contact tracing and partner notification (or lack thereof), and the decision in 2000 on the mandatory reporting of all HIV-positive cases.

The state AIDS Institute was at the center of much of the state's HIV/AIDS activities. One of their major functions was educational. The institute produced materials promoting prevention and listing the availability of services. For hospitals and clinics, the institute served as a clearinghouse for materials on AIDS prevention. The State Department of Education also participated in prevention education and, along with the city, cooperated in the production of and HIV/AIDS Prevention Curriculum Guide for the schools. The AIDS Institute funded prevention programs targeted at women and adolescents. The state, cooperating with the city, was also involved in creating supportive housing programs for those with HIV/AIDS.

Obesity is another public health issue where the state engaged in educating the public. The state's Just Say Yes to Fruits and Vegetables program was targeted to food stamp recipients. The state, along with the city, implemented the Eat Well Play Hard Program in childcare centers and in the early elementary grades. Similarly, the state's Active8Kids program attempts to educate children about eating well and engaging in physical activity.

HIV/AIDS forced the state and city to involve themselves in the direct provision of services. The state was able to modify Medicaid funding in order to better address the service needs of AIDS patients. Ultimately, the state established a pool of funds for those uninsured persons with AIDS. For eligible children with asthma, Medicaid and the complementary State Child Health Insurance Program (SCHIP) pay for spacers and peak flow meters.

Some of the state's HIV/AIDS service provision activities were subsidized by federal Ryan White funding. The state used these funds to establish networks of community-based organizations that could deliver services to those in need. Following a somewhat similar strategy, the state established regional asthma coalitions. The purpose of theses coalitions was to develop better methods at the community level to improve the delivery of asthma care.

New York State's Department of Health maintains laboratory facilities for testing the presence of diseases and conditions. The city does as well, but there has been an attempt to reduce redundancy, especially during times of budgetary scarcity. During the initial West Nile virus outbreak, the state lab tested specimens for the presence of the virus.

One of the more unique public health policy roles for the state is training. The state has traditionally held the responsibility for the licensing of occupations in the health and allied health professions. The state coordinates and licenses the training for contractors and subcontractors who engage in household lead paint abatement. Similarly, the state environmental authorities control permitting for the use of substances that are considered toxic or hazardous to the environment. To this effect, the city had to obtain permission from the state to use larvacide in its attempt to eradicate West Nile virus. The State Department of Environmental Conservation both issued the permit and monitored the spraying.

Is New York Unique?

Historians of public health in the United States have long noted the leading role played by New York City in the development of U.S. public health policy. While the city was not the first city to adopt each and every public health policy innovation, it was noteworthy for its comprehensive public health policies dealing with multiple public health problems. Some cities adopted responses to childhood lead paint poisoning long before New York. In responding to the rise of HIV/AIDS, San Francisco's efforts predate some of those developed by New York. Nevertheless, in looking across the array of public health problems, New York stands out as a city that has adopted a comprehensive policy response to public health issues. Because of New York's size and density, any public health problem that exists in densely populated urban areas is going to be present in New York, probably with greater intensity and prevalence than in most other cities. In addition, the city's age can explain the existence of some public health problems as well. Aging housing stock has contributed to the lead paint and asthma problems.

A second reason for New York's status as a public health leader is the city's political culture and liberal attitudes toward the use of government to solve problems. Fed by waves of immigrants, many of whom have arrived with liberal, if not socialist, ideals about the role of government, the city's political establishment has never questioned the necessity of government intervention in the lives of its citizens to achieve positive ends. Just as important, public health policy has served as one example, if not the most visible example, of how successful government intervention can be.

New York City's strong-mayor form of government has also allowed the city's leaders to move expeditiously in attending to public health problems. Strong mayors have the ability move their executive branches to respond to public health problems without being hampered by legislatures or constituency politics. The public health leadership of Mayor Bloomberg has been one of the significant hallmarks of his three terms. Under his leadership the city has initiated a major campaign against obesity and has furthered the city's fight against childhood asthma. Without his leadership, it is likely that the policy tools employed by the city against obesity and asthma would be much fewer than they are.

But on occasion strong mayors in New York have used their powers to block public health responses. Mayor Koch failed to implement the existing lead paint poison policy and was accused of delaying the city's response to AIDS. Mayors Giuliani and Bloomberg both used their position to block comprehensive lead paint poisoning legislation. While Mayor Giuliani moved rapidly to stop the spread of West Nile virus and initiated the city's campaign against childhood asthma, budgetary politics during both his administration and the administration of Mayor Bloomberg resulted in setbacks in the delivery of needed services to persons with HIV/AIDS.

Have the forces that influence the adoption of public health policy tools in New York City had a similar affect on other cities? There is little reason to believe that those forces discussed in this study, the availability of knowledge, the need of cities to promote economic development, racial and ethnic diversity, and the impact of the state and federal levels of government have not had the same impact on other cities' adoption of public health policy tools. Knowledge is ubiquitous. Information about public health research and policy innovations is disseminated through professional journals, professional societies, organizations that represent the interests of cities, and federal public health officials. Moreover, big-city public health officials frequently change jobs moving from one large city to another. In addition, these cities' public health establishments are constantly monitoring each other looking for ways in which to respond to current public health problems.

Because the same forces that affect New York City influence all large cities in the United States, their influence, to the extent that these forces influence public health policy, should be similar in all cities. With regard to economic development, all large cities in the United States experienced declining federal aid over the past decades. As a result, toward the end of the twentieth century these cities were increasingly left to fend for themselves. And the promotion of economic development became one of the primary strategies for securing a positive revenue flow. At the same time, in promoting economic development, these cities faced an emerging global market in which they had to compete for economic development. All cities have to deal with the negative externalities of development success: larger, more dense populations, increased traffic, more waste, and housing issues. But some cities, such as New York, succeeded in attracting more economic development than others, giving them the revenue to respond to the public health problems created by economic development.

With regard to intergovernmental relations, most large U.S. cities experienced decreased federal assistance in the final decades of the twentieth century. New York City's aggressive pursuit of federal funding in the middle of the twentieth century made it more vulnerable to federal cuts later on. Another major difference among these cities is that states differ to the extent to which they divide public policy responsibilities, including public health, between themselves and their local governments. So while New York State was an equal partner to New York City in combating HIV/AIDS and has played a significant role in the campaign against obesity, it is not known what role other states play in assisting their respective large cities in responding to public health problems.

Finally, urban racial and ethnic diversity does not so much create public health problems or even influence the choice of public policy tool, but it does challenge, if not complicate, the way in which the tools are implemented. All cities with diverse racial and ethnic populations should be experiencing the same challenges. Public health education programs must be presented in the languages that will allow racial and ethnic minorities to receive the appropriate message. And regulations and services must be employed in a culturally competent manner if they are to be utilized correctly. Presently, New York is the most racially and ethnically diverse city in the country. As a result, the challenges in implementing public health policy in New York City are greater than other cities. Because of the growing diversity of many large cities in the country, however, this difference is one of degree, not of approach.

Chapter 1 · Introduction

Allison, Graham. 1971. *Essence of Decision: Explaining the Cuban Missile Crisis.* Chicago: University of Chicago Press.

Bautista, Eddie. 2010. Making fair share fairer. *Gotham Gazette,* October 5. www.gotham gazette.com/article/20101005/203/3378.

Berg, Bruce. 2007. *New York City Politics: Governing Gotham.* New Brunswick: Rutgers University Press.

Birkland, Thomas. 2005. *An Introduction to the Study of Public Policy* (2nd edition). New York: M. E. Sharpe.

Braybrooke, David, and Charles Lindblom. 1963. *A Strategy of Decision: Policy Evaluation as a Social Process.* New York: Free Press.

Clinton, Hillary Rodham. 2004. Now can we talk about health care? *New York Times,* April 18.

Duffy, John. 1968a. *A History of Public Health in New York City, 1625–1866.* New York: Russell Sage Foundation.

———. 1968b. *A History of Public Health in New York City, 1866–1966.* New York: Russell Sage Foundation.

———. 1990. *The Sanitarians.* Urbana: University of Illinois Press.

Elkin, Stephen. 1985. Pluralism in its place: state and regime in liberal democracy. In Roger Benjamin and Stephen Elkin (eds.), *The Democratic State,* 179–212. Lawrence: University Press of Kansas.

Fee, Elizabeth. 1993. Public health, past, present and future: a shared social vision. Introduction to George Rosen, *A History of Public Health,* ix–lxvii. Baltimore: Johns Hopkins University Press.

Fritschler, A. Lee. 1975. *Smoking and Politics: Policymaking and the Federal Bureaucracy.* Englewood Cliffs: Prentice Hall.

Joseph, Stephen. 1992. *Dragon within the Gates: The Once and Future AIDS Epidemic.* New York: Carroll and Graf.

Kirk, Krishna. 2002. *The 2002–03 Green Book: Official Directory of the City of New York.* New York City: City of New York Department of Citywide Administrative Services (Martha Hirst, Commissioner; Michael Bloomberg, Mayor).

Koch, Edward I. 1980. The mandate millstone. *Public Interest* 61, 42–57.

Leavitt, Judith Walzer. 1995. Be safe, be sure: epidemic smallpox. In David Rosner (ed.), *Hives of Sickness: Public Health and Epidemics in New York City,* 95–114. New Brunswick: Rutgers University Press.

Lieber, Joseph, and Sandra Opdycke. 1995. Public health. In Kenneth Jackson (ed.), *The Encyclopedia of New York City,* 910–914. New Haven: Yale University Press.

Logan, John, and Harvey Molotch. 1996. The city as growth machine. In Susan Fainstein and Scott Campbell (eds.), *Readings in Urban Theory*, 291–337. Cambridge, MA: Blackwell.

Markel, Howard. 2010. Tuberculosis. In Kenneth Jackson (ed.), *The Encyclopedia of New York City* (2nd edition), 1337. New Haven: Yale University Press.

New York City Department of Health and Mental Hygiene. 2004. *Health Disparities in New York City* (supported by the Commonwealth Fund).

New York City Health and Hospitals Corporation. 2003. Facility Directory. NYC Health and Hospitals Corporation Website: www.nyc.gov/html/hhc/html/directory.html. (accessed April 12, 2003).

Patel, Kant, and Mark E. Rushefsky. 2005. *The Politics of Public Health in the United States*. New York: M. E. Sharpe.

Rosen, George. 1993. *A History of Public Health*. Baltimore: Johns Hopkins University Press.

Rosner, David. 1995. Introduction: "Hives of Sickness and Vice." In David Rosner (ed.), *Hives of Sickness: Public Health and Epidemics in New York City*, 1–22. New Brunswick: Rutgers University Press.

Sassen, Saskia. 2001. *The Global City* (2nd edition). Princeton: Princeton University Press.

Savitch. H. V. 1988. *Post Industrial Cities: Politics and Planning in New York, Paris and London*. Princeton: Princeton University Press.

Schneider, Mary-Jane. 2011. *Introduction to Pubic Health* (3rd edition). Boston: Jones and Bartlett Publishers.

Simon, Herbert. 1965. *Administrative Behavior: A Study of Decision Making Processes in Administrative Organizations*. New York: Free Press.

Stone, Clarence. 1989. *Regime Politics: Governing Atlanta*. Lawrence: University Press of Kansas.

Stone, Deborah. 2002. *The Policy Paradox: The Art of Political Decision Making-Revised Edition*. New York: W. W. Norton.

Thacker, S. B., and D. F. Stroup. 1994. Future direction for comprehensive public health surveillance and health information systems in the United States. *American Journal of Epidemiology* 140, 383–397.

Thaler, Richard, and Cass Sunstein. 2008. *Nudge*. London: Penguin Books.

Wildavsky, Aaron. 1979. *Speaking Truth to Power: The Art and Craft of Policy Analysis*. New York: Little, Brown.

World Health Organization. 2010. Adelaide Statement on Health in All Policies. www.who .int/social_determinants/hiap_statement_who_sa_final.pdf.

Chapter 2 · Lead Poisoning in Children

Alfaro, Jose, Sally Kohn, and Nicholas Freudenberg. 1982. New law on lead poisoning isn't enough (letter to the editor). *New York Times*, January 30.

American Academy of Pediatrics Committee on Environmental Health. 2005. Lead exposure in children: prevention, detection and management. *Pediatrics* 116, no. 4, October, 21–23.

Archibold, Randall C. 2003. Council speaker is accused of stalling lead paint bill. *New York Times*, July 16.

Arena, Salvatore. 1995. Court tells city to explain lead lag. *Daily News*, July 4.

Baker, Al, and Randall C. Archibald. 2003. Appeals court strikes down city's law on lead-based paint. *New York Times*, July 2.

Basler, Barbara. 1986. City will close family shelter for renovation. *New York Times*, March 29.

Beller, Margo D. 1994. Lead looms as next threat facing property insurers potential seen as rival asbestos. *Journal of Commerce*, June 16. www.joc.com/lead-looms-next-threat-facing-property-insurers-potential-seen-rival-asbestos_19940616.html (accessed June 24, 2014).

Bellinger, David C., and Andrew M. Bellinger. 2006. Childhood lead poisoning: the tortuous path from science to policy. *Journal of Clinical Investigation* 116, no. 4, April 3, 853–857.

Berney, Barbara. 1993. Round and round it goes: the epidemiology of childhood lead poisoning, 1950–1990. *Milbank Quarterly* 71, no. 1, 3–39.

Bluemel, Erik, Perry Chen, and Cary Hirschstein. 2005. Assessing the impacts of New York City's lead-based paint legislation (Local Law 1 of 2004) on the housing market. *New York University Environmental Law Journal*, 13, 199–297.

Brody, Jane E. 2006. Dally no longer: get the lead out. *New York Times*, January 17.

Cardwell, Diane. 2002. Study says many children are still poisoned by lead. *New York Times*, June 14.

Chachere, Matthew, and Andrea Rodriguez. 2004. A bill that helps end lead poisoning. *Gotham Gazette*, February 4. www.gothamgazette.com/print/857.

Chen, David W. 2003. Council, ignoring veto threat, approves tough lead-based paint bill. *New York Times*, December 16.

Citylaw. 1996. Current developments: court orders against the city: city held in contempt for failure to issue lead-based paint regulations. February–March.

———. 1997. Current developments: institutional reform litigation: city in contempt over lead regs. May–June.

Cooper, Michael. 2003. City council spars with Bloomberg over lead-based paint legislation. *New York Times*, December 17.

Dell'Antonia, K. J. 2012. Drastic cuts to lead poisoning and prevention funds. *New York Times*, March 7.

Eidsvold, Gary, Anthony Mustalish, and Lloyd F. Novick. 1974. The New York City Department of Health: lessons in a lead poisoning control program. *American Journal of Public Health* 64, no. 10, October, 956–962.

Florini, Karen L., and Ellen K. Silbergeld. 1993. Getting the lead out. *Issues in Science and Technology*, Summer, 33–39.

Freudenberg, Nicholas, and Carol Steinsapir. 1986. Two ways new city could enforce its lead-based paint law. *New York Times*, October 15.

Gaiter, Dorothy J. 1981. Despite U.S. cutbacks, city fights lead poisoning. *New York Times*, August 27.

Goldstein, Eric A. 2003. A letter about lead poisoning. *Gotham Gazette*, May 5.

Hartocollis, Anemona. 2012. C.D.C. lowers recommended lead-level limits in children. *New York Times*, May 16.

Herszenhorn, David M. 1999. Lead-based paint bill is expected to pass in vote Wednesday. *New York Times*, June 30.

Hevesi, Dennis. 1989. Judge orders lead-based paint removal expanded. *New York Times*, July 23.

———. 1991. Bronx home offers refuge from danger of lead-based paint. *New York Times*, May 6.

Hsu, Karen. 1997. Neighborhood report: East New York/Brownsville; lead chips from el make parents look up with worry. *New York Times*, September 8.

Hu, Winnie. 1999. Despite hisses, mayor signs lead-paint bill. *New York Times*, July 16.

———. 2003. In the council, leader treads delicate line on lead-based paint. *New York Times*, September 13.

———. 2004. Over veto, council passes tougher law on lead-based paint. *New York Times*, February 5.

Johnson, Kirk. 2003a. For a changing city, new pieces in a lead poisoning puzzle. *New York Times*, September 30.

———. 2003b. Looking outside for lead danger: finding it overhead and underfoot. *New York Times*, November 2.

Kennedy, Randy. 1996. Bill reignites a debate on lead risk. *New York Times*, April 30.

Lambert, Bruce. 2000a. E.P.A. says lead-based paint law may increase risks to children. *New York Times*, September 23.

———. 2000b. Judge overturns lead-based paint control law, citing "perfunctory" review by city council. *New York Times*, October 14.

Lombardi, Frank. 1999. Suit filed to reverse lead-paint legislation. *New York Daily News*, October 22.

Make the Road New York Staff. 2009. If walls could talk: how landlords fail to obey childhood lead poisoning prevention laws in Bushwick. July 28. www.maketheroad.org.

McIntire, Mike. 2003. Mayor's office objects to bill on lead abatement. *New York Times*, November 18.

McKinley, James C. 1992a. Mayor seeks relaxation of lead law. *New York Times*, September 5.

———. 1992b. City Council debates plan on lead-based paint. *New York Times*, October 11.

McLaughlin, Mary Culhane. 1956. Lead poisoning in children in New York City, 1950–1954. *New York State Journal of Medicine* 56, no. 23, December 1, 3711–3714.

Medley, Sara Sullivan. 1982. Childhood lead toxicity: a paradox of modern technology. *Annals of the American Academy of Political and Social Science* 461, May, 63–73.

Middlekauff, Tracey. 2001. Lead poisoning. *Gotham Gazette*, April 16. www.gothamgazette.com/iotw/lead/ (accessed April 4, 2003).

Molloy, Laurence. 1992. Lead in schools contributes to low test scores (letter to the editor). *New York Times*, August 22.

Morrison, Dorothy. 1998. Lead-based paint hazards: funding opportunities provide control. *Public Management* 80, no. 1, January, 16–19.

Needleman, Herbert L. 1998. Childhood lead poisoning: the promise and abandonment of primary prevention. *American Journal of Public Health* 88, no. 12, December, 1871–1877.

New York City Coalition to End Lead Poisoning. 1999. What's wrong with the current law (Local Law 38)? www.nmic.org/nyccelp/Documents/Wrong.htm (accessed November 16, 2009).

———. 2003a. A Comparison between the New York City Childhood Lead Poisoning Prevention Act of 2003 (Intro 101A) and Local Laws 1 and 50. www.nmic.org/nyccelp/Documents/101-vs-1.htm (accessed November 16, 2009).

———. 2003b. Summary of Intro 101A (N.Y. City Childhood Lead Poisoning Prevention Act). November 7. www.nmic.org/nyccelp/laws/Summary-of-Intro-101.pdf (accessed November 16, 2009).

———. 2003c. A comparison between the New York City Childhood Lead Poisoning Prevention Act of 2003 (Intro 101A) and the recently nullified Local Law 38 (accessed November 16, 2009).

New York City Department of Health. 1954. News Release. October 29.

———. 1969. Lead poisoning issue study. December 15.

———. 1970a. Project plan for lead poisoning control. March 13.

———. 1970b. Health Services Administrator Gordon Chase announced . . . (press release). Office of the Administrator, Office of Public Information, September 23.

New York City Department of Health and Mental Hygiene. 2002. Preventing Lead Poisoning in New York City: Annual Report, 2001.

———. 2004a. New York City Childhood Lead Poisoning Prevention Program: Annual Report, 2002. April.

———. 2004b. New York City Childhood Lead Poisoning Prevention Program: Annual Report, 2003. December.

———. 2005a. Health Warning: Do Not Use Litargirio.

———. 2005b. New York City Plan to Eliminate Childhood Lead Poisoning. Lead Poisoning Prevention Program, December.

———. 2008. Preventing Lead Poisoning in New York City: Annual Report, 2006. March.

———. 2009a. Preventing Lead Poisoning in New York City: Annual Report, 2007. June.

———. 2009b. Lead Poisoning in New York City: Annual Report, 2008. September.

———. 2011. Report to the New York City Council on Progress in Preventing Childhood Lead Poisoning in New York City. September 30.

New York City Department of Housing Preservation and Development. 2004. Local Law 1/2004—section-by-section analysis.

———. 2005. $7.5 Million in federal funds to combat lead-based paint poisoning in Brooklyn communities (press release), October 4. www.nyc/html/hpd/html/pr2005/pr-10-04-05.shtml.

New York City Independent Budget Office. 2006. First year finds lead-based paint law not as costly as predicted. January.

New York City Office of Chronic Disease Services. 1969. Ten month report: lead poisoning control program. December 22.

New York City Office of Management and Budget. 2009. Fiscal Year 2010 adopted budget revenue. June 19.

New York City Office of the Mayor. 2003. Introductory Number 101-A. Veto message to Victor L. Robles, City Clerk and Clerk of the Council. December 19.

New York Daily News. 2004. Law and order: special schools unit. February 9.

New York Public Interest Research Group. 1999. Brooklyn and Queens 1997 lead belt confirmed (press release). January 14.

New York State Comptroller. 2007. Childhood lead poisoning. Deputy Comptroller Mary Louise Mallick, Office of Budget and Policy Analysis. June.

New York State Department of Health. 2004. Eliminating childhood lead poisoning in New York State by 2010. June.

———. 2008. New York State's Primary prevention of childhood lead poisoning pilot program: preliminary results of year one implementation.

———. 2009. New York State Medicaid Update Special Edition. Vol. 25, no. 8.

New York Times. 1985. Families sue over lead-based paint. May 9.

———. 1995. New York is fined over lead hazard. December 15.

———. 1999. Get the lead out (editorial). June 21.

Northern Manhattan Improvement Corporation. 2011. Environmental justice: lead paint poisoning legal efforts. www.nmic.org/environmentaljustice.html (accessed June 21, 2011).

Northern Manhattan Improvement Corporation—Lead Poisoning. 2011. Lead poisoning prevention workshops—lead safe housing. www.nmic.org/lead.html (accessed June 22, 2011).

O'Neil, John. 2004. Unlikely sources of lead poison. *New York Times*, July 20.

Oser, Alan S. 2004. Lead-based paint law frustrates plans for low-income housing. *New York Times*, May 28.

Pedro, Verne A. 2000. Still hazy after all these years: New York City's local law 38 and the legislative debate over landlord liability in lead-based paint poisoning cases. *Seton Hall Legislative Journal* 24, 542–577.

Perez-Pena, Richard. 2003. Dominican-made powder remedy is poisonous, health officials say. *New York Times*, November 6.

Public Advocate for the City of New York. 1998. Lead and kids: why are 3,000 New York City children contaminated? New York City. Public Advocate for the City of New York. Public Advocate Mark Green. www.pubadvocate.nyc.gov/padcdetail.cfm?id1=7&id2=1 (accessed August 10, 1999).

Purdy, Matthew. 1994. Cost of lead clean puts more poor children at risk. *New York Times*, August 25.

Rabin, Richard. 1989. Warnings unheeded: a history of child lead poisoning. *American Journal of Public Health* 79, no. 12, December, 1668–1674.

Rechtschaffen, Clifford L. 1997. The lead poisoning challenge: an approach for California and other states. *Harvard Environmental Law Review* 21, 387–455.

Romano, Jay. 2003. Your home: lead-based paint regulation is in limbo. *New York Times*, July 13.

———. 2004. New rules that govern lead-based paint. *New York Times*, February 22.

Sengupta, Somini. 1995. Neighborhood report: Sunnyside; city found in violation on lead-based paint. *New York Times*, December 17.

Steinhauer, Jennifer. 2004. Gladly taking the blame for health in the city. *New York Times*, February 14.

Strasburg, Joseph. 2002. Lead paint ruling for tenants (letter to the editor). *New York Times*, January 20.

Tinker, Tim L., and Niki Keiser. 1997. Childhood lead poisoning prevention: an overview of federal education programs and resources. *Journal of Primary Prevention* 18, no. 1, 129–143.

United States Catalog of Federal Domestic Assistance. 2009. www.cfda.gov/index (accessed November 18, 2009).

United States Centers for Disease Control and Prevention. 2007. Interpreting and Managing BLLs < 10ug/dL in children and reducing childhood exposure to lead: recommendations of CDC's Advisory Committee on Childhood Lead Poisoning Prevention. *Morbidity and Mortality Weekly Report* 56, no. RR-6, November 2.

Vitullo-Martin, Julia. 2003. The lead-based paint bill. *Gotham Gazette*, December 13. www.gothamgazette.com/article/20021213/202/805.

Wasserman, Joanne. 2003. Lead law gets dusting: court KO's '99 rule, criticizes council. *New York Daily News*, July 2.

Chapter 3 · *Managing Asthma*

Akinbami, Lara J. 2006. The state of childhood asthma, United States, 1980–2005. Advance data from vital and health statistics; no. 381. Hyattsville, Md.: National Center for Health Statistics. July.

Akinbami, Lara J., and Kenneth C. Schoendorf. 2002. Trends in childhood asthma: prevalence, health care utilization and mortality. *Pediatrics* 110, no. 2, August, 315–322.

Asthma Free School Zones. 2010. About us. www.afsz.org/html_major/about.html (accessed February 21, 2010).

Belluck, Pam. 1996. With asthma rising, expanded health sessions for pupils, parents. *New York Times*, September 29.

Bernstein, Nina. 2004. Study shows health benefit for immigrants. *New York Times*, October 6.

Bonforte, Richard J., and Jacqueline D. Mc Leod. 1995. Allergic to latex; it's also in the air to manage asthma (letter to the editor). *New York Times*, September 13.

Bowen, Shawn. 2001. Testimony at Bronx Borough President Fernando Ferrer Press Conference. July 20.

Bowen, William, et al. 1995. Toward environmental justice: spatial equity in Ohio and Cleveland. *Annals of the Association of American Geographers* 85, no. 4, December, 641–663.

Braiker, Brian. 2003. Q&A: stealth attack. *Newsweek*, November 27.

Brauer, Michael, Gerard Hoek, Patricia Van Vilet, Kees Mielifste, et al. 2002. Air pollution from traffic and the development of respiratory infections and asthmatic and allergic symptoms in children. *American Journal of Respiratory and Critical Care Medicine* 166, 1092–1098.

Brown, Clive M., Henry A. Anderson, and Ruth A. Etzel. 1997. Asthma: the states' challenge. *Public Health Reports* 112, no. 3, May–June, 198–205.

Calderone, Joe. 1998a. Asthmatics to be given vital devices. *Daily News*, March 19.

———. 1998b. City forms a battle plan: schools are key in fight versus disease. *Daily News*, March 30.

———. 1998c. Rudy unveils campaign to aid asthma kids. *Daily News*, July 30.

Calderone, Joe, et al. 1998a. Simple tools every child should have. *Daily News*, February 22.

———. 1998b. The South Bronx—asthma's battleground. *Daily News*, February 22.

———. 1998c. Taking our breath away—asthma: the silent epidemic. *Daily News*, February 22.

Carr, Willine, Lisa Zeitel, and Kevin Weiss. 1992. Variations in asthma hospitalizations and deaths in New York City. *American Journal of Public Health* 82, no. 1, January, 59–65.

Catalog of Federal Domestic Assistance. 2010. Preventive Health and Health Services Block Grant. www.cdfa.gov/index (accessed December 28, 2009).

Clougherty, Jane E., Jonathan Levy, Laura D. Kubzansky, P. Barry Ryan, et al. 2007. Synergistic effects of traffic-related air pollution and exposure to violence on urban asthma etiology. *Environmental Health Perspectives* 115, no. 8, August, 1140–1146.

Cohen, Neil. 1998. City Council Committee on Health (Testimony). March 31.

Collin, Robert W., Timothy Beatley, and William Harris. 1995. Environmental racism: a challenge to community development. *Journal of Black Studies* 25, no. 3, January, 354–376.

Collins, Glenn. 1985. Parents of asthmatics offer helping hands. *New York Times*, December 23.

Corburn, Jason, Jeffrey Osleeb, and Michael Porter. 2006. Urban asthma and the neighborhood environment in New York City. *Health and Place* 12, 167–179.

Dao, James. 1997. Bronx Lebanon hospital to shut waste incinerator. *New York Times*, June 27.

Das, Alina. 2007. The asthma crisis in low income communities of color: using the law as a tool for promoting public health. *New York University Review of Law and Social Change* 31, 273–314.

Davis, Lorna. 2010. Phone interview with Lorna Davis, director, New York City Department of Mental Health and Hygiene Asthma Initiative. February 19.

DePalma, Anthony. 2004. Bus companies agree to cut engine idling near schools. *New York Times*, January 24.

———. 2005a. State leads in ill effects from diesels, report says. *New York Times*, February 23.

———. 2005b. City, looking to health and costs, is to pass emissions laws for its fleet. *New York Times*, April 20.

De Palo, Vera A., Paul Mayor, Patricia Friedman, and Mark J. Rosen. 1993. Demographic influences on asthma hospital admission rates in New York City. *Chest* 106, no. 2, August, 447–451.

Diette, Gregory B., Nadia Hansel, Timothy Buckley, Jean Curtin-Brosnan, et al. 2007. Home indoor pollutant exposures among inner-city children with and without asthma. *Environmental Health Perspectives* 115, no. 11, November, 1665–1669.

Edwards, Randall. 1999. 2 states seek to join suit vs. AEP: air-pollution problems are being blamed on Midwest power plants. *Columbus Dispatch*, November 30.

Egbert, Bill. 2005. Bus firms ok clean air pact no idling near schools. *New York Daily News*, September 27.

Ellin, Abby. 2003. A family problem prompts a career. *New York Times*, October 19.

Environmental Defense Fund. 2007. All choked up: heavy traffic, dirty air and the risk to New Yorkers. March.

Feinberg, Marian. 2001. Victory in the South Bronx: what it took to win. South Bronx Clean Air Coalition. www.crp.cornell.edu/projects/southbronx/history/victory.html (accessed June 7, 2001).

Fernandez, Manny. 2006. A study links trucks' exhaust to Bronx schoolchildren asthma. *New York Times*, October 29.

Frankel, Bruce. 1992. Raising a stink over incinerator. *USA Today*, August 13.

Gergen, Peter J., Daniel I. Mullally, and Richard Evans. 1988. National survey of prevalence of asthma among children in the United States, 1976 to 1980. *Pediatrics* 81, no. 1, January, 1–7.

Gilmour, M. Ian, Maritta S. Jaakkola, Stephanie J. London, Andre E. Nei, et al. 2006. How exposure to environmental tobacco smoke, outdoor air pollutants, and increased pollen burdens influences the incidence of asthma. *Environmental Health Perspectives* 114, no. 4, April, 627–634.

Gonen, Yoav. 2003. Hundreds protest vs. bus depot. *New York Daily News*, September 7.

Gotham Gazette. 2010a. City government: city laws: bus idling. www.gothamgazette.com /city.vote_records (accessed January 25, 2010).

———. 2010b. City government: city laws: new taxis. www.gothamgazette/com/city.vote _records (accessed January 25, 2010).

———. 2010c. City government: city laws: promoting the use of clean air and accessible taxicabs and for hire vehicles. www.gothamgazette/com/city.vote_records (accessed January 25, 2010).

———. 2010d. City government: city laws: replacement cycles for taxicabs. www.gotham gazette/com/city.vote_records (accessed January 25, 2010).

Grant, Roy, et al. 2010. Health care savings attributable to integrating guidelines-based asthma care in the Pediatric Medical Home. *Journal of Health Care for the Poor and Underserved* 21, no. 2, May supplement, 82–92.

Hakim, Danny. 2007. Silver challenges health benefits promised in Manhattan toll plan. *New York Times*, June 12.

Hayes, Roger. 2014. Building Healthy Communities: Promoting Health Equity in Harlem (PowerPoint). Presentation at the Fourth Annual National Urban Health Conference, New York Academy of Medicine, New York City, April 25.

Heigel, Marianne. 2010. Phone interview with Marianne Heigel, Asthma Coalition Coordinators, NYS Department of Health, Bureau of Community Chronic Disease Prevention. February 17.

Hernandez, Javier. 2010. Program to combat asthma would lean on landlords. *New York Times*, May 11.

Holloway, Lynette. 1999. Reading, writing and runny noses; for those without insurance, school clinics fill in. *New York Times*, April 21.

Hsu, Karen. 2000. Boston will get 1.9M to prevent asthma grant from HUD to help renovate 500 residences. *Boston Globe*, February 24.

Institute of Medicine. 2000. Clearing the air: asthma and indoor air exposures. Committee on the Assessment of Asthma and Indoor Air, Division of Health Promotion and Disease Prevention.

Jean-Louis, Bettina. 2003. Harlem Children's Zone Asthma Initiative (presentation at Sarah Lawrence College-Childhood Asthma and the Community), December 3.

Jones, Charisse. 2006. Activists use research to win pollution battles. *USA Today*, December 6.

Kassel, Rich. 2008a. Next steps for congestion pricing. *Gotham Gazette*, January 23. www .gothamgazette.com/article/environment/20080123/7/2411.

———. 2008b. How the city has reduced soot. *Gotham Gazette*, July 3. www.gotham gazette.com/article/environment/20080703/7/2572.

———. 2009. Moving the city along the road to sustainability. *Gotham Gazette*, October 29. www.gothamgazette.com/article/environment/20091029/7/3077.

Kassel, Richard, and Katherine Kennedy. 1996. Asthma and air (letter to the editor). *New York Times*, October 7.

Kaufman, Leslie. 2012. Pressured, E.P.A. proposes soot limit. *New York Times*, June 14.

Kiely, Kathy. 1998. Centers to target asthma enviro diseases up. *Daily News*, August 10.

Kinney, Patrick L., Mary E. Northridge, Ginger L. Chew, Erik Gronning, et al. 2002. On the front lines: an environmental asthma intervention in New York City. *American Journal of Public Health* 92, no. 1, January, 24–26.

Koenig, Jane Q. 1999. Air pollution and asthma. *Journal of Allergy and Clinical Immunology*, October, 717–722.

Koutsavlis, Anthanasios Tom, Tom Kosatsky, Joseph Cox, and Eric Goyer. 2001. Reporting childhood asthma: why? why not? what else? *Journal of Public Health Policy* 22, no. 3, 311–319.

Kugel, Seth. 2003. Neighborhood report: East Harlem; a bus depot will reopen and residents worry. *New York Times*, August 24.

Larsen, Gary L., Craig Beskid, and Lat Shirname-More. 2002. Environmental air toxics: role in asthma occurrence. *Environmental Health Perspectives* 110, supplement 4, August, 501–504.

Leonnig, Carol D. 2005. Easing of pollution rules heightens health worries: seeking to keep regulations strict, Sierra Club sues EPA. *Washington Post*, September 4.

Liff, Bob. 2000. Pols waging war on waste—fed probes of transfer stations eyed. *New York Daily News*, July 25.

Little, Amanda Griscom. 2007. Not in whose backyard. *New York Times*, September 2.

Lobach, Katherine S. 1996. Childhood asthma: providing a "medical home." *City Health Information*. NYC Department of Health, vol. 15, no. 3, December. www.ci.nyc.us/html /doh/html/chi/v15-3.html (accessed November 22, 1999).

Lombardi, Frank. 2003. Pollution solution law to curb diesel construction machines. *New York Daily News*, December 22.

Lovasi, G. S., J. W. Quinn, K. M. Neckerman, M. S. Perzanowski, et al. 2008. Children living in areas with more street trees have lower prevalence of asthma. *Journal of Epidemiology and Community Health* 62, 647–649.

Lueck, Thomas J. 2000. Environmentalists assail plan to add diesel buses. *New York Times*, January 2.

Maantay, Julianna, Juan Carlos Saborio, Dellis Stanberry, and Holly Porter-Morgan. 1999. Mapping asthma hot spots: the geography of asthma and air pollution in the Bronx, New York City. CUNY and National Oceanographic and Atmospheric Agency Cooperative Remote Science and Technology Center.

Maher, Timothy. 1998. Environmental oppression: who is targeted for toxic exposure? *Journal of Black Studies* 28, no. 3, January, 357–367.

Marks, Alexandra. 2003. For a change, good news about health insurance. *Christian Science Monitor*, August 1.

Matusui, Elizabeth C., Peyton Eggleston, Timothy Buckley, Jerry A Krishnan, et al. 2006. Household mouse allergen exposure and asthma morbidity in inner city preschool children. *Annals of Allergy, Asthma and Immunology* 97, October, 514–520.

McLean, Diane E., Shawn Bowen, Karen Drezner, Amy Rowe, et al. 2004. Asthma among homeless children. *Archives of Pediatric and Adolescent Medicine* 138, March, 244–249.

New York City Childhood Asthma Initiative. 2001a. What is the "public health" approach to asthma? *Asthma Initiative Info*. New York City: A Project of Community Health Works, New York City Department of Health. Winter.

———. 2001b. Asthma SMART: people and technology working together. *Asthma Initiative Info*. New York City: A Project of Community Health Works, New York City Department of Health. Spring.

———. 2002. Spreading the work about asthma action plans. *Asthma Initiative Info*. New York City: A Project of Community Health Works, New York City Department of Health. Winter.

New York City Clean Heat. 2013. About NYC Clean Heat. www.nyccleanheat.org/content /what-nyc-clean-heat (accessed October 2, 2013).

New York City Council. 1998. Committee on Health. Hearing on the Asthma Initiative. March 31.

———. 2000. Committee on Transportation. Hearing on bus depots in Northern Manhattan. March 23.

———. 2006. Committee on Sanitation and Solid Waste Management. Hearing on mayor's solid waste management plan. Crosswalks Network, New York City Department of Information Technology and Telecommunications. June 26.

———. 2009. Committee on Environmental Protection. Hearing on Diesel Powered School Buses. September 9.

New York City Department of City Planning. 1995. Fair Share: An Assessment of New York City's Facility Siting Process. New York City: New York City Department of City Planning.

New York City Department of Environmental Protection. 2012. DEP announces "Stop Idling" enforcement and public education campaign at city schools in neighborhoods with high asthma rates (press release). May 22.

New York City Department of Health and Mental Hygiene. 2003. Asthma Facts (2nd edition). New York City Childhood Asthma Initiative. May.

———. 2008. Childhood Asthma in New York City (NYC Vital Statistics) 7, no. 1, May.

———. 2009. The New York City Community Air Survey. December 15.

———. 2010a. School Health: open airways for schools. www.nyc.gov/html/doh/html/scah /openair.shtml (accessed February 1, 2010).

———. 2010b. Asthma Initiative. www.nyc.gov/html/doh/html/asthma/asthma.shtml (accessed February 2, 2010).

———. 2010c. Creating a medical home for asthma: introduction. www.nyc.gov/html/doh /html/cmha/introduction.htlm (accessed February 2, 2010).

———. 2010d. Asthma Initiative: what everyone should know. www.nyc.gov/html/doh /html/asthma/asthma1.shtml (accessed February 9, 2010).

———. 2014. District Public Health Offices. www.nyc.gov/html/doh/html/diseases/dpho -homepage.shtml (accessed June 23, 2014).

New York City Office of the Mayor. 1998a. Mayor Giuliani launches citywide asthma education campaign and asthma action line (press release #369-98). July 29. www.ci.nyc.ny .us/html/om/html/98b/pr369-98.html.

———. 1998b. Mayoral press conference announcing Asthma Initiative. Crosswalks Network. July 29.

———. 1999. Mayoral press conference announcing publication of asthma services directory. Crosswalks Network. July 22.

———. 2000. Press conference dealing with the Asthma Initiative's progress. Crosswalks Network. August 2.

———. 2007. East Harlem Asthma Center (press conference). May 30.

———. 2009a. Mayor Bloomberg and Agriculture Secretary Vilsack announce $2 million federal grant to create green jobs as part of the Million Trees NYC campaign. News from the Blue Room, April 8.

———. 2009b. East Harlem Asthma Center (press conference). August 12.

———. 2011. Mayor Bloomberg signs legislation modifying the alternative enforcement program at the Department of Housing, Preservation and Development. News from the Blue Room. January 13.

———. 2013. Mayor Bloomberg announces New York City's air quality has reached the cleanest levels in more than 50 years (press release PR 311-13). September 26.

New York City PlaNYC. 2014. Green buildings and energy efficiency. www.nyc.gov/html /gbee/html/codes/heating/shtml (accessed June 16, 2014).

New York State Department of Health. 2005. RFA FAU Control no. 0502100917. Center for Community Health, Division of Family Health, Bureau of Child and Adolescent Health.

———. 2007. New York State Asthma Surveillance Summary Report. October.

———. 2009. New York State Asthma Surveillance Summary Report (Public Health Information Group Center for Community Health). October.

New York Times. 2006. Black soot and asthma. November 19.

Noble, Holcomb B. 1999. Study shows big asthma risk for children in poor areas. *New York Times,* July 27.

Pear, Robert. 1999. States criticized on lax lead tests for poor youths. *New York Times,* August 21.

Perez-Pena, Richard. 2003a. Study finds asthma in 25% of children in central Harlem. *New York Times,* April 19.

———. 2003b. Program to cut air pollution by school buses is stalled. *New York Times,* May 25.

Phua, Chelsea. 2003. It's 11th hour at 12 clinics pediatric health centers facing doom of budget ax. *New York Daily News,* June 26.

Rabin, Roni Caryn. 2010. Enlisting patients in the fight to cut costs. *New York Times,* June 7.

———. 2011. Asthma rate rises sharply in U.S., government says. *New York Times,* May 3.

Rauh, Virginia A., Ginger L. Chew, and Robin Garfinkel. 2002. Deteriorated housing contributes to high cockroach allergen levels in inner city households. *Environmental Health Perspectives* 110, supplement 2, April, 323–327.

Redd, Stephen C. 2002. Asthma in the United States: burden and current theories. *Environmental Health Perspectives* 110, supplement 4, August, 557–560.

Richardson, Lynda. 1993. Too ill to learn: health system fails to meet students' needs, educators say. *New York Times,* October 10.

Rosenstreich, David L., Peyton Eggleston, Meyer Kattan, and Dean Baker. 1997. The role of cockroach allergy and exposure to cockroach allergen in causing morbidity among inner city children. *New England Journal of Medicine* 336, no. 19, May 8, 1356–1364.

Santora, Marc. 2005. U.S. praises program in city for children with asthma. *New York Times,* January 14.

Sengupta, Somini. 2000. Care for homeless children with asthma topic of lawsuit. *New York Times,* March 17.

Shankardass, Ketan, Rob McConnell, Michael Jerrett, Joel Milam, et al. 2009. Parental stress increases the effect of traffic-related air pollution on childhood asthma incidence. *Proceedings of the National Academy of Sciences* 106, July 28, 12406–12411.

Sheridan, Dick. 1998. War on childhood asthma. *New York Daily News,* May 10.

Shipp, E. R. 2000. Don't let fumes cloud Harlem development. *New York Daily News,* December 26.

Singleton, Don. 1996. Docs cite roaches in child asthma surge. *New York Daily News,* June 9.

Snow, Reva E., Marian Larkin, Sarah Kimball, Kelechi Iheagwara, et al. 2005. Evaluation of asthma management policies in New York City public schools. *Journal of Asthma,* no. 1, 51–55.

Stevenson, Lori. 2003. Childhood asthma in New York City. What does it look like? Where do we find it? (presentation at Sarah Lawrence College, Health Advocacy Program). December 3.

Stewart, Barbara. 2000. Complaint says 3 neighborhoods bear brunt of city garbage. *New York Times*, July 25.

Stolberg, Sheryl Gay. 1999. Poor fight baffling surge in asthma. *New York Times*, October 18.

Strouse, Kevin. 2001. Asthma. *Gotham Gazette*, May 14. www.gothamgazette.com/iotw /asthma/ (accessed June 6, 2001).

Sugarman, Raphael. 1998. Asthma info on tap spring program is set in all city school districts. *New York Daily News*, December 31.

Sustainable Cleveland Partnership. 2010. Environmental justice. www.nhlink.net/enviro/scp /ej.html (accessed January 10, 2010).

Sykes, Annmarie, and Sebastian Johnston. 2008. Etiology of asthma exacerbations. *Journal of Allergy and Clinical Immunology* 122, no. 4, October, 685–688.

Sze, Julie. 2007. *Noxious New York: The Racial Politics of Urban Health and Environmental Justice*. Cambridge, MA: MIT Press.

U.S. Centers for Disease Control and Prevention. 2011. Vital signs: asthma prevalence, disease characteristics, and self-management education—United States, 2001–2009. *Morbidity and Mortality Week Report* 60, no. 17, May 6.

Wakin, Daniel J. 2001. Breathless. *New York Times*, May 13.

WE ACT for Environmental Justice. 2006a. Sheila Foster, Testimony to the New York City Council Committee on Transportation. October 18.

———. 2006b. Peggy Shepard and Cecil Corbin Mark, Testimony to the New York City Council Committee on Transportation. October 18.

———. 2009. The MTA Accountability Campaign. August 1.

Webber, Mayris P., Anne-Marie-Hosie, Michelle Odium, Tosan Oruwariye, et al. 2005. Impact of asthma intervention in two elementary school-based health centers in the Bronx, New York City. *Pediatric Pulmonology*. www.ncbi.nim.nih.gov/pubmed /16193475.

Weiss, Kevin B., and Diane K. Wagener. 1990. Changing patterns of asthma mortality. *Journal of the American Medical Association* 264, no. 13, October 3, 1683–1687.

Weisskopf, Michael. 1992. EPA study addressed "environmental racism." *Washington Post*, January 19.

World Health Organization. 2010. Adelaide Statement on Health in All Policies. www.who .int/social_determinants/hiap_statement_who_sa_final.pdf.

Yeatts, Karin, Peter Sly, Stephanie Sore, and Scott Weis. 2006. A brief targeted review of susceptibility factors, environmental exposures, asthma incidence, and recommendations for future asthma incidence research. *Environmental Health Perspectives* 114, no. 4, April, 634–641.

Chapter 4 · *Living with HIV/AIDS*

Adler, Jerry. 1985. The AIDS conflict. *Newsweek*, September 23.

Aidala, Angela, et al. 2005. Housing status and HIV risk behaviors: implications for prevention and policy. *AIDS and Behavior* 9, no. 3, September, 251–265.

AIDS United. 2011. HIV/AIDS Funding in New York, 2008–2010 (Policy and Advocacy State Facts).

Allon, Janet. 1998. Neighborhood report: New York up close; new tension for city and AIDS group. *New York Times*, March 1.

Altman, Lawrence K. 1982. New homosexual disorder worries health officials. *New York Times*, May 11.

———. 1983. Debate grows on U.S. listing of Haitians in AIDS category. *New York Times*, July 31.

———. 1985. Drug users try to cut AIDS risk. *New York Times*, April 18.

———. 1997. Deaths from AIDS decline sharply in New York City. *New York Times*, January 25.

———. 1999a. New York study finds gay men use safer sex. *New York Times*, June 28.

———. 1999b. Fewer gay men in New York are contracting AIDS. *New York Times*, July 4.

———. 2004. Nationwide H.I.V. reporting to bring trends into focus. *New York Times*, February 17.

Anderson, Warwick. 1991. The New York needle trial: the politics of public health in the age of AIDS. *American Journal of Public Health* 81, no. 11, November, 1506–1517.

Arno, Peter S., and Karyn Feiden. 1986. Ignoring the epidemic: how the Reagan administration failed on AIDS. *Health PAC Bulletin*, December, 7–11.

Arno, Peter S., and Robert G. Hughes. 1987. Local policy responses to the AIDS epidemic: New York and San Francisco. *New York State Journal of Medicine*, May, 264–272.

Barbanel, Josh. 1985a. Koch to request more U.S. help on AIDS costs. *New York Times*, October 21.

———. 1985b. To combat AIDS, Koch urges anti drug effort. *New York Times*, December 17.

Barron, James. 1993. AIDS message in subway comic strip: New York City health agency teaches about the disease in a soap with a sober focus. *New York Times*, November 9.

Batchelor, Walter F. 1988. AIDS 1988: the science and the limits of science. *American Psychologist* 43, no. 11, 853–858.

Bayer, Ronald. 1991. AIDS: the politics of prevention and neglect. *Health Affairs*, Spring, 87–97.

———. 1995. The Dependent Center: the first decade of the AIDS epidemic in New York City. In David Rosner (ed.), *Hive of Sickness: Public Health and Epidemics in New York City*, 131–150. New Brunswick: Rutgers University Press.

Bayer, Ronald, and Amy L. Fairchild. 2006. Changing the paradigm for HIV testing—the end of exceptionalism. *New England Journal of Medicine*, August 17, 647–649.

Berger, Joseph. 1990. New York City school board members clash on condom proposal. *New York Times*, December 20.

———. 1991. Dinkins shores up power in condom vote. *New York Times*, September 13.

Bertozzi, Stefano, Tyler E. Martz, and Peter Piot. 2009. The evolving HIV/AIDS response and the urgent tasks ahead. *Health Affairs*, November–December, 2009, 1578–1589.

Blake, John. 1999. Black churches to target AIDS epidemic. *Atlanta Constitution*, October 2.

Blumenthal, Ralph. 1985. At homosexual establishments, a new climate of caution. *New York Times*, November 9.

Boyle, Christina. 2008. City teen HIV rate highest since 2001. *New York Daily News*, May 18.

Bronstein, Scott. 1987. 4 New York bathhouses still operate under city's program of inspections. *New York Times*, May 3.

Burr, Chandler. 1997. The AIDS exception: privacy vs. public health. *Atlantic Monthly*, June.

Cardwell, Diane. 2010. More rent relief for AIDS patients is vetoed. *New York Times*, September 10.

Chambre, Susan M. 2006. *Fighting for Our Lives: New York's AIDS Community and the Politics of Disease*. New Brunswick: Rutgers University Press.

Chan, Sewell. 2006a. H.I.V. is spreading in New York City at three times the national rate, a study finds. *New York Times*, August 28.

———. 2006b. Rifts emerge on push to end written consent for H.I.V. tests. *New York Times*, December 25.

———. 2009. City unveils Facebook page to encourage condom use. *New York Times*, February 12.

Chiasson, Mary Ann. 2000. Using AIDS data (letter to the editor). *New York Times*, January 21.

Clark, Matt. 1985. AIDS: the blood-bank scare. *Newsweek*. January 28.

Cohen, Neil. 2000. Testimony before the New York City Council Committee on Health. April 25.

Collins, Huntly. 1997. AIDS deaths leveling off for the first time; New York rate falls 30%; better medicine credited. *New Orleans Times Picayune*, January 25.

Connelly, Mary. 1985. Privacy versus the risk to the public; opportunities for education. *New York Times*, December 15.

Cooper, Gail. 2000. In the news: AIDS peril for people of color. *Gotham Gazette*, May. www.gothamgazette.com/socialservices/may.00.shtml (accessed April 23, 2003).

Dao, James. 1993. New York State overturns rule of AIDS study. *New York Times*, February 9.

Davis, Henry L. 1993. Local stations slow to show AIDS message; N.Y. also lags in airing ads pushing condom use. *Buffalo News*, November 17.

Donovan, Mark. 1996. The politics of deservedness: The Ryan White Act and the social construction of people with AIDS. In Stella Z. Theodoulou (ed.), *AIDS: The Politics and Policy of Disease*, 68–87. Upper Saddle River: Prentice Hall.

Dowd, Maureen. 1983. For victims of AIDS, support in a lonely siege. *New York Times*, December 5.

Drucker, Ernest. 1986. AIDS and addiction in New York City. *American Journal of Drug and Alcoholism Abuse* 12, nos. 1–2, March, 165–181.

Dudley, Jacqueline. 2012. Testimony before the New York City Council Committee on General Welfare. February 8.

Dunlap, David W. 1987. For homeless with AIDS, a new home. *New York Times*, January 5.

———. 1995a. Crackdown on gay theaters and clubs. *New York Times*, April 16.

———. 1995b. Closing of a gay theater, the site if high-risk sex, is upheld. *New York Times*, April 19.

———. 1996. Three Black members quit AIDS organization board. *New York Times*, January 11.

———. 1997. Building blocks in the battle on AIDS. *New York Times*, March 30.

Economist. 1987. The awful cost of AIDS. April 11.

Eisenman, David. 1985. We need safer blood: and the way to get it is to screen out the risky donors. *Washington Post*, April 10.

Fallik, Dawn. 2006. Almost one in 10 straight men on the "down-low" study finds. *Philadelphia Inquirer*, September 19.

Fein, Esther B. 1995. Report says plan could hurt AIDS care. *New York Times*, October 4.

Ferraro, Susan. 1998a. The face of AIDS/HIV hits some groups hard, but new weapons are coming. *New York Daily News*, June 22.

———. 1998b. Living with HIV—families struggle to survive in the face of a deadly disease. *New York Daily News*, November 30.

Ferraro, Susan, and Jon R. Sorenson. 1997. Feds ok Pataki Medicaid plan. *New York Daily News*, July 16.

Finder, Alan, and Mary Connelly. 1985. The region: Dr. Sencer steps down. *New York Times*, December 8.

Fineberg, Harvey V. 1988. Education to prevent AIDS: prospects and obstacles. *Science* 239, February 5, 592–596.

Firestone, David. 1996. Life span dips for men born in New York. *New York Times*, April 27.

Foreman, Judy. 1989. N.Y. study finds infection rate stable for addicts. *Boston Globe*, February 17.

Freedman, Samuel. 1987. New AIDS battlefield: addicts' world. *New York Times*, April 8.

Frieden, Thomas R., Moupali Das Douglas, Scott E. Kellerman, and Kelly J. Henning. 2005. Applying public health principles to the HIV epidemic. *New England Journal of Medicine*, December 1, 2397–2402.

Gardner, Tracie M. 2008. The spread of H.I.V. among Black and Latina women. *New York Times*, September 10.

Gay Men's Health Crisis. 2010. HIV/AIDS Basics. www.gmhc.org/learn/hivaids-basics (accessed March 9, 2010).

Goldman, Ari. 1987. AIDS patients in dire need find some solace. *New York Times*, December 12.

Gonzalez, David. 2007. For smaller fighters of H.I.V., weapons dwindle. *New York Times*, March 27.

Grace, Melissa. 2006. Fighting new AIDS tide, Brklyn drive starts today. *New York Daily News*, July 31.

Gross, Jane. 1985. Homosexuals stepping up AIDS education. *New York Times*, September 22.

———. 1987a. Explicit AIDS ads expect to spark debate in New York. *New York Times*, May 11.

———. 1987b. The most tragic of victims of AIDS: thousands of youngsters. *New York Times*, July 17.

Gruson, Lindsey. 1987. Condoms: experts fear false sense of security. *New York Times*, August 18.

Hamilton, Johann. 2011. AIDS program cuts stir protest. *City Limits*, June 1.

Hansell, David. 2000. Testimony before the New York City Council Committee on Health. April 25.

Hartocollis, Anemona. 2008. Push in Bronx for H.I.V. test for all adults. *New York Times*, June 26.

———. 2011. City's graphic ad on the dangers of H.I.V. is dividing activists. *New York Times*, January 3.

Havlir, Diane, and Chris Bayer. 2012. The beginning of the end of aids? *New England Journal of Medicine* 367, August 23, 685–687.

Hays, Elizabeth. 2006. Boros shorted on AIDS funds, Thompson says. *New York Daily News*, April 28.

Henig, Robin Marantz. 1983. AIDS: a new disease's deadly odyssey. *New York Times*, February 6.

Hentoff, Nat. 1987. AIDS: mandatory testing would help. *Washington Post*, May 30.

Herman, Robin. 1982. A disease's spread provokes anxiety. *New York Times*, August 8.

Hernandez, Raymond. 1999. State court rejects Giuliani's policy on AIDS benefits. *New York Times*, October 20.

Hilts, Philip J. 1990. U.S. to alter screening of those giving blood. *New York Times*, December 5.

Howe, Marvine. 1984. Homosexuals call for assurances on confidentiality of AIDS tests. *New York Times*, October 12.

Jacobs, Andrew. 1996. East Harlem: misery compounded; life in El Barrio, life with AIDS. *New York Times*, June 9.

Jaccarino, Mike. 2009. HIV group: just say know, Bronx program cheers rise in testing to help thwart disease. *New York Daily News*, June 28.

Joseph, Stephen G. 1992. *Dragon within the Gates: The Once and Future AIDS Epidemic*. New York: Carroll and Graff.

Kaiser Family Foundation. 2008. HIV testing for mothers and newborns. www.statehealth facts.org (accessed April 26, 2010).

Kaiser State Health Facts. 2012. Ryan White Program total funding. FY 2010. www.state healthfacts.org (accessed March 8, 2012).

Kennedy, Randy. 2001. Gay health ads in bus shelters are pulled after complaints. *New York Times*, June 27.

Kerr, Peter. 1988. Ideas and trends: free needles for addicts; experts find fault in New City AIDS plan. *New York Times*, February 7.

King, Wayne. 1986. Doctors cite stigma of AIDS in declining to report cases. *New York Times*, May 27.

Knox, Richard A. 1998. Needle programs cut AIDS; studies. *Boston Globe*, July 5.

Kolata, Gina. 1994. Discovery that AIDS can be prevented. *New York Times*, November 3.

Lambert, Bruce. 1987. AIDS rise spurs debate on testing of victim's sex partners. *New York Times*, January 27.

———. 1988a. New York called unprepared on AIDS. *New York Times*, July 14.

———. 1988b. A nursing home ward is approved for AIDS. *New York Times*, August 12.

———. 1988c. The region: the free needle program is under way and under fire. *New York Times*, November 13.

———. 1989a. New York officials reject joint AIDS group. *New York Times*, April 5.

———. 1989b. Koch to seek $40 million more for AIDS. *New York Times*, May 15.

———. 1989c. Black clergy set to preach about AIDS. *New York Times*, June 10.

———. 1989d. New York report on AIDS assails inadequate financing. *New York Times*, August 1.

———. 1989e. In shift, gay men's group endorses testing for AIDS virus. *New York Times*, August 16.

———. 1989f. Protests greet removal of top AIDS officials. *New York Times*, November 12.

———. 1989g. New York City will test for AIDS in autopsies to trace its spread. *New York Times*, December 15.

———. 1990a. Now, no Haitians can donate blood. *New York Times*, March 14.

———. 1990b. Health chief is criticized on AIDS shift. *New York Times*, May 10.

———. 1990c. As AIDS spreads, so do warnings for partners. *New York Times*, May 13.

———. 1990d. New York hospitals to urge AIDS tests for patients. *New York Times*, July 27.

———. 1990e. New York recommends a broader policy on AIDS testing. *New York Times*, August 28.

———. 1991. AIDS protesters test state needle laws. *New York Times*, April 14.

Lee, Felicia R. 1994. Needle exchange programs shown to slow H.I.V. rates. *New York Times*, November 11.

———. 1995. Blacks' dollars seem scarce in AIDS fight. *New York Times*, August 20.

Levine, Carol, and Ronald Bayer. 1985. Screening blood: public health and medical uncertainty. *Hastings Center Report*, August 8.

Levitt, Miriam, and Donald B. Rosenthal. 1999. The third wave: a symposium on AIDS politics and policy in the United States in the 1990s. *Policy Studies Journal* 27, no. 4, 783–795.

Lindsey, Robert. 1985. Bathhouse curbs called help in coast AIDS fight. *New York Times*, October 24.

Link, Derek. 1998. H.I.V. testing access (letter to the editor). *New York Times*, April 2.

———. 2005. Tackling a taboo. HIV/AIDS is growing among the city's Asians, but the clergy steers clear of any sex talk. *New York Daily News*, November 30.

Lite, Jordan. 2006a. Once-bleak outlook shining with hope, city babies beat odds. *New York Daily News*, May 29.

———. 2006b. Don't cut city's AIDS money! Hil and Chuck fight plan to shift funds. *New York Daily News*, September 28.

Mansnerus, Laura. 2000. Judge's ruling puts city AIDS under U.S. monitor. *New York Times*, September 20.

Markey, Eileen. 2010. City pulls back from AIDS services cuts. *City Limits*, June 24. www.citylimits.org/news/article_print.cfm?article_id=4080 (accessed August 3, 2010).

Marks, Peter. 1993. The vote against Fernandez; Fernandez silently sits in real-life people's court. *New York Times*, February 11.

Marriott, Michel. 1988. New York City asks state and U.S. for AIDS help. *New York Times*, May 17.

Mays, Vickie M., and Susan D. Cochran. 1988. Issues in perception of AIDS risk and risk reduction activities by Black and Hispanic/Latina women. *American Psychologist* 43, no. 11, 949–957.

McNeil, Donald G., Jr. 2006. U.S. urges H.I.V. Tests for adults and teenagers. *New York Times*, September 22.

———. 2010a. New lines of attack in H.I.V prevention. *New York Times*, November 8.

———. 2010b. An AIDS advance, hiding in the open. *New York Times*, November 27.

———. 2011a. Early H.I.V. therapy sharply cuts transmission. *New York Times*, May 12.

———. 2011b. New HIV cases steady despite better treatment. *New York Times*, August 3.

———. 2012. Another use for rapid home HIV test: screening sexual partners. *New York Times*, October 5.

McQuiston, John T. 1986. AIDS test centers are set for city. *New York Times*, March 30.

Mechanic, David, and Linda H. Aiken. 1989. Lessons from the past: responding to the AIDS crisis. *Health Affairs*, Fall, 16–32.

Meyer, Kate, and Lisa Colangelo. 2005. Blanket city in latex? Public condom giveaway urged. *New York Daily News*, May 24.

Mooney, Mark. 1995. City ends some free, no-name HIV tests. *New York Daily News*, July 17.

Moynihan, Colin. 1999. Neighborhood report: Staten Island up close; fight over needle exchange. *New York Times*, April 18.

Myers, Steven Lee. 1994. Adult movie theater is shut as a health hazard. *New York Times*, January 23.

Navarro, Mireya. 1991a. AIDS definition is widened to include blood cell count. *New York Times*, August 8.

———. 1991b. 3 Black church groups to house AIDS patients. *New York Times*, October 13.

———. 1991c. Dinkins panel is moving to revive needle exchange to combat AIDS. *New York Times*, October 29.

———. 1991d. Dinkins endorses privately financed needle swap plan. *New York Times*, November 5.

———. 1991e. Epidemic changes all at inner-city medical center. *New York Times*, November 11.

———. 1993a. In the age of AIDS, sex clubs proliferate again; unable to eliminate high-risk activities, New York City considers closer monitoring. *New York Times*, March 5.

———. 1993b. AIDS numbers increase under new federal rules. *New York Times*, March 22.

———. 1993c. Testing newborns for AIDS virus raises issue of mothers' privacy. *New York Times*, August 8.

———. 1994a. Group begins new AIDS ads in subways. *New York Times*, January 14.

———. 1994b. AIDS plan for poor seen as model for other ills. *New York Times*, February 22.

Newman, Maria. 1995. Board adopts a curriculum about AIDS. *New York Times*, January 19.

New York City Commission on HIV/AIDS. 2005. Report of the New York City Commission on HIV/AIDS. October 31.

New York City Council. 1999. Council Committee on General Welfare (hearing). June 23.

———. 2000a. Council Committee on Health (hearing). April 25.

———. 2000b. Council Committee on General Welfare (hearing). September 7.

———. 2002. Council Committee on General Welfare (hearing). November 6.

———. 2007. Council Committee on Health (hearing). December 13.

———. 2008. Council Committee on Health (hearing). May 1.

———. 2009. Council Committee on Health (hearing). September 23.

———. 2012. Council Committee on General Welfare (hearing). February 8.

New York City Department of Education. 2005a. Lesson Guide: Grade 7.

———. 2005b. Lesson Guide: Grade 12.

———. 2006. HIV/AIDS Education (pamphlet). February 21.

———. 2009. Condom Availability Program. September 9.

———. 2010. Dear Parent of Guardian (letter template).

New York City Department of Health. 1985. AIDS. July 1.

———. 1986. For facts about AIDS call: (wallet size). October.

———. 1987a. Shooting up and AIDS. February.

———. 1987b. AIDS, the straight facts. May.

———. 1987c. Women and AIDS. February.

———. 1987d. AIDS and drugs: the best protection is no injection. May.

New York City Department of Health and Mental Hygiene. 2001. Understanding the Basics—Ryan White Care Services. New York City: New York City Department of Health and Mental Hygiene.

———. 2005. Report of the New York City Commission on HIV/AIDS. October 31.

———. 2010a. NYC Condom. www.nyc.gov/html/doh/html/condoms/condoms-more .shtml (accessed April 11, 2010).

———. 2010b. HIV/AIDS Information: HIV Reporting/Partner Notification Law. www .nyc.gov/html.doh/ah/ahn1.shtml (accessed February 19, 2010).

———. 2011. HIV Epidemiological and Field Services Semiannual Report. Vol. 6, no. 1, April.

———. 2012. Health department announces 41% drop in deaths among Black New Yorkers living with HIV/AIDS (press release). February 7. www.nyc.gov/html/doh/html /pr2012/pr002-12.shtml (accessed February 9, 2012).

New York City Department of Health and Mental Hygiene HIV Epidemiology and Field Services Program. 2009. Reported AIDS Diagnoses and Deaths in 1981–2000 and Reported Persons Living with AIDS as of 12/31/81–2008, New York City.

New York City Human Resources Administration. 2010a. Department of Social Services, HASA Services (accessed May 4, 2010). www.nyc.gov/html/hra/html/directory_services .shtml.

———. 2010b. HIV/AIDS Services Administration: HASA Facts (accessed May 4, 2010). www.nyc.gov/html/hra/html/directory_hasafact.shtml.

———. 2013. HIV/AIDS Services Administration Program Overview.

New York City Mayor's Office of Operations. 1988. *The Mayor's Management Report*. New York City: New York City Mayors Office of Operations, Director, Barbara Gunn; Mayor Edward Koch. September 15.

———. 1992. *The Mayor's Management Report*. New York City. New York City Mayor's Office of Operations, Director, Harvey Robbins, Mayor David Dinkins. September 17.

New York City Office of the Mayor. 1983. Statement by Mayor Edward I Koch. June 6.

———. 1985. Statement by Mayor Edward I. Koch (523–85). December 16.

New York City Panel Convened to Review the Cases of AIDS in School Aged Children. 1985. Statement.

New York State Department of Health AIDS Institute. 2009. About the AIDS Institute 2009.

———. 2010. HIV Special Needs Plans (HIV SNPS). www.health.state.ny.us/diseases/aids /resources/snps/index/htm (accessed May 10, 2010).

———. 2012. Chapter 308 of the Laws of 2010 HIV Testing Law Mandated Report. August.

New York State Office of the Governor. 2010. Governor Paterson signs bills to promote HIV testing and remove barriers to needle exchange and syringe access. July 30.

New York Times. 1985. Axelrod says hotels are subject to curbs on sex linked to AIDS. November 18.

———. 1986. Metro Datelines: city to prepare plan for addicts. November 10.

———. 1987. AIDS: the next phase; an ever-widening epidemic tears at the city's life and spirit. March 6.

———. 1992. City council's poor health (editorial). May 2.

———. 1997. Bill on AIDS services is passed by council. June 26.

———. 1999. Spreading the word on AIDS. May 9.

———. 2006. Modifying the AIDS law. February 6.

———. 2010. Sensible rules, soon. July 2, 2010.

Nicholson, Joe. 1995. The changing face of AIDS. *Daily News*, August 30.

Nix, Crystal. 1985. More and more cases found among drug users. *New York Times*, October 20.

Norwood, Chris. 2007. Follow the money: AIDS funding and AIDS deaths in the Bloomberg years. New York: Community Preventive Health Institute.

O'Grady, Jim. 2004. A scorned plan seeks to undo needles and the damage done. *New York Times*, February 15.

Paul, Ari. 2010. Pressure builds to lift ban on gay men giving blood. *Gotham Gazette*, June 29. www.gothamgazette.com/print/3302.

Perez-Pena, Richard. 2001. State overlooks minority run AIDS groups, a report finds. *New York Times*, January 23.

———. 2006a. Federal policy on H.I.V. testing poses unique local challenge. *New York Times*, October 2.

———. 2006b. H.I.V. testing increases in city jails and hospitals. *New York Times*, October 3.

Perrow, Charles, and Mauro F. Guillen. 1990. *The AIDS Disaster: The Failure of Organizations in New York and the Nation.* New Haven: Yale University Press.

Peterson, John L., and Gerardo Marin. 1988. Issues in the prevention of AIDS among Black and Hispanic Men. *American Psychologist* 43, no. 11, 871–877.

Ports, Suki Terada. 2000. Testimony before the New York City Council Committee on Health. April 25.

Purnick, Joyce. 1985a. AIDS and the state. *New York Times*, October 30.

———. 1985b. City shuts a bathhouse as site of unsafe sex. *New York Times*, December 7.

Quimby, Ernest, and Samuel R. Friedman. 1989. Dynamics of black mobilization against AIDS in New York City. *Social Problems* 36, no. 4, 403–415.

Rangel, Jesus. 1985. City expanding its plan to help victims of AIDS. *New York Times*, March 30.

Richardson, Lynda. 1997a. An AIDS nursing home finds it is no longer the last stop. *New York Times*, January 25.

———. 1997b. White patients have more access to new AIDS drugs, a survey shows. *New York Times*, July 27.

———. 1997c. Condoms in school said not to affect teen-age sex rate. *New York Times*, September 30.

———. 1997d. Hospital opens clinic at AIDS agency in Chelsea. *New York Times*, December 15.

———. 1998. AIDS agency, in policy reversal, to call for reporting HIV cases to state. *New York Times*, January 13.

———. 1999. Study finds H.I.V. infection is high for young gay men. *New York Times*, February 16.

———. 2000. Bureaucracy and bitterness. *New York Times*, September 24.

Roberts, Katherine. 1985. Ideas and trends: New York curbs bathhouses. *New York Times*, October 27.

Rohter, Larry. 1985. Quinones sets a policy on AIDS, citing illness among 6 employees. *New York Times*, September 12.

Rosenthal, Elisabeth. 1996. Managed care has trouble treating AIDS, patients say. *New York Times*, January 15.

Ruiz, Albor. 2005a. Language barrier brick wall at hosps. *New York Daily News*, January 13.

———. 2005b. Bill aims to clean up AIDS housing mess. *New York Daily News*, January 20.

Sack, Kevin. 1991. Shift in care for Medicaid in budget deal. *New York Times*, May 31.

Santora, Marc. 2005. U.S. is close to eliminating AIDS in infants, officials say. *New York Times*, January 30.

———. 2006a. Overhaul urged for laws on AIDS tests and data. *New York Times*, February 2.

———. 2006b. City AIDS report highlights risk to Black men and women. *New York Times*, February 4.

Sengupta, Somini. 1997. Students fault Board of Education on AIDS classes. *New York Times*, March 13.

Shilts, Randy. 1987. *And the Band Played On: Politics, People and the AIDS Epidemic*. New York: St. Martins Griffin.

Siegel, Joel. 1995. City cuts off some poor AIDS patients. *New York Daily News*, December 25.

Sisk, Jane E., Maria Hewitt, and Kelly L. Metcalf. 1988. The effectiveness of AIDS education. *Health Affair*, Winter, 37–51.

Smith, James Monroe. 1996. *AIDS and Society*. Upper Saddle River: Prentice Hall.

Sontag, Deborah. 1997. H.I.V. testing for newborns debate anew. *New York Times*, February 10.

Staley, Peter. 2006. Why it's right to test. *New York Times*, June 4.

Steinhauer, Jennifer. 2001. AIDS at 20: a city transformed. *New York Times*, June 4.

Stolberg, Sheryl Gay. 1997. Identity crisis; gay culture weights sense and sexuality. *New York Times*, November 23.

Sullivan, Ronald. 1983a. City takes Haitians off list of high risk groups. *New York Times*, July 29.

———. 1983b. Cuomo signs a law subsidizing AIDS research. *New York Times*, August 6.

———. 1985. State to propose centers for AIDS. *New York Times*, December 24.

———. 1987a. New York will start giving out condoms in bars and movies. *New York Times*, May 31.

———. 1987b. Warn AIDS patients' partners, health official urges. *New York Times*, October 15.

Supportive Housing Network of New York. 2013. Housing Opportunities for Persons with AIDS (HOPWA) Competitive Grants. shnny.org/fundingguide/housing-opportunities-for-persons-with-aids-hopwa-competitive-grants/ (accessed September 15, 2013).

Sweeney, Monica. 2009. Testimony before New York City Council Committee on Health. September 23.

Sweeney, Patricia, et al. 2013. Shifting the paradigm: using HIV surveillance data as a foundation for improving HIV and preventing HIV infection. *Milbank Quarterly* 91, no. 3, 558–603.

United States Catalog of Federal Domestic Assistance. 2010. www.cfda.gov.

United States Centers for Disease Control. 1988. Understanding AIDS. HHS Publication No (CDC) HHS-88-8404.

———. 2002. CDC's HIV/AIDS prevention activities. May.

———. 2006. Evolution of HIV/AIDS prevention programs—United States, 1981–2006. *Morbidity and Mortality Weekly Review*, June 2, 597–603.

———. 2008. New HIV incidence estimates: CDC responds. September.

———. 2010a. HIV/AIDS—Basic Information. www.cdc.gov/hiv/topics/basic/index.htm #origin (accessed March 2, 2010).

———. 2010b. Public Health Law Program. www2a.cdc.gov/phlp/PHlawreadings.asp (accessed April 19, 2010).

United States Department of Health and Human Services. 1998. HHS Fact Sheet—The Ryan White Comprehensive AIDS Resources Emergency Care Act. Department of Health and Human Services Press Office, December 18. www.hhs.gov/news/press/1998pres/981218 .html.

———. 2001. Eligible Metropolitan Area Reports-2001 Grantee Allocations. Washington, D.C.: United States Department of Health and Human Services, Health Resources and Services Administration, HIV/AIDS Bureau. ftp://hrsa.gov/hab/2001titlei.pdf (accessed April 14, 2003).

———. 2002. CARE Act Overview and Funding. Washington, D.C.: United States Department of Health and Human Services, Health Resources and Services Administration, HIV/AIDS Bureau. January. ftp://ftp.hrsa.gov/hab/fundhistory.pdf (accessed April 14, 2003).

Valdiserri, Ronald. 2011. Evolutions in the minority AIDS initiative secretary's fund. AIDS blog. May 12. blog.aids.gov/2011/5/evolutions-in-the-minority-aids-initiative-secretary's-fund.html.

Washington Post. 1990. 50,000 protest ban on blood donations by Haitians, Africans. April 21.

———. 2000. New York loses welfare lawsuit; city violated disabilities act in AIDS cases judge rules. September 20.

Welsh, Tracy. 2006. H.I.V. tests in the Bronx (letter to the editor). *New York Times,* July 5.

White House Office of National AIDS Strategy. 2011. National HIV/AIDS Strategy: Implementation Update. July.

Whitmore, George. 1985. Reaching our to some with AIDS. *New York Times,* May 19.

Chapter 5 · Helping a City Lose Weight

Adams, Elisabeth, Laurence Grummer-Strawn, and Gilberto Chavez. 2003. Food insecurity is associated with increased risk of obesity in California women. *Journal of Nutrition* 1070–1074.

Amar, Natalie. 2009. Restaurants swallow New York City calorie posting rules. *City Law* 15, May–June, 54–55.

Associated Press. 2006. Study of children with diabetes suggests obesity is affecting life expectancy. *New York Times,* July 26.

Bakalar, Nicholas. 2005a. Nutrition: dubious results for "Clean Your Plate" syndrome. *New York Times,* June 28.

———. 2005b. On the scales: the road to obesity begins at your TV. *New York Times,* September 20.

Berg, Joel. 2008. Taking questions. *New York Times* (blog). November 28.

Better Business Bureau. 2014. Children's Food and Beverage Advertising Initiative. www .bbb.org/council/the-national-partner-program/national-advertising-review-services /children<#213>s-food-and-beverage-advertising-initiative/.

Booth, William. 1991. Americans fail to see the "lite"; quarter of population overweight, same as in the 60s, CDC says. *Washington Post,* July 13.

Bor, Jonathan. 2010. The science of childhood obesity. *Health Affairs* 29, no. 3, March, 393–397.

Brody, Jane. 2003. Major study erases doubt on link between excess weight and cancer. *New York Times,* May 6.

———. 2004a. The widening of America, or how size 4 became a size 0. *New York Times*, January 20.

———. 2004b. In an obese world, sweet nothings add up. *New York Times*, March 9.

———. 2005. Personal health: sparing the calories won't spoil the child. *New York Times*, April 5.

———. 2009. America's diet: too sweet by the spoonful. *New York Times*, February 10.

———. 2011. A simple map to the land of wholesome. *New York Times*, February 14.

Brownell, Kelly D., Rogan Kersh, David Ludwig, et al. 2010. Personal responsibility and obesity: a constructive approach to a controversial issue. *Health Affairs* 29, no. 3, March, 379–387.

Brustein, Joshua, and Gail Robinson. 2006. The challenge of eating health. *Gotham Gazette*, November 20. www.gothamgazette.com/article//20061120/2041.

Burros, Marian. 1994. Despite awareness of risks, more in U.S. are getting fat. *New York Times*, July 17.

———. 1996. Federal report promotes commonplace exercise. *New York Times*, July 12.

Campanile, Carl. 2006. Trans fats are out—fruits and veggies are in. *New York Post*, December 8.

Chan, Sewell. 2009. Court upholds the city's rule requiring some restaurants to post calorie counts. *New York Times*, February 18.

Charbonneau, Nicolle. 2002. Kids' obesity tied to mom's feeding approach. *Health Scout News Reporter*, February 22.

Cohen, Nevin. 2013. Urban Food Policy: Foodworks Update, September 9. www.urban food-policy.com (accessed June 24, 2014).

Cohen, Stephen L. 2000. PE programs sag out of shape. *USA Today*, October 9.

Collins, Glenn. 2009. Customers prove there's a market for fresh produce. *New York Times*, June 11.

Community Health Care Association of New York State. 2014. New York City Childhood Obesity Initiative. www.chcanys.org.index.php?src=gendocs&ref=NYC-Childhood -Obesity (accessed June 24, 2014).

Connelly, Marjorie. 2003. More children are obese, and more Americans know it. *New York Times*, May 13.

Crawford, Lynda. 2005. Hunger and obesity in the two New Yorks. *Gotham Gazette*, October 12. www.gothamgazette.com/article/socialservice/20051012/15/1615.

Danis, Kirsten. 2008. City scales back plan to put more fruit, vegetable vendors in poor areas. *New York Daily News*, February 21.

Diet and Fitness. 2010. Body Mass Index (BMI) FAQ. www.dietandfitnesstoday.com/bmi faq.php (accessed July 2, 2010).

Duenwald, Mary. 2002. An "Eat More" message for a fattened America. *New York Times*, February 19.

Dumanovsky, Tamara, Cathy A. Nonas, Christina Y. Huang, et al. 2009. What people buy from fast-food restaurants: caloric content and menu item selection, New York City, 2007. *Obesity* 17, no. 7, July, 1369–1374.

Ebbeling, Cara B., Dorota B. Pawlak, and David S. Ludwig. 2002. Childhood obesity: public health crisis, common sense cure. *Lancet* 360, August 10, 473–482.

Eichel, Joanne De Simone. 2011. Prevention—Promoting health education to prevent disease in New York City (lecture). New York Academy of Medicine, October 13.

Elbel, Brian, Rogan Kersh, Vincent Brescoli, et al. 2009. Calorie labeling and food choices: a first look at the effects on low income people in New York City. *Health Affairs* (web exclusive), October 6, w1110–w1121. Content.healthaffairs.org/content/28/6/w1110.long.

Emerson, Christopher. 2009. A food policy for New York. *Gotham Gazette*, March 4. www.gothamgazette.com/article/health/20090304/9/2846.

Farely, Thomas A., Anna Caffarelli, Mary T. Bassett, et al. 2009. New York City's fight over calorie labeling. *Health Affairs* (web exclusive, October 6, w1098–w1109. Content.healthaffairs.org/content/28/6/w1098.full.pdf+html.

Finholm, Valerie. 1997. Overweight kids need better diet and more exercise. *Montreal Gazette*, May 28.

Flegal, Katherine M., Margaret D. Carroll, and Cynthia Ogden. 2002. Prevalence and trends in obesity among adults, 1999–2000. *Journal of the American Medical Association* 288, no. 14, October 9, 1723–1727.

Flegal, Katherine M., Margaret D. Carroll, Cynthia Ogden, et al. 2010. Prevalence and trends in obesity among U.S. adults. *Journal of the American Medical Association* 303, no. 3, January 20, 235–241.

Frazier, Sara Kugler. 2010. NY seeks to ban sugary drinks from food stamp buys. *Yahoo News*, October 7. www.yahoo.com/s/ap/20101007/ap_on_re_us/us_food_stamps_sugary_drinks.

Grady, Denise. 2000. Diabetes rises: doctors foresee a harsh impact. *New York Times*, August 24.

Gross, Courtney. 2008. Creating healthy bodegas. *Gotham Gazette*, March 3. www.gothamgazette.com/article/health/20080303/9/2451.

Grynbaum, Michael M. 2012a. Health panel approves restriction on sale of large sugary drinks. *New York Times*, September 13.

———. 2012b. Soda industry sues to stop a sales ban on big drinks. *New York Times*, October 12.

Hartocollis, Anemona. 2010a. Calorie postings no match for holiday gluttony. *New York Times*, January 14.

———. 2010b. Failure of the state soda tax plan reflects power of an antitax message. *New York Times*, July 2.

———. 2010c. City's efforts fail to dent child obesity. *New York Times*, September 4.

———. 2010d. New York asks to bar use of food stamps to buy sodas. *New York Times*, October 6.

———. 2010e. Plan to ban food stamps for sodas has hurdles. *New York Times*, October 7.

———. 2011. Obesity rate falls for New York schoolchildren. *New York Times*, December 15.

Hayes, Roger. 2014. Building Healthy Communities: Promoting Health Equity in Harlem (PowerPoint). Presentation at the Fourth Annual National Urban Health Conference, New York Academy of Medicine, April 25.

Healthy Food Access Portal. 2014. Healthyfoodaccess.org/find-money/hffi/federal (accessed: June 23, 2014).

Henig, Robin Marantz. 2006. Fat factors. *New York Times*, August 13.

Hillier, Amy. 2008. Childhood overweight and the built environment: making technology part of the solution rather than part of the problem. *Annals of the American Academy of Political and Social Science* 615, January, 56–82.

Huang, Christina, and Tamara Dumanovsky. 2009. Evaluating New York City's calorie labeling regulation: assessing calorie content and consumer awareness. American Public Health Association Annual Meeting and Expo (Philadelphia), November 7–11. www.apha .confex/apha/137am/webprogram/Paper210918.htm (accessed August 2, 2010).

Ives, Nat. 2004. A report on childhood obesity. *New York Times*, February 25.

Jerome, Sara. 2008. Those restaurant calorie counts: too good to be true? *Gotham Gazette*, August 4. www.gothamgazette.com/article/20080804/202/2601 (accessed June 26, 2010).

Kakutani, Michiko. 2003. Land of the free. Home of the fat. *New York Times*, January 7.

Kolata, Gina. 2002. Asking if obesity is a disease or just a symptom. *New York Times*, April 16.

———. 2003. What we don't know about obesity. *New York Time,* June 22.

———. 2007. Genes take charge, and diets fall by the wayside. *New York Times*, May 8.

Kopelman. P. 2007. Health risks associated with overweight and obesity. *Obesity Reviews* 8, supplement 1, 13–17.

Krucoff, Carol. 1997. Get moving: stop trying to be thin and start trying to be healthy. *Washington Post*, August 12.

Larkin, Marilynn. 2007. The limits of willpower. *New York Times*, August 29.

Lennard, Natasha, and Patrick McGeehan. 2010. Where produce is scared, supermarkets will grow. *New York Times*, February 9.

Let's Move. 2010. www.letsmove.gov.

Lopez, Russell P., and H. Patricia Hynes. 2006. Obesity, physical activity, and the urban environment: public research needs. *Environmental Health: A Global Access Science Source* 5, no. 25, 1–10.

McGeehan, Patrick. 2011. U.S. rejects mayor's plan to ban use of food stamps to buy soda. *New York Times*, August 20.

McMillan, Tracie. 2004. The action diet: get better food in your neighborhood. *City Limits*, July 15.

Mokdad, Ali H., Mark K Serdula, William Dietz, et al. 1999. The spread of the obesity epidemic in the United States, 1991–1998. *Journal of the American Medical Association* 282, no. 16, October 27, 1519–1522.

Moore, Toby. 1999. The United States of obesity. *Express*, October 29.

Morland, Kimberly, Ana V. Diez, and Steve Wing. 2006. Supermarkets, other food stores, and obesity: the atherosclerosis risk in communities study. *American Journal of Preventive Medicine* 30, no. 4, 333–339.

Moss, Michael. 2010. While warning about fat, U.S. pushes cheese sales. *New York Times*, November 6.

Nagourney, Eric. 2004. Measurements: US widens lead over Europe. *New York Times*, January 13.

Nestle, Marion. 2003. Increasing portion sizes in American diets: more calories, more obesity. *Journal of the American Dietetic Association* 103, no. 1, January, 39–40.

———. 2006. Food industry and health: mostly promises, little action. *Lancet* 368, August 12, 564–565.

Neuman, William. 2010. Ad rules stall, keeping cereal a cartoon staple. *New York Times*, July 23.

New York Academy of Medicine. 2013. DASH-NY (fact sheet).

New York City Council. 2008. Proposed law dealing with green carts (public hearing). January 31.

New York City Department of Education. 2010a. Chancellor Klein asks parents to review school fitness reports with their children. June 16. Schools.nyc.gov/Offices/mediarelations /NewsandSpeeches/2009-2010/fitnessgram061610.htm.

———. 2010b. NYC Fitnessgram Assessment. Schools.nyc.gov/Academics/Fitnessand Health/StandardsCurriculum/NYCFitnessgram.htm.

———. 2010c. Wellness Policies on Physical Activity and Nutrition. June.

———. 2013. NYC Fitnessgram Assessments. Schools.nyc.gov/Academics/Fitnessand Health/NycFitnessgram/NYCFITNESSGRAM.htm (accessed September 25, 2013).

New York City Department of Health and Mental Hygiene. 2003. NYC Vital Signs: Obesity Begins Early. Vol. 2, no. 5, June.

———. 2006. NYC Vital Statistics: Obesity in Early Childhood. Vol. 5, no. 2, March.

———. 2007. Eating well in Harlem: how available is health food?

———. 2009a. NYC Vital Statistics: Childhood Obesity Is a Serious Concern in New York City. Vol. 8, no. 1, June.

———. 2009b. Report to the New York City Council on Green Carts, FY2008-2009. September 10.

———. 2009c. Health Department's anti-obesity poster inspires a video sequel (press release 083-09). December 14.

———. 2010a. Epidemiology Services: NYC Youth Risk Behavior Survey. www.nyc.gov /html/doh/html/episrv-youthriskbehavior.shtml (accessed July 12, 2010).

———. 2010b. Epiquery: NYC Heath and Nutrition Examination Survey (HANES). a816-healthspi-nyc.gov/epiquery (accessed July 12, 2010).

———. 2010c. Epiquery: NYC Community Health Survey (CHS). a816-healthpsi-nyc.gov /epiquery (accessed July 12, 2010).

———. 2010d. Epiquery: NYC Youth Risk Behavior Study. a816-healthspi.nyc.gov/epiquery (accessed July 13, 2010).

———. 2010e. New York City Healthy Bodegas Initiative: 2010 Report.

———. 2010f. NYC Green Cart.

———. 2010g. Working with farmers' markets. www.nyc.gov.html/doh/html/cdp/cdp_pan _health_bucks.shtml (accessed June 13, 2010).

———. 2010h. Health Bucks Program 2010 Community Based Organization Application.

———. 2010i. Farmers' Markets Initiatives: Promoting Fresh Fruits and Vegetables in Underserved Communities—2010 Report.

———. 2010j. Health Department launches new effort to wean New Yorkers from sugary beverages (press release 036-10). August 2.

———. 2010k. What's required in group child care centers. www.nyc.gov/html/doh/html /cdp/cdp_pan_gcc.shtml (accessed June 14, 2010).

———. 2010l. Trainings on nutrition and physical activity for staff in child care centers and elementary schools. www.nyc.gov/html.doh/html.cdp/cdp_pan_staff.shtml (accessed June 13, 2010).

———. 2010m. Shape Up New York: a free family fitness program. www.nyc.gov/html/doh /html/cdp/shapeupny.shtml (accessed June 13, 2010).

———. 2013. Health Department expands Shop Healthy NYC to three new neighborhoods in the Bronx (press release 020-13). June 26.

New York City Department of Health and Mental Hygiene and New York City Department of Education. 2009. Letter regarding low fat milk. April.

New York City Economic Development Corporation. 2009. Mayor Bloomberg, Governor Paterson and Speaker Quinn announce comprehensive strategies to increase and retain grocery stores in New York City (press release). May 20.

———. 2010. NYCIDA approves FRESH incentives for supermarket in the Bronx (press release). August 3.

New York City Five Borough Economic Opportunity Plan. 2009. Food retail expansion to support health.

New York City Food. 2013. Shop Healthy. www.nyc.gov/html/nycfood/html/shop/shop .shtml.

New York City Obesity Task Force. 2012. Reversing the epidemic: the New York City obesity task force plan to prevent and control obesity. May 31.

New York City Office of the Mayor. 2007. Schoolyards to playgrounds announcement (press release PR 223-07). July 2.

———. 2008. Mayor Bloomberg signs legislations establishing 1,000 new "Green Cart" permits (press release PR 086-08).

———. 2009a. New York City beverage vending machine standards. May.

———. 2009b. Combating early childhood obesity (press conference). October 23.

———. 2010. New York City Agency Food Standards.

———. 2011. FRESH Zoning (press conference). November 21.

———. 2012. Anti-obesity program (press conference). July 23.

———. 2013. Mayor Bloomberg announces first ever Center of Active Design to promote physical activity and health in buildings and public spaces through building code design and standard changes (press release PR 250-13). July 17.

New York State Department of Health. 2005. Activ8Kids!—Associated Programs and Activities. www.health.state.ny.us/prevention/obesity/activ8kids/associated_programs_ activities.htm (accessed September 3, 2010).

———. 2006. New York State Strategic Plan for Overweight and Obesity Prevention.

———. 2007. Activ8Kids! New York State School Nutrition and Physical Activity Best Practices Toolkit.

———. 2008. Healthy Kids, Healthy New York–After School Initiative Toolkit. www.health .state.ny.us/prevention/obesity/active8kids/ (accessed September 3, 2010).

———. 2010a. Just Say Yes: Resources. www.jsyfruitsveggies.org/jsyresources (accessed September 3, 2010).

———. 2010b. Just Say Yes: New York Region 1. www.jsyfruitsveggies.org/Calendar/index .cfm.

New York Times. 1995. Study finds a soaring rate of obesity in U.S. children. October 8.

———. 2008. Does fructose make you fatter? July 24.

Nixon, Ron. 2014. House panel advances bill on school lunch options. *New York Times*, May 29.

Norton, Jennifer. 2010. Phone interview with Jennifer Norton, Epidemiological Services, New York City Department of Health. July 8.

Ogden, Cynthia L., Margaret D. Carroll, Lester R. Curtin, et al. 2006. Prevalence of overweight and obesity in the United States, 1999–2004. *Journal of the American Medical Association* 295, no. 13, April 5, 1549–1555.

———. 2010. Prevalence of high body mass index in US children and adolescents, 2007–2008. *Journal of the American Medical Association* 303, no. 3, January 30, 242–249.

Ogden, Cynthia L., Margaret D. Carroll, and Katherine M. Flegal. 2008. High body mass index for age among US children and adolescents, 2003–2006. *Journal of the American Medical Association* 299. no. 20, May 28, 2401–2405.

Ogden, Cynthia L., Katherine M. Flegal, Margaret D. Carroll, et al. 2002. Prevalence and trends in overweight among US children and adolescents, 1999–2000. *Journal of the American Medical Association* 288, no. 14, October 9, 1728–1732.

Parker-Pope, Tara. 2008. Hint of hope as child obesity rate hits plateau. *New York Times*, May 28.

Perdue, Wendy. 2008. Obesity, poverty, and the built environment: challenges and opportunities. *Georgetown Journal on Poverty, Law and Policy* 15, Fall, 821–832.

Perez-Pena, Richard. 2003. Obesity on rise in New York public schools. *New York Times*, July 9.

Piernas Carmen, and Barry M. Popkin. 2010. Trends in snacking among U.S. children. *Health Affairs* 29, no. 3, March, 398–404.

Rabin, Roni Caryn. 2009. Regimens: click off the TV, and burn more calories. *New York Times*, December 22.

———. 2010. Childhood: obesity in young subjects drops in study. *New York Times*, July 12.

Reuters Health. 2002. Obese kids in U. S. often have prediabetic condition. March 13.

Robinson, Gail. 2005. New York's grocery gap. *Gotham Gazette*, November 21. www.gothamgazette.com/article//20551121/200/1658.

Robinson, Thomas N. 1999. Reducing children's television viewing to prevent obesity. *Journal of the American Medical Association* 282, no. 16, October 27, 1561–1567.

Rothstein, Caroline, and Cecile Dehesdin. 2010. A tale of two bodegas. *City Limits*, August 16.

Rundle, Andrew, Ana V. Diez Roux, Lance M. Freeman, et al. 2007. The urban built environment and obesity in New York City: a multilevel analysis. *American Journal of Health Promotion* 21, no. 4 supplement, December 1, 326–334.

Russell, Cristine. 1994. More adolescents are overweight; federal studies find one in five too heavy. *Washington Post*, November 15.

Rutkow, Lainie, Jon S. Vernick, James Hodge Jr., et al. 2008. Preemption and the obesity epidemic: state and local menu labeling laws and the Nutrition Labeling and Education Act. *Journal of Law, Medicine and Ethics* 36, Winter, 772–789.

Santora, Marc. 2006. New York pushing better diet in poorer neighborhoods. *New York Times*, January 20.

Singer, Natasha. 2010. Fixing a world that fosters fat. *New York Times*, August 21.

Singh, Gopal K., Mohammad Siapush, and Michael Kagan. 2010. Neighborhood socioeconomic conditions, built environments, and childhood obesity. *Health Affairs* 29, no. 3, March, 503–512.

Squires, Sally. 1998. Obesity-linked diabetes rising in children; experts attending Agriculture Dept. forum call for new strategies to reverse trend. *Washington Post*, November 3.

Strom, Stephanie. 2007. $500 million pledged to fight childhood obesity. *New York Times*, April 4.

———. 2011. McDonalds trims its Happy Meal. *New York Times*, July 27.

United States American Recovery and Reinvestment Act Prevention and Wellness Initiative. 2010. Communities Putting Prevention to Work (Fact Sheet). March 19.

United States Centers for Disease Control. 2010a. Defining Overweight and Obesity. www.cdc.gov/obesity/defining.html (accessed July 2, 2010).

———. 2010b. About BMI for Adults. www.cdc.gov/healthyweight/assessing/bmi/adult _bmi/index.html (accessed July 2, 2010).

———. 2010c. About BMI for Children and Teens. www.cdc.gov/healthyweight/assessing /bmi/children_bmi/about_childrens_bmi.html (accessed July 2, 2010).

———. 2010d. Defining Childhood Overweight and Obesity. www.cdc.gov/obesity/child hood/defining.html (accessed July 2, 2010).

———. 2010e. Childhood: Consequences-Obesity and Overweight for Professionals. www .cdc.gov/obesity/childhood/consequences.html (accessed July 1, 2010).

———. 2013. *Morbidity and Mortality Weekly Report.* August 6.

United States Department of Agriculture. 2014. Food and Nutrition Service: School Meals: Health Hunger Free Kids Act. www.fns.usda.gov/school-meals-hunger-free-kids-act (accessed June 24, 2014).

United States Department of Health and Human Services. 2010. The Surgeon General's Call to Action to Prevent Overweight and Obesity.

United States National Heart, Lung and Blood Institute. 2013. About We Can. www.nhlbi .nih.gov/health/public/heart/obesity/wecan/about-wecan/index.htm (accessed October 30, 2013).

Van Wye, Gretchen. 2010. Phone interview with Gretchen Van Wye, director, NYC Communities Putting Prevention to Work-Obesity, NYC DOHMH, Bureau of Chronic Disease Prevention and Control. July 28.

Warner, Melanie. 2005a. Snack makers use a calorie count to appeal to dieters. *New York Times*, May 30.

———. 2005b. Coke is urging youths to get physical. *New York Times*, July 12.

———. 2006. Industry urged to offer more nutritious foods for children. *New York Times*, May 3.

Web MD. 2010. Cholesterol Management Health Center-Weight Loss: health risks associated with obesity. www.webmd.com/cholesterol-management/obesity-health-risks (accessed July 3, 2010).

Wetzstein, Cheryl. 1997. Health club memberships getting bigger, members too. *Washington Times*, June 10.

White House. 2010. First Lady Michelle Obama launches Let's Move: America's move to raise a healthier generation (press release). February 9.

World Health Organization (WHO). 2000. Obesity: Preventing and Managing the Global Epidemic (WHO Technical Report Series 894). Geneva.

———. 2010. Adelaide Statement on Health in All Policies. www.who.int/social_determi nants/hiap_statement_who_sa_final.pdf.

Young, Lisa R., and Marion Nestle. 2003. Expanding portion sizes in the US marketplace: implications for nutrition counseling. *Journal of the American Dietetic Association* 103, no. 2, February, 231–234.

Zimmer, Amy. 2008. Mean green, veggie fight. *Metro New York*, February 2.

Chapter 6 · The First Appearance of West Nile Virus

Altman, Lawrence K. 2002. West Nile and its lessons for doctors. *New York Times*, August 13.

Cardwell, Diane. 2001. City to look beyond spraying for West Nile. *New York Times*, May 4.

Chen, David. 2000. City expands spraying of mosquitoes on ground. *New York Times*, August 18.

———. 2002. West Nile case in Queens shows virus is enduring. *New York Times*, August 17.

Cohen, Neil. 1999.Testimony before New York City Council Committee on Health. Crosswalks Network, New York City, October 12.

———. 2000a. Testimony before New York City Council Committee on Health. Crosswalks Network, New York City, January 18.

———. 2000b. Statement at Mayoral Press Conference. Crosswalks Network, New York City. April 13.

———. 2001. Testimony before the New York City Council Committee on Health. Crosswalks Network, New York City, May 31.

Colangelo, Lisa L. 2000. Cloud hangs over spraying health concerns despite city assurance. *New York Daily News*, August 21.

———. 2003. '02 deadliest year for West Nile Virus in city. *New York Daily News*, January 23.

Colangelo, Lisa, et al. 2001. W. Nile found in City—Queens, S. I. critters have traces of virus. *New York Daily News*, July 20.

DePalma, Anthony. 2005. Metro briefing New York: council breaks pesticide notice. *New York Times*, April 21.

Duenwald, Mary. 2005. Preventing West Nile infection could be just a spray away. *New York Times*, July 19.

Fish, Durland. 2007. Back to bite us. *New York Times*, May 27.

Hayes, Curtis G. 2001. West Nile Virus: Uganda 1937, to New York City, 1999. *Annals of the New York Academy of Medicine* 951, December, 25–37.

Jacobs, Andrew. 1999. Exotic virus is identified in 3 deaths. *New York Times*, September 26.

Kelley, Tina. 2002. Lawsuit over West Nile spraying dismissed by judge, city says. *New York Times*, December 3.

Kershaw, Sarah. 2000. Federal judge allows spraying to continue. *New York Times*, July 27.

Lipton, Eric. 2000a. Nile virus found again in the city. *New York Times*, July 18.

———. 2000b. Central Park shut to spray for virus. *New York Times*, July 25.

———. 2000c. A fight against fear as well as mosquitoes. *New York Times*, July 26.

Lombardi, Frank. 1999a. 2nd virus strain eyed city's encephalitis may be from Africa. *New York Daily News*, September 25.

———. 1999b. Fed aid for spray costs eyed. *New York Daily News*, October 16.

Lueck, Thomas J. 2000. Questions about where, and whether, to spray pesticides. *New York Times*, July 22.

———. 2002. Spraying for West Nile Virus. *New York Times*, July 23.

Mahoney, Joe. 2000. Girding for fight vs. skeeter virus. *Daily News*, February 19, 6.

Marfin, Anthony A., Lyle R. Peterson, Millicent Eldson, et al. 2001. Widespread West Nile Virus activity, Eastern United States, 2000. *Emerging Infections Diseases* 7, no. 4, July–August, 730–735.

Mostashari, Farzad, Michael L. Burning, Paul T. Kitsutani, et al. 2001. Epidemic West Nile encephalitis, New York, 1999: results of a household based seroepidemiological survey. *Lancet* 358, July 28, 261–264.

Nasci, Roger S. 1999. Testimony, New York City Council Committee on Health. Crosswalks Network, New York City, October 12.

Nash, Denis, Farzad Mostashari, Annie Fine, et al. 2001. The outbreak of West Nile Virus infection in the New York City area in 1999. *New England Journal of Medicine* 344, no. 24, June 14, 1807–1814.

Newman, Andy. 2002. Queens man is city's first West Nile fatality of 2002. *New York Times*, September 3.

New York City Council. 1999. Committee on Health hearing on West Nile Virus and the City's Use of Pesticides. October 12.

New York City Department of Health. 2001. Questions & Answers on Serosurvey, 2000. www.nyc.gov/html/wnv/wnvs/2000.shtml (accessed September 12, 2010).

New York City Department of Health and Mental Hygiene. 2003. Comprehensive Mosquito Surveillance and Control Plan.

———. 2010a. Comprehensive Mosquito Surveillance and Control Plan.

———. 2010b. Dead Bird Monitoring Report Form. www.nyc.gov/html/doh/html/wnv /wnvbird.shtml (accessed September 12, 2010).

———. 2010c. Guidelines for West Nile Virus Testing and Reporting Cases of Viral Encephalitis and Meningitis. June.

———. 2010d. Reducing mosquitoes around your home and community. www.nyc.gov /html/doh/html/wnv/wnvfaq2.shtml (accessed September 13, 2010).

———. 2010e. Standing Water Monitoring Report Form. www.nyc.gov/html/doh/html /wnv/wnvwater.shtml (accessed September 12, 2010).

———. 2010f. West Nile Virus Questions & Answers. www.nyc.gov/html/doh/html/wnv /wnvfaq1.shtml (accessed September 13, 2010).

New York City Office of the Mayor. 1999. Mayoral Press Conference. Crosswalks Network, New York City, September 9.

Perez-Pena, Richard. 2003. Who's afraid of this little fellow? *New York Times*, September 21.

Petersen, Lyle R., and Anthony A. Marfin. 2002. West Nile Virus: a primer for the clinician. *Annals of Internal Medicine* 137, no. 3, August 6, E173–E179.

Petersen, Lyle R., Anthony A. Marfin, and Duane J. Gubler. 2003. West Nile Virus. *Journal of the American Medical Association* 290, no. 4, July 23, 524–527.

Petersen, Lyle R., and John T. Roehrig. 2001. West Nile Virus: a reemerging global pathogen. *Revista Biomedica* 12, no. 3, July–September, 208–216.

Quinn, Christine. 2003. Press conference with environmental advocates on pesticide use. Crosswalks Network, New York City, January 16.

Revkin, Andrew C. 2000. Latest battle with virus to be fought in backyards. *New York Times*, March 24.

Steinhauer, Jennifer. 1999. Viral outbreak highlights city-state tensions. *New York Times*, October 16.

———. 2000a. Mosquito program favors prevention over pesticide use. *New York Times*, April 14.

———. 2000b. Tests rule out West Nile Virus in death of man, 71. *New York Times*, July 21.

Toy, Vivian. 2000. Nassau unfazed by mosquitoes, so far. *New York Times*, August 13.

United States Centers for Disease Control and Prevention. 2010. Final 2009 West Nile Virus Activity in the United States. www.cdc.gov/ncidod/dvbid/westnile/surv&control CaseCount09_detailed.htm (accessed September 13, 2010).

Weiss, Don, Darcy Carr, Jacqueline Kellachan, et al. 2001. Clinical findings of West Nile virus infection in hospitalized patients in New York and New Jersey, 2000. *Emerging Infection Diseases* 7, no. 4, July–August, 654–658.

Chapter 7 · Conclusion

Joseph, Stephen. 1992. *Dragon within the Gates: The Once and Future AIDS Epidemic.* New York: Carroll and Graf.

Rein, Andrew. 2013. Maintaining a Public Health Agenda Political Change (conference discussion). New York Academy of Medicine. September 20.

Stevenson, Lori. 2003. Childhood asthma in New York City. What does it look like? Where do we find it? (presentation at Sarah Lawrence College, Health Advocacy Program). December 3.

United States Centers for Disease Control and Prevention. 2013. Community Transformation Grant Program Fact Sheet. www.cdc.gov/communitytransformation/funds/index .htm (accessed September 29, 2013).

quarantine, 9, 20, 23, 26, 235–36
Queens, 39, 68, 137, 206, 210, 213

race and ethnicity: and asthma, 74, 76–77,
78, 80, 81, 93, 99–102; and diversity, 15, 18,
25–29, 30, 248–49; and enclaves, 26; and
HIV/AIDS, 144–48, 156–57, 160; and lead
poisoning, 32, 39, 67–70; and obesity, 165,
166, 167, 168, 195–96; and public health
policy, 11, 15, 16, 220, 241–42; and urban
politics, 237; and West Nile virus, 203, 217.
See also environmental racism; minority
groups
rational model, in public policy, 11, 12–15,
237–38
Reagan administration, 61
real estate interests and industry, 239;
campaign contributions and electoral
support by, 66; and childhood lead
poisoning, 238; and lead paint regulations,
229; and lead poisoning, 32, 45, 48, 62,
66–67, 69, 240; and lead poisoning
programs, 56, 65. *See also* developers;
housing; landlords
Red Hook, Brooklyn, 68, 102
Reducing Indoor Allergens Study Team, 97,
100, 228
Rent Stabilization Association, 66
reporting, 4, 5–6, 231, 232, 243, 245; and
HIV/AIDS, 123–24, 128, 231; and lead
poisoning, 37, 58, 243; and West Nile virus,
211, 212–13, 214, 215–16, 224, 243
Residential Lead-Based Paint Hazard
Reduction Act, 63
restaurants, 180–81, 241; calorie posting in, 7,
181–83, 189, 224, 229, 238–39; fast food,
173, 181–83, 184, 189, 195, 201
Reversing the Epidemic report, 176
rodents, 73, 75, 89, 90, 97
Roosevelt, Franklin D., 23
Ryan White Comprehensive AIDS Resources
Emergency Act (CARE), 148, 152, 155–56,
157, 233, 234, 244, 246

safe sex, 129, 131, 132, 224, 225
San Francisco, 137–38, 159–60, 240, 247
SARS. *See* severe acute respiratory
syndrome

Satcher, David, 162, 198, 201
school buses, 86–87, 98, 105, 107, 230
School Nutrition Association, 200
schools, 4, 52; and absences from asthma, 71,
72, 82, 91, 92, 106, 107; and asthma, 102,
105; and asthma management, 94–95, 96,
97–98, 227; and asthma reporting, 94,
222; clinics in, 91, 92; condoms in, 135,
147; and engine idling, 87, 105; food and
nutrition in, 174, 175, 184, 190–93, 199,
232, 235; and HIV/AIDS, 122, 133–35, 153,
154, 226, 246; and obesity, 190–93, 198–99,
232, 235; and obesity education, 227, 246;
and obesity rates, 167, 168–69, 170, 176,
222; and physical education, 170, 175,
191–93, 235
Schoolyards to Playgrounds program,
192–93, 235
Schumer, Charles, 101, 156
screening, 4; and asthma, 107, 222; consent
for, 221; and federal government, 62, 63,
65–66; and Fitnessgram Program, 4, 169,
192, 222; and intergovernmental relations,
243; of newborns, 4; and obesity, 222; as
public policy tool, 3; and state government,
59; universal mandate for, 59; and West
Nile virus, 222. *See also under* HIV/AIDS;
under lead-based paint poisoning,
childhood
Sencer, David, 136, 153
seniors, 186, 196
September 11 terrorist attacks, 25, 98
severe acute respiratory syndrome (SARS),
26, 241
sex, and HIV/AIDS, 110, 127, 129, 133, 134,
226
sexually transmitted diseases (STDs), 123,
127, 132, 236
Shape Up New York Program, 190
shelter, right to, 11
Shepherd-Towner Act, 23
Shop Healthy NYC, 186, 235
Sierra Club, 207
Simon, Herbert, 12
Small Business Congress, 186
smallpox, 26; vaccine for, 9
smoking, 8, 30, 195, 237; and asthma, 73, 93,
95, 97, 231; and cessation programs, 93; and

United States (*cont.*)
　Office of Women's Health, 157; Public
　　Health Service, 10, 23, 243; Social Security
　　Administration, 155; Substance Abuse and
　　Mental Health Services Administration,
　　157; Supreme Court, 17
United Way of New York City, 194
urban political systems, 15, 237
urban political theory, 11, 15–18
US Department of Agriculture (USDA),
　　88, 193, 200; and Child and Adult Care
　　Food Program, 196; Dairy Management,
　　199; and food stamps for sugary beverages,
　　194; and obesity, 172, 175, 194, 197, 198, 199,
　　200; and research, 243
US government: and aid to state and local
　　governments, 10, 16; and air and water
　　quality, 24, 90; assistance and regulatory
　　guidance from, 21–25; and asthma,
　　76–77, 82, 94, 100–101, 103–6, 105; 221;
　　and cigarette smoking, 24; city policy
　　choices dictated by, 17; and community
　　as focus of public health, 21; Congestion
　　Mitigation and Air Quality grant, 105;
　　conservative-neoliberal regimes in, 16–17;
　　Consumer Product Safety Commission,
　　61; decline in aid from, 248; and
　　education and child nutrition, 198; and
　　emergency preparedness, 25; Farmers
　　Market Nutrition Program, 198; and
　　food, 188, 194, 197, 198–99, 200; funding
　　by, 10, 16–17, 23, 24, 59, 60, 62, 63,
　　64–65, 94, 104–5, 146, 154–57, 243, 248;
　　Healthy Communities Grant Program,
　　64; Healthy Homes Initiative, 105;
　　Healthy People 2010 initiative, 63; and
　　HIV/AIDS, 124, 125, 131, 132, 141, 142,
　　143, 146, 148, 150–51, 152–57, 159, 221, 224,
　　231, 233, 234, 244; and hospital construc-
　　tion funds, 24; and immigrant health,
　　25–26; impact of, 25, 248; and intergov-
　　ernmental relations, 20; and interstate
　　commerce, 24; Lead-Based Paint Hazard
　　Control, 64; Lead Hazard Reduction
　　program, 64; and lead poisoning, 34, 37,
　　38, 39, 46, 49, 55, 57, 58, 59, 61–66, 68,
　　221, 243, 244; Let's Move campaign,
　　199–200, 244; and needle exchange

programs, 136–37; and nutritional
　labeling, 181–82, 183; and obesity, 22,
　162, 172, 191, 192, 197–201, 224; policy
　tools of, 242–45; Preventive Health and
　Health Services Block Grant, 60, 105;
　as primary purchaser of health care, 22;
　and public policy, 220; and quarantine
　laws, 21; Task Force on Childhood
　Obesity, 200; We Can program, 200;
　and West Nile virus, 203, 207, 210, 211,
　217, 218

vaccines, 9–10, 29
Vacco, Dennis, 101, 107
Velazquez, Nydia, 102

waste management, solid, 86, 89–90
waste transfer/disposal, 30, 75, 89–90, 98,
　102
water, standing, 211, 214–15, 216, 219, 224,
　230
WE ACT, 100–101
West Nile virus, 2, 30, 204–5; action taken
　against, 207–16; and birds, 204, 206, 210,
　214, 215, 216, 221, 224; controversy about,
　221; death from, 203; diagnosis of, 205; and
　economic development, 216–17; education
　about, 212, 215, 216, 217, 219, 223, 224, 225;
　and ethnicity, 217; and federal govern-
　ment, 203, 210, 211, 217, 218; incidence of,
　203, 207, 222; and intergovernmental
　relations, 10, 217–18, 243; knowledge of,
　238; larvacides for, 214–15, 219, 246; and
　mayors, 247; medical treatment of, 214,
　218–19, 222; and mosquitoes, 203, 204,
　206–7, 210, 214, 215, 216, 219, 221, 224, 230;
　and NYS, 245, 246; pesticide spraying for,
　203, 207, 210–12, 217, 219, 223; prevalence
　of, 205–7, 213–14, 215, 218; and race, 217;
　and regulation, 230; and screening, 222;
　symptoms of, 205; testing for, 205, 212, 213,
　221, 222, 230
whites, 145, 241; and asthma, 76, 78, 80,
　81, 101; and HIV/AIDS, 146, 147, 148;
　and lead poisoning, 68; and obesity,
　166, 167, 168, 169; and waste transfer
　stations, 89
Williams, Enoch, 147